Atlas of Genitourinary Pathology

Gregory T. MacLennan • Liang Cheng

Atlas of Genitourinary Pathology

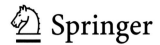
Springer

Authors
Gregory T. MacLennan, M.D
Professor of Pathology, Urology and Oncology
Director of Surgical Pathology
University Hospitals Case Medical Center
Case Western Reserve University
Cleveland, Ohio
USA
gtm2@case.edu

Liang Cheng, M.D
Professor of Pathology and Urology
Director of Molecular Diagnostics Service
Chief of Genitourinary Pathology Division
Director, Fellowship in Urologic Pathology
Indiana University School of Medicine
Indianapolis, Indiana
USA
liang_cheng@yahoo.com

ISBN 978-1-84882-394-5   e-ISBN 978-1-84882-395-2
DOI 10.1007/978-1-84882-395-2
Springer London Dordrecht Heidelberg New York

British Library Cataloguing in Publication Data
A catalogue record for this book is available from the British Library

Library of Congress Control Number: 2010937969

Cover design: eStudioCalamar, Figueres/Berlin

Printed on acid-free paper

Springer is part of Springer Science+Business Media (www.springer.com)

To my wife, Carrol MacLennan, in appreciation of your endless good humor, patience, and support for my endeavors, which you make possible.

Gregory T. MacLennan

This book is dedicated to our friend and mentor, Dr. David G. Bostwick.

Liang Cheng

Preface

This *Atlas* is presented to the reader as a quick reference guide to the diagnosis and classification of a wide spectrum of congenital, acquired, and neoplastic pathologic conditions that occur in the adrenal gland, the urinary tract, and the male genital tract. The *Atlas* is organized to provide quick access to lesions that arise in specific organs or sites, recognizing that certain disease entities, such as malakoplakia, may develop in more than one site. We have endeavored to conform to well-known and widely accepted classification schemes and staging algorithms in our descriptions of these entities.

The *Atlas* is not intended to serve as a comprehensive source of detailed information concerning the entities shown, or to provide an exhaustive list of references to enhance one's knowledge about specific topics. Those functions are served admirably by a large number of excellent textbooks that have become available in recent years in the fields of adrenal and genitourinary pathology; these textbooks are listed at the end of the *Atlas* as suggested reading materials.

For their entire careers in pathology, the authors have been devoted collectors of interesting case material related to the pathologic conditions presented in this *Atlas*, and have published their findings extensively in other venues in the pathology literature. Indeed, many of the images shown in this *Atlas* have been presented in other publications, and are reproduced here with permission. We have included a large number of gross photographs in the *Atlas* because we believe that careful gross assessment of pathologic specimens is very important. We have also included a number of endoscopic images, as well as a few relevant radiologic images, in hopes that the reader will enjoy seeing a different aspect of certain cases. The great majority of the material in this *Atlas* deals with entities that are quite familiar to pathologists, urologists, medical oncologists, and radiation oncologists. However, the *Atlas* also contains images of pathologic entities that are quite uncommon, such as leiomyosarcoma arising in a renal angiomyolipoma, or even entirely unique and astonishingly rare, such as mesodermal adenosarcoma of the testis. We hope that the reader shares our interest in exploring the complexities of pathologic conditions in humans, and our delight in learning new things about these diseases.

Cleveland, OH, USA
Indianapolis, IN, USA

Gregory T. MacLennan
Liang Cheng

Acknowledgments

The authors wish to express their profound appreciation for the assistance they have received from the many colleagues in pathology, urology, and radiology who have generously provided material for presentation in this *Atlas*, or have given us permission to reproduce certain images, some of which are arguably almost impossible to replace. We are also very appreciative of the technical assistance provided by the pathology residents and other support staff at our respective institutions for their invaluable help in preparing this material.

Our thanks are also extended to Lisa Dickason for her stellar administrative assistance, and to Christine Lemyre and Ryan P. Christy, whose assistance in preparing and photographing many of the beautiful gross specimens in this *Atlas* is gratefully acknowledged.

Contents

Table of Images

5   Prostate

8   Penis and Scrotum

Neoplastic Scrotal Lesions

The adrenal gland is an interesting organ with a wide spectrum of unique and challenging pathologic disorders, some acquired in the absence of a neoplastic process, and others that represent neoplasms of diverse origin. Certain entities, such as the adrenal findings in Waterhouse–Friderichsen syndrome, or diffuse and nodular hyperplasia of the adrenal cortex, are encountered exclusively or most frequently in the autopsy suite. Surgical pathologists are presented with a variety of neoplasms of diverse origin, as well as lesions that cannot be distinguished from neoplasms clinically or radiologically, such as myelolipoma and adrenal hemorrhage. In some cases, an entirely accurate clinical diagnosis is made before surgical resection, as in the case of aldosteronoma or pheochromocytoma.

1.1 Nonneoplastic Entities

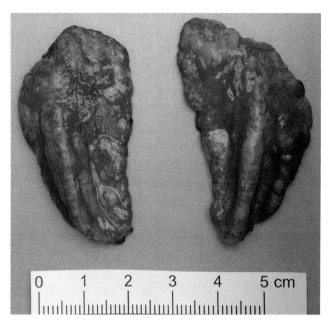

Fig. 1.1 Normal adrenal glands from an adult, with a combined weight of 11 g. Both are elongate and semilunar. Often, the right adrenal is flattened and triangular (*Image courtesy of* Linda Ho, MD)

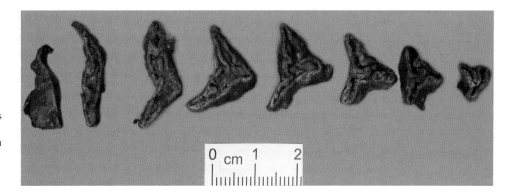

Fig. 1.2 Adrenal glands in cross section. The peripheral cortex is uniformly thin and bright golden yellow. The central medulla is pale gray-white (*Image courtesy of* Linda Ho, MD)

G. MacLennan and L. Cheng, *Atlas of Genitourinary Pathology*, DOI: 10.1007/978-1-84882-395-2_1,
© Springer-Verlag London Limited 2011

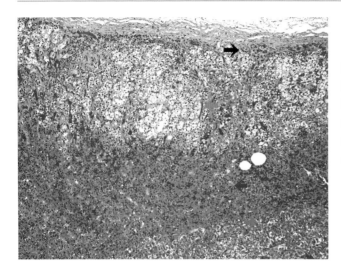

Fig. 1.3 Normal histology of adrenal gland. Zona glomerulosa (*black arrow*) lies beneath the capsule. It is thin, indistinct, and focally incomplete, consisting of cells with minimal eosinophilic cytoplasm and small round dark nuclei. Beneath it lies the zona fasciculata (*green arrow*), which consists of long columns of large cells with pale vacuolated cytoplasm. The zona reticularis (*blue arrow*) lies innermost, and consists of short anastomosing cords of eosinophilic cells. Zona fasciculata and zona reticularis are richly supplied with sinusoids and capillaries. The medulla (*orange arrow*) comprises about 10% of adrenal mass. It is composed of polyhedral cells with granular basophilic cytoplasm, uniform round to oval nuclei, and inconspicuous nucleoli, arranged in nests and short cords intermingled with numerous capillaries

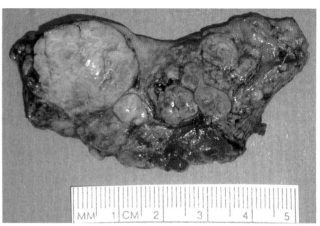

Fig. 1.5 Adrenal cortical hyperplasia, diffuse and nodular. Cortical hyperplasia is defined as a nonneoplastic increase in the number of cortical cells. It is usually bilateral, and may be diffuse, nodular, or both. Multiple nodules are noted in 1.5–2.9% of autopsies. Nodular adrenal glands contain multiple (and usually bilateral) discrete or confluent nodules that can be greater than 2 cm in diameter. Extrusion of the nodules into surrounding fat is common. Some nodules are composed only of cortical tissue whereas others show fibrosis, cyst formation, fatty change, myeloid metaplasia, or rarely, osseous metaplastic change (*Image courtesy of* Shams Halat, MD)

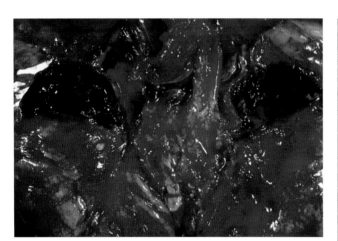

Fig. 1.4 Waterhouse–Friderichsen syndrome. Adrenal glands at autopsy (posterior aspect of retroperitoneum) in a patient who succumbed to meningococcal septicemia. Both adrenals are diffusely hemorrhagic. Adrenal hemorrhage tends to occur in adrenocorticotropic-stimulated glands that are challenged by endotoxin or hypovolemia in a clinical setting associated with low cortisol levels, such as sepsis (*see* MacLennan GT, Resnick MI, Bostwick DG 2003. With permission)

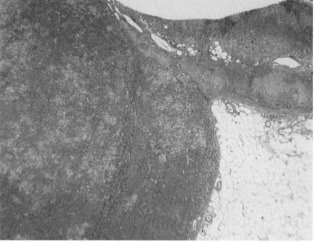

Fig. 1.6 Adrenal cortical hyperplasia, diffuse and nodular. The hyperplastic nodule at left appears to be composed of cells of fasciculata and reticularis type. The cells are arranged in nests, sheets, cords or ribbons, and sometimes, glands

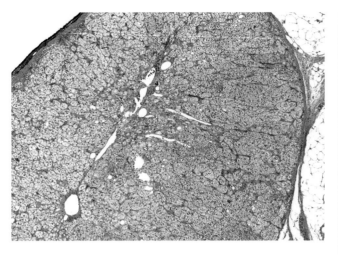

Fig. 1.7 Adrenal cortical hyperplasia, diffuse and nodular. The zona fasciculata appears to be markedly expanded. No medullary tissue is present in this section

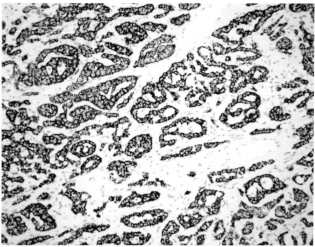

Fig. 1.10 Pseudoglandular adrenocortical hyperplasia. The adrenocortical cells show appropriately positive immunostaining for Melan A

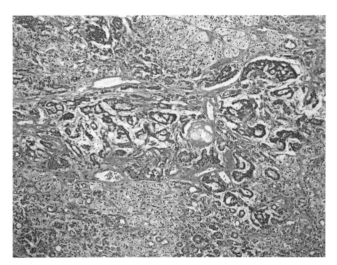

Fig. 1.8 Pseudoglandular adrenocortical hyperplasia. In this case, a focal area of pseudogland formation raised concern for metastatic adenocarcinoma

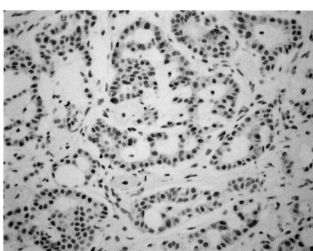

Fig. 1.11 Pseudoglandular adrenocortical hyperplasia. The adrenocortical cells show appropriately positive immunostaining for inhibin

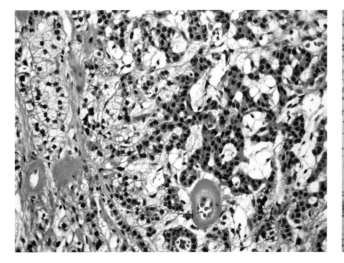

Fig. 1.9 Pseudoglandular adrenocortical hyperplasia. Wispy blue mucinous material is evident in the stroma

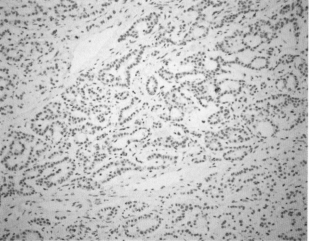

Fig. 1.12 Pseudoglandular adrenocortical hyperplasia. The adrenocortical cells show appropriately negative immunostaining for keratin AE1/AE3

Fig. 1.13 Macronodular hyperplasia with marked adrenal enlargement. Clinically, autonomous hypercortisolism (independent of pituitary or extrapituitary adrenocorticotropic hormone stimulation), resulting from aberrant expression of hormone receptors in adrenal cortical cells. In this condition, both adrenals are greatly enlarged. In the example shown, the smaller adrenal, sectioned at top, weighed 39 g, and the larger adrenal, sectioned at bottom, weighed 79 g. The adrenal cortex is composed of innumerable, variably sized hyperplastic nodules

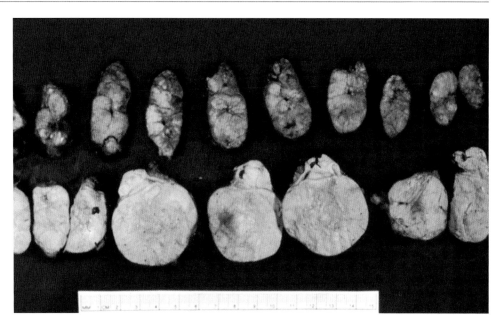

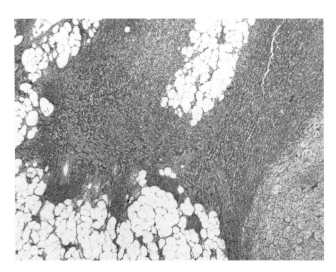

Fig. 1.14 Macronodular hyperplasia with marked adrenal enlargement. The amount of lipid-rich pale-staining cytoplasm is variable in adjacent regions of the hyperplastic nodules. Some of the fat within the cortical tissue may represent lipomatous metaplasia. Irregular extensions of cortical cells into periadrenal adipose tissue are sometimes noted, as in this case

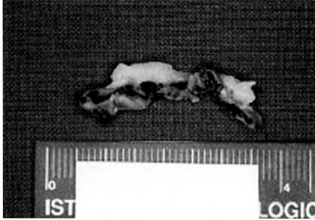

Fig. 1.15 Primary pigmented nodular adrenal cortical disease (PPNAD). Clinically, autonomous hypercortisolism (independent of pituitary or extrapituitary adrenocorticotropic hormone stimulation) of uncertain pathogenesis, typically occurring in young persons, most often females. PPNAD is observed in 45% of cases of Carney's complex. This patient was a 27-year-old female with hypercortisolism and other features consistent with Carney's complex. The left adrenal gland was radiologically abnormal and was removed; it weighed 4.8 g, and contained multiple dark brown nodules (*Image and case courtesy of Marina Scarpelli, MD*)

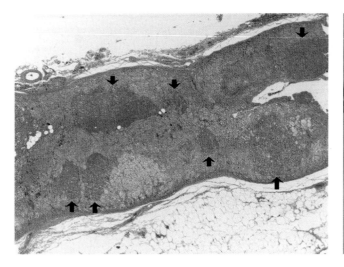

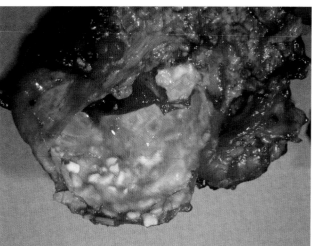

Fig. 1.16 Primary pigmented nodular adrenal cortical disease. Numerous small round to oval unencapsulated nodules of darkly eosinophilic cortical cells are randomly dispersed within the cortex (*arrows*) (*Image and case courtesy of* Marina Scarpelli, MD)

Fig. 1.18 Adrenal cyst, with extensive mural calcifications. Most adrenal cysts (about 85%) result from hemorrhage in normal or abnormal adrenals, and are designated "pseudocysts" or "endothelial cysts," depending upon whether an endothelial lining is present. Vascular malformations are often implicated in the formation of these lesions. A small number are parasitic in origin, usually secondary to echinococcus infestation. About 9% of adrenal cysts have an epithelial lining, reflecting cystic change in entrapped mesothelium or in heterotopic urogenital tissue; others represent cystic change within adrenal neoplasms, including cortical adenoma, cortical carcinoma, or pheochromocytoma (*Image courtesy of* Stacy Kim, MD)

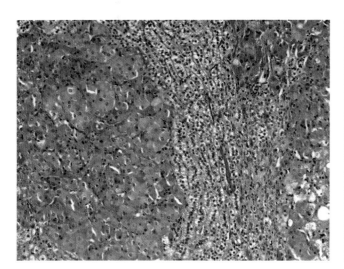

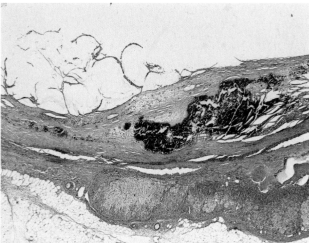

Fig. 1.17 Primary pigmented nodular adrenal cortical disease. The cortical cells forming the nodules possess abundant eosinophilic cytoplasm. Although not evident in this image, the cells in such nodules often contain coarse granular pigment that resembles lipofuscin (*Image and case courtesy of* Marina Scarpelli, MD)

Fig. 1.19 Adrenal cyst. The upper half of the image is a fibrous-walled cystic space containing amorphous material. Adipose and normal adrenal tissues are present in the lower half of the image

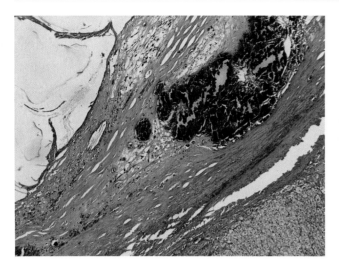

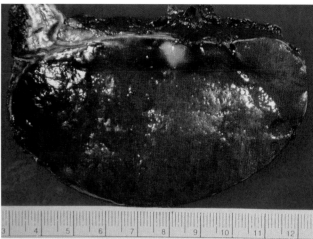

Fig. 1.20 Adrenal cyst. Calcific deposits are present in the fibrous wall. No lining epithelial or endothelial cells are evident in the cystic space at left; immunostains for keratin and epithelial markers were negative

Fig. 1.22 Myelolipoma. This example was almost entirely composed of red-brown myeloid tissue, with only a small nodule of adipose tissue at center top

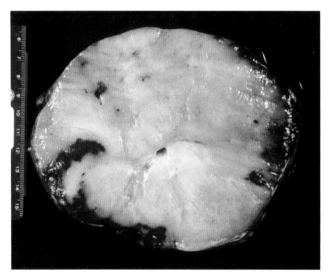

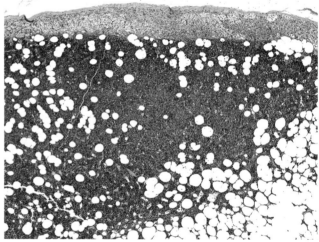

Fig. 1.21 Myelolipoma. Myelolipoma is a benign tumor, usually discovered incidentally. Myelolipoma is usually unilateral and solitary, varying in size up to 34 cm, and weighing up to 5,900 g. It is smooth, well circumscribed, and yellow to red-brown, depending upon the amount of adipose or myeloid tissue present. This example was predominantly adipose tissue; the small peripheral red-brown areas are myeloid tissue

Fig. 1.23 Myelolipoma. A thin rim of normal adrenal cortex is seen at top. The tumor tissue in this case is an almost equal mix of adipose tissue and myeloid tissue

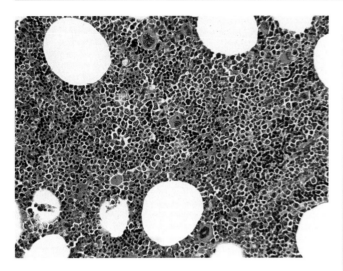

Fig. 1.24 Myelolipoma. Microscopically, it is composed of mature adipose tissue and hematopoietic tissue, including myeloid and erythroid cells and megakaryocytes (trilinear hematopoiesis). Trabeculae of bone may be present

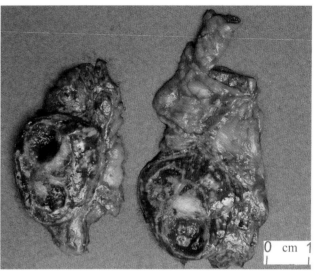

Fig. 1.26 Myelolipoma and hemangioma. There appears to be an irregular but somewhat circumscribed central portion, surrounded peripherally by organizing hematoma (*Image courtesy of* Paul Grabenstetter, MD)

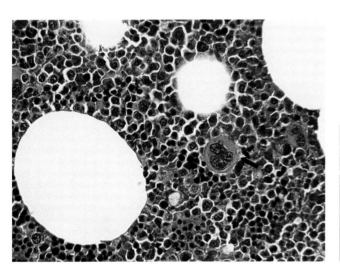

Fig. 1.25 Myelolipoma. Identification of the multilobed nuclei of megakaryocytes (*arrow*) is often the first clue to the diagnosis

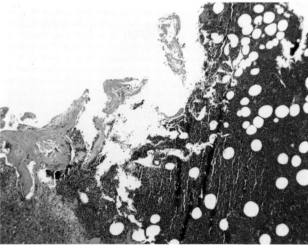

Fig. 1.27 Myelolipoma and hemangioma. Normal adrenal cortex appears at the lower left, myelolipoma on the right, and portions of a cavernous hemangioma at mid-to-upper left

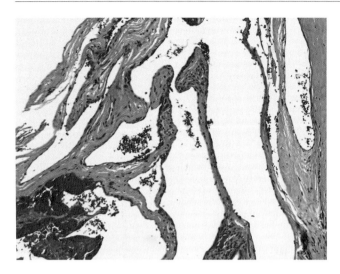

Fig. 1.28 Myelolipoma and hemangioma. High-power view of the cavernous hemangioma component, which may have been responsible for the presence of the peripherally located organizing hematoma

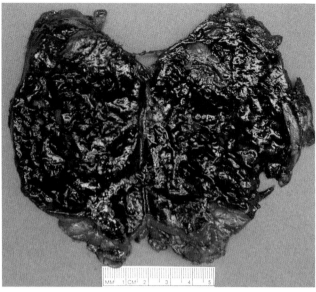

Fig. 1.30 Hematoma. This lesion was clinically of recent origin, and the gross findings suggest recent bleeding. No etiology was apparent, clinically or pathologically (*Image courtesy of* Shams Halat, MD)

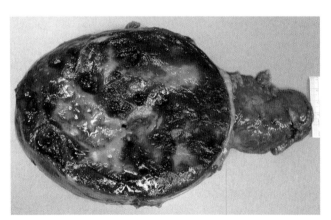

Fig. 1.29 Hematoma. Radiologically, this lesion was thought to be a very large renal cancer, but ultimately proved to be a very large organizing hematoma of the adrenal. No etiology was apparent, clinically or pathologically (*Image courtesy of* Amber Petrolla, MD)

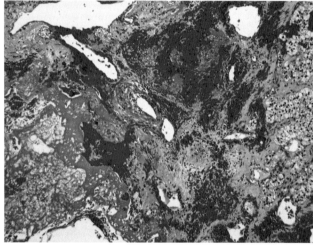

Fig. 1.31 Hematoma. Blood, fibrin, and cortical tissue at right. The etiology of the bleeding is not evident

Fig. 1.32 Adrenal medullary hyperplasia. This lesion can occur sporadically or as part of multiple endocrine neoplasin (MEN) types 2a or 2b; in either case, it may be symmetric or asymmetric. The clinical scenario is that of pheochromocytoma. It is an accepted cause of pseudopheochromocytoma, in which the clinical scenario suggests pheochromocytoma but none can be readily identified. The adrenal shown here was from a 43-year-old female with severe drug-resistant hypertension. ^{131}I-MIBG scan showed abnormal uptake in this adrenal, and it was excised. The gland weighed 5.9 g; notably, the medullary compartment extends into both alae, but no distinct nodules are present (*Image and case courtesy of* Marina Scarpelli, MD)

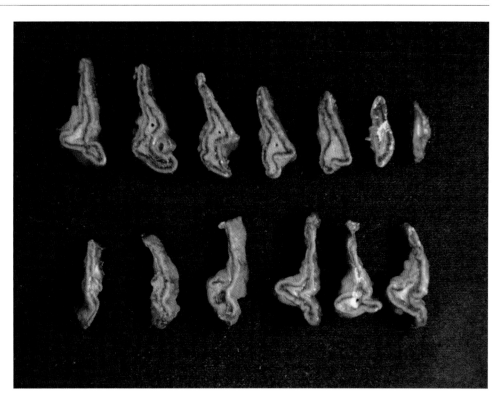

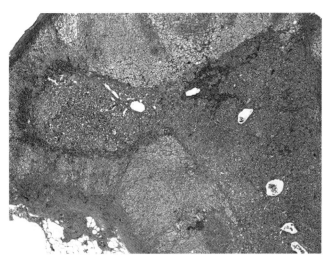
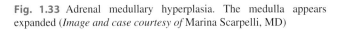

Fig. 1.33 Adrenal medullary hyperplasia. The medulla appears expanded (*Image and case courtesy of* Marina Scarpelli, MD)

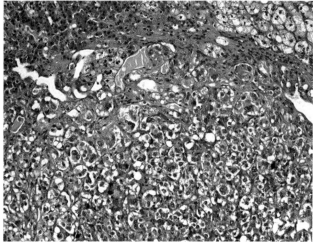

Fig. 1.34 Adrenal medullary hyperplasia. Section from the medulla shows a diffuse growth of hyperplastic chromaffin cells. After adrenalectomy, patient's blood pressure reverted to normal (*Image and case courtesy of* Marina Scarpelli, MD)

1.2 Adrenal Cortical Neoplasms

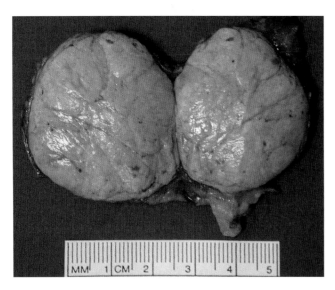

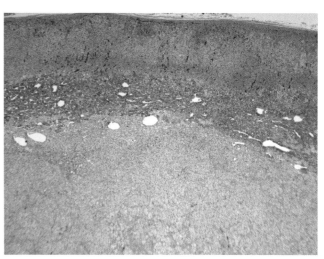

Fig. 1.37 Adrenal cortical adenoma. A large expansile nodule of pale cells at bottom stands out in contrast to the normal adrenal medullary tissue and normal cortical tissue at top

Fig. 1.35 Adrenal cortical adenoma. A benign neoplasm derived from cortical cells, usually solitary and unilateral, and more frequently in women. Most adrenal cortical adenomas associated with hypercortisolism are less than 6 cm in diameter (average 3.6 cm) and weigh less than 40 g. Adenomas are typically yellow or golden-yellow, and are circumscribed but unencapsulated. Small areas of hemorrhage, fibrosis, or cystic degeneration may be present (*Image courtesy of* Philip Bomeisl, MD)

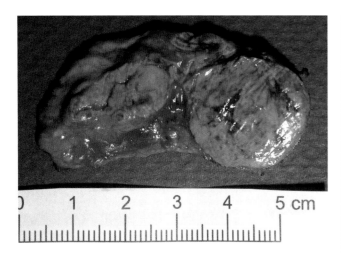

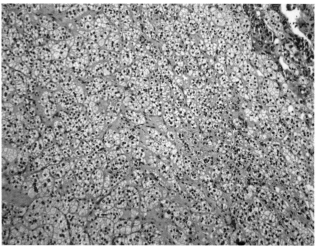

Fig. 1.36 Adrenal cortical adenoma, multiple. This adrenal gland from a patient with hypercortisolism appeared to harbor two distinct adenomas. The uninvolved cortex did not show the diffuse thickening and nodularity typical of diffuse and nodular hyperplasia (compare with findings in Fig. 1.5). There is considerable overlap between the pathologic findings in cortical adenoma and hyperplastic macronodule. Cortical tissue adjacent to an adrenal cortical adenoma is usually atrophic, rather than hyperplastic (*Image courtesy of* M. Carmen Frias-Kletecka, MD)

Fig. 1.38 Adrenal cortical adenoma. Tumor cells are arranged in nests or short cords. Most cells contain abundant lipid and are pale-staining. Minor components of smaller cells with dense eosinophilic cytoplasm are usually present. In some adenomas, large pale "balloon cells," or clusters of spindle cells are seen

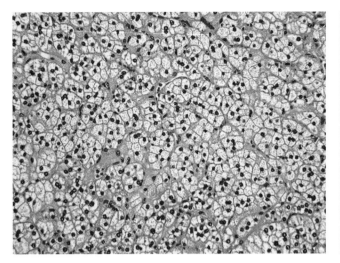

Fig. 1.39 Adrenal cortical adenoma. Cell nuclei are fairly uniform, with inconspicuous nucleoli. Mitotic figures are infrequent and necrosis is unusual

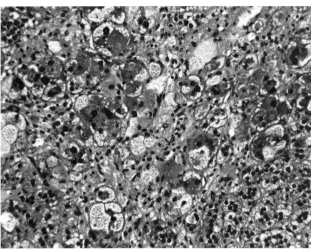

Fig. 1.41 Adrenal cortical adenoma, pigmented. The adenoma shown in Fig. 1.40 was partially composed of large lipid-poor cells with dark eosinophilic cytoplasm containing abundant brown pigment, which imparts the dark color of the tumor

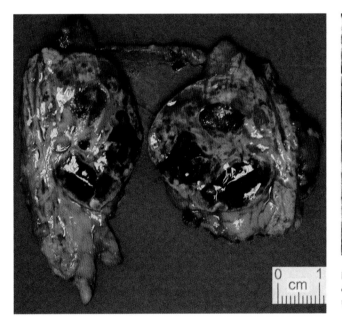

Fig. 1.40 Adrenal cortical adenoma, pigmented. Some cortical adenomas exhibit widespread brown or black discoloration, to the extent that they sometimes merit the term "black adenoma." Pigmented adenomas are most often associated with hypercortisolism, or less often, hyperaldosteronism; the lesion shown here was nonfunctional, and was an incidental finding in a patient with colon cancer (*Image courtesy of Douglas Hartman, MD*)

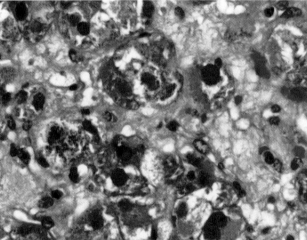

Fig. 1.42 Adrenal cortical adenoma, pigmented. The brown granular cytoplasmic pigment is believed to be lipofuscin, a notion supported by ultrastructural studies

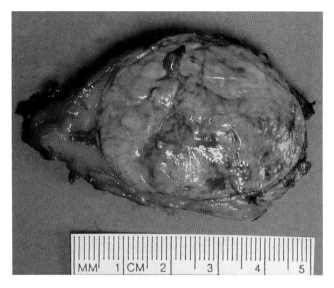

Fig. 1.43 Aldosteronoma (adrenal cortical adenoma with hyperaldosteronism). Aldosteronoma is usually unilateral and solitary, with gross findings indistinguishable from those of other forms of adrenal cortical adenoma. Although their median diameter is 1.7 cm, and nearly all weigh less than 10 g, some are quite large, as in this example. Most are bright yellow or yellow-orange, and sharply circumscribed, to an extent that may mimic encapsulation. Cystic degeneration or hemorrhage may be seen in larger tumors (*Image courtesy of* Shams Halat, MD)

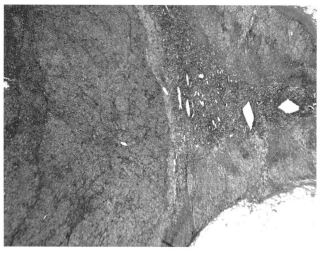

Fig. 1.45 Aldosteronoma. Tumor forms a large expansile nodule at left, in marked contrast to the normal adrenal tissue on the right

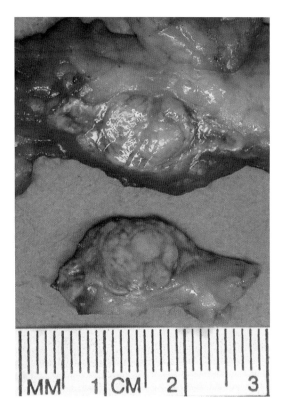

Fig. 1.44 Aldosteronoma. In some instances, the adrenal lesion is small and difficult to identify radiologically. This adenoma in a patient with well-documented hyperaldosteronism and associated hypertension was only about 1 cm in diameter (*Image courtesy of* Richard Naturale, MD)

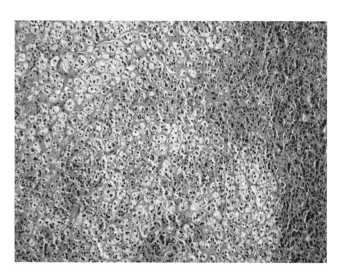

Fig. 1.46 Aldosteronoma. Tumor cells are arranged in nests, cords, or interconnecting ribbons. Tumors consist of a mixture of large vacuolated lipid-rich cells, smaller cells with dark eosinophilic cytoplasm, and "hybrid cells" with lightly eosinophilic cytoplasm

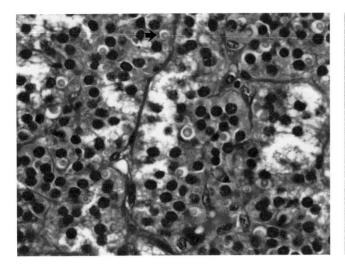

Fig. 1.47 Aldosteronoma. Spironolactone bodies (*arrow*) are sometimes evident in normal zona glomerulosa cells, or in the cells of aldosteronoma, in patients treated with spironolactone, an aldosterone antagonist. They are laminated pink cytoplasmic inclusions, 2–12 μm in diameter, surrounded by a clear halo

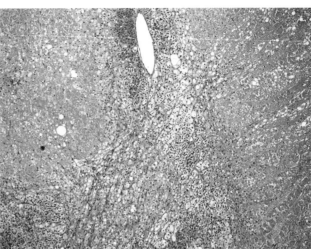

Fig. 1.49 Atypical adrenal cortical adenoma. The lesion showed extensive areas of necrosis. It had none of the other features that have been associated with malignant biologic behavior in adrenal cortical neoplasms

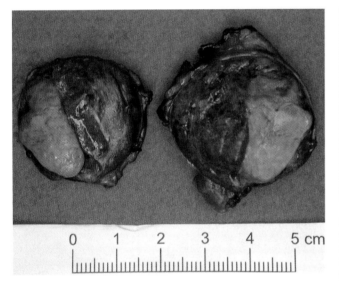

Fig. 1.48 Atypical adrenal cortical adenoma. This lesion was identified in a 16-year-old female with Cushing syndrome. It weighed 8.5 g and is remarkable for the presence of an unusual area of yellow discoloration (*Image courtesy of* Shunyou Gong, MD)

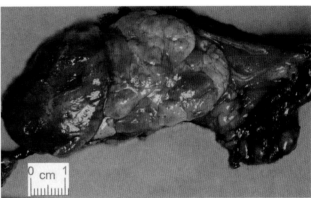

Fig. 1.50 Pediatric adrenal cortical neoplasm. Adrenal cortical neoplasms in the pediatric age group, particularly in those younger than 5 years old, are not strictly comparable to those in adults. Such neoplasms occurring in children under age 5, completely resectable, weighing less than 400 g, with fewer than 15 mitotic figures/high-power field, and with minimal necrosis, have an excellent prognosis. The tumor shown here was from a 2-year-old boy. This tumor was 7.5 cm in diameter and weighed 67 g (*Image* courtesy of Diane Kidric, MD)

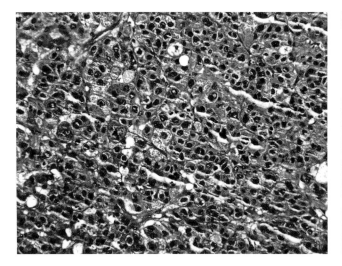

Fig. 1.51 Pediatric adrenal cortical neoplasm. Tumor grows in sheets, with readily evident mitotic figures

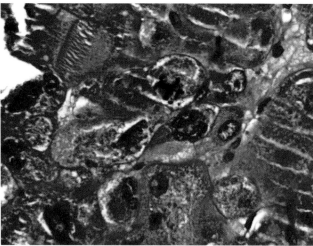

Fig. 1.53 Pediatric adrenal cortical neoplasm. Atypical mitotic figures are included in the list of malignant criteria in children, along with tumor weight of more than 400 g, tumor size larger than 10.5 cm, involvement of periadrenal soft tissues and/or adjacent organs, extension into vena cava, venous invasion, capsular invasion, tumor necrosis, and more than 15 mitotic figures per 20 high-power fields

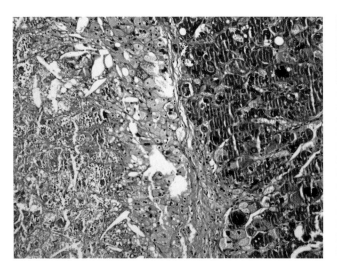

Fig. 1.52 Pediatric adrenal cortical neoplasm. Necrosis is evident at left but was minimal in this case. Pronounced nuclear atypia is evident at right, but this finding in a young child has no predictive value

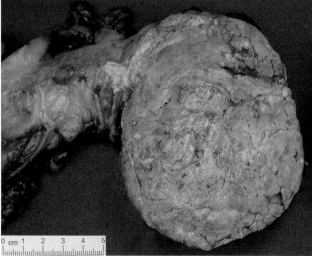

Fig. 1.54 Adrenal cortical carcinoma. Cortical carcinoma, derived from cells of the adrenal cortex, averages 12–16 cm in diameter, and most weigh between 700 and 1,200 g. Tumors consist of expansile tan to yellow-orange nodules intersected by thick fibrous bands. Necrosis, hemorrhage, and areas of cystic degeneration are commonly present. Extension of tumor into surrounding tissues or into large veins may be noted. The tumor shown in this illustration was hormonally nonfunctional and both radiologically and grossly was initially thought to represent an upper pole renal cell carcinoma, and surgical excision included the kidney, at left (*Image courtesy of* Huankai Hu, MD)

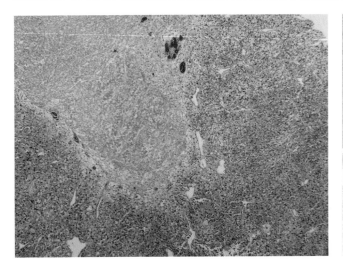

Fig. 1.55 Adrenal cortical carcinoma. Extensive necrosis is readily apparent. The distinction between cortical adenoma and carcinoma is sometimes challenging. Statistically, the most reliable microscopic criteria of malignancy include (1) more than five mitotic figures per 50 high-power fields; (2) less than 25% of the tumor is composed of clear or vacuolated cells resembling the normal zona fasciculata; (3) presence of atypical mitotic figures; (4) necrosis in confluent nests of cells; and (5) presence of capsular invasion. Tumor invasion into an adjacent organ is observed only in malignant neoplasms. In some instances, the ultimate diagnosis is determined by the patient's clinical course

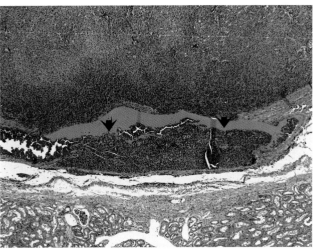

Fig. 1.57 Adrenal cortical carcinoma. Vascular invasion (*arrows*) has been implicated as an adverse histologic finding associated with aggressive tumor behavior, but there is considerable interobserver variability in its identification

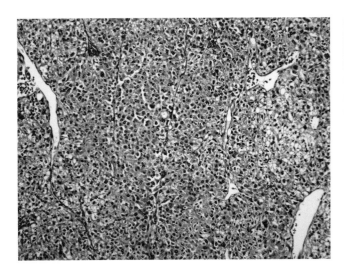

Fig. 1.56 Adrenal cortical carcinoma. Tumor cells are arranged in sheets and broad columns, separated by prominent sinusoidal vascular spaces. Mixtures of lipid-rich cells and cells with compact eosinophilic cytoplasm are usually present. Adrenal neoplasms composed of less than 25% of lipid-rich cells are more likely to behave aggressively

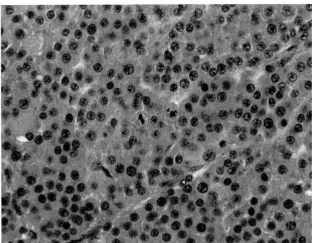

Fig. 1.58 Adrenal cortical carcinoma. The presence of more than five mitotic figures per 50 high-power fields is an adverse histologic finding. Mitotic figures are rarely seen in cortical adenoma or hyperplasia

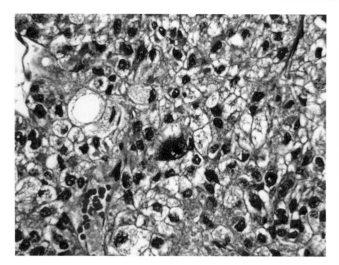

Fig. 1.59 Adrenal cortical carcinoma. Pronounced nuclear atypia in tumor cells, although commonly seen in cortical carcinoma, may also be seen in cortical adenomas, and therefore cannot be used to make a reliable distinction between these entities

1.3 Adrenal Medullary Neoplasms

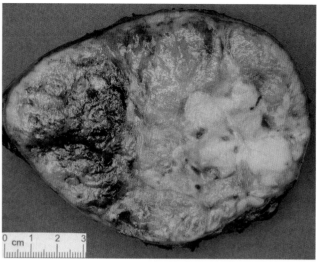

Fig. 1.61 Pheochromocytoma. This is a paraganglioma derived from chromaffin cells in a specific anatomic site – the adrenal medulla. Pheochromocytoma is round to oval, and sharply circumscribed but unencapsulated. It averages 3–5 cm in diameter, with weight ranging from 75 to 150 g. It may be tan, brown, or gray-white, and may have areas of hemorrhage, necrosis or cystic degeneration (*Image courtesy of* Jason Rarick, MD)

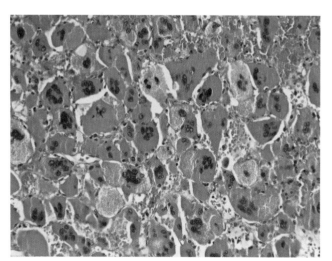

Fig. 1.60 Oncocytic adrenal cortical carcinoma. In this rare variant, the tumor is diffusely composed of rather dyscohesive cells with abundant intensely eosinophilic granular cytoplasm

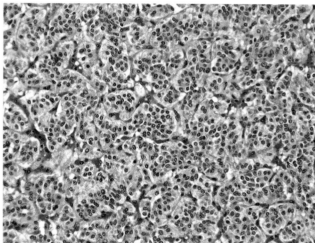

Fig. 1.62 Pheochromocytoma. Tumor cells are arranged in nests ("zell-ballen") surrounded by a network of blood vessels and other supporting cells. Tumor cells are round or polygonal, with limited amounts of basophilic cytoplasm. Intracytoplasmic hyaline globules are sometimes present. Nuclei are usually round to oval with small nucleoli

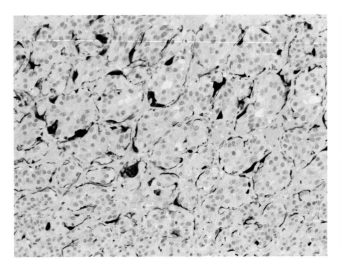

Fig. 1.63 Pheochromocytoma. Sustentacular cells form part of the network of supporting cells around cell nests. They are inconspicuous on routinely stained sections, but can be demonstrated with immunostain for S100 protein

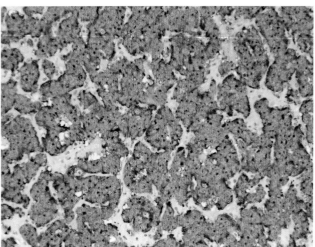

Fig. 1.65 Pheochromocytoma. Tumor cells show positive immunostaining for synaptophysin

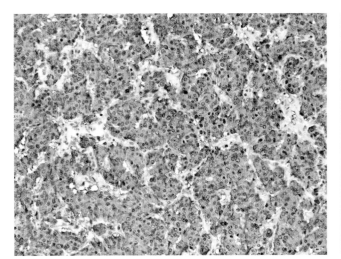

Fig. 1.64 Pheochromocytoma. Tumor cells show positive immunostaining for chromogranin

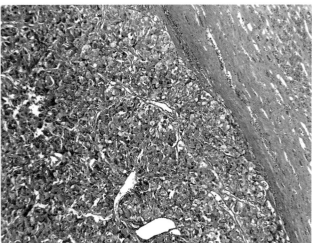

Fig. 1.66 Pheochromocytoma. In contrast to the nested architecture typically seen, pheochromocytoma may grow in diffuse sheets, with more prominent sinusoidal vasculature. A fibrous pseudocapsule may be present at the interface between tumor and normal adrenal tissue, as in this case

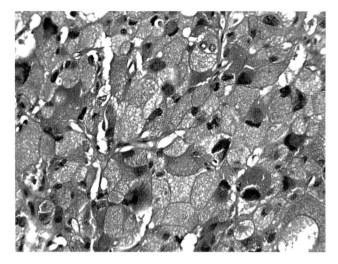

Fig. 1.67 Pheochromocytoma. In the diffuse growth pattern, tumor cells may exhibit abundant amphophilic cytoplasm

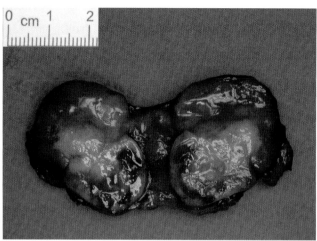

Fig. 1.69 Pheochromocytoma. This is an image of a local recurrence of pheochromocytoma in the surgical bed of a previously resected adrenal pheochromocytoma. Malignancy in pheochromocytoma is defined by the identification of metastasis, which occurs in up to 14% of pheochromocytomas; currently there are no other clear-cut morphologic assessments that allow a reliable diagnosis of malignancy in this neoplasm. Metastasis is uncommon in children, and is more often seen in cases of extra-adrenal intra-abdominal paraganglioma than in adrenal pheochromocytoma. Features associated with malignancy include large size, local invasion, coarse tumor nodularity, mitotic activity, widespread necrosis, and lack of intracellular hyaline globules (*Image courtesy of* Anna Balog, MD)

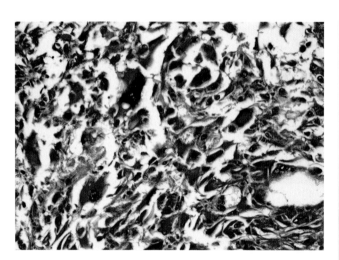

Fig. 1.68 Pheochromocytoma. Marked nuclear atypia and hyperchromasia, focal necrosis, and increased mitotic activity are noted in some tumors. However, nuclear atypia is not predictive of malignant behavior

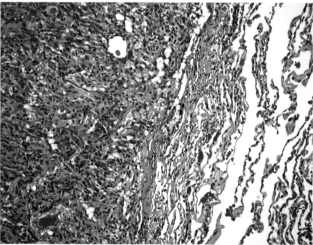

Fig. 1.70 Pheochromocytoma. Image shows metastatic pheochromocytoma in lung. Patient had undergone adrenalectomy 10 years previously for pheochromocytoma. Three months after the wedge resection of the lung nodule, a nodule of recurrent pheochromocytoma was excised from the site of the original adrenalectomy

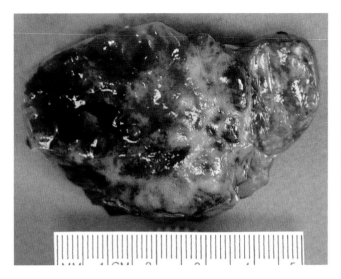

Fig. 1.71 Concurrent pheochromocytoma and adrenal cortical adenoma. When examined in the fresh state, pheochromocytoma (*left*) is often an admixture of plum-colored and pink-white tissue. A golden yellow cortical adenoma is on the right (*Image courtesy of* Stacy Kim, MD)

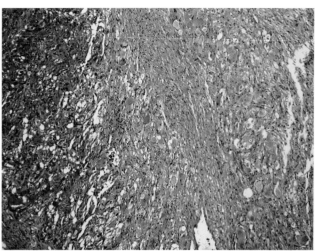

Fig. 1.73 Composite pheochromocytoma. This term denotes pheochromocytomas with components that resemble ganglioneuroma, ganglioneuroblastoma, neuroblastoma, or malignant peripheral nerve sheath tumor. At left is a typical pheochromocytoma. At right is an admixture of ganglion cells in a background of mature Schwann cells, typical of ganglioneuroma

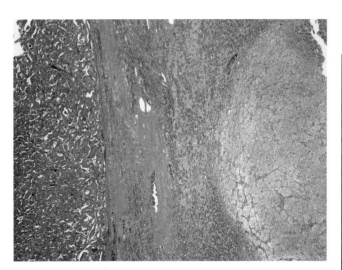

Fig. 1.72 Concurrent pheochromocytoma and adrenal cortical adenoma. A central zone of fibrous tissue separates the pheochromocytoma (*left*) from the cortical adenoma (*right*)

1.4 Neuroblastic Neoplasms

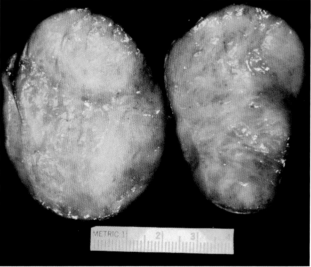

Fig. 1.74 Ganglioneuroma. This is a benign neoplasm of the sympathetic nervous system, up to 30% of which occur primarily in the adrenal, which is thought to arise from neuroblasts in the adrenal medulla. Those that arise in the adrenal are found in patients in the fourth and fifth decades of life. Some represent maturation of preexisting neuroblastoma, but the majority arise de novo. Although it can be as large as 18 cm in diameter, average diameter is about 8 cm. It is typically smooth, gray-white or tan-yellow, well-circumscribed but nonencapsulated, and rubbery, without necrosis or hemorrhage

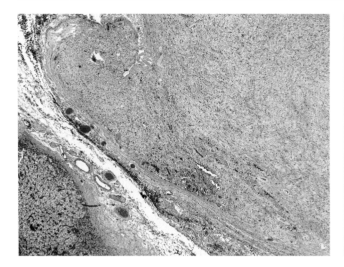

Fig. 1.75 Ganglioneuroma. It is composed of a predominance of neurofibroma-like areas composed of Schwann cells, admixed with ganglion cells in varying proportions. Necrosis, mitotic figures, and cellular atypia are absent

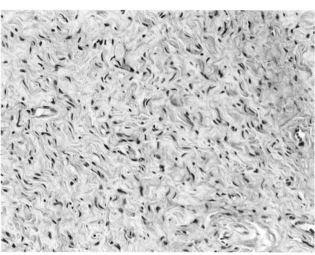

Fig. 1.77 Ganglioneuroma. Schwann cells exhibit scant spindled cytoplasm, wavy dark nuclei, and inconspicuous nucleoli

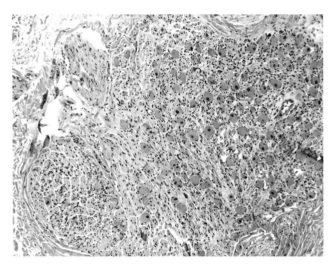

Fig. 1.76 Ganglioneuroma. Ganglion cells, at right, possess abundant eosinophilic cytoplasm, large vesicular nuclei and prominent nucleoli; they are scattered throughout the tumor, often as small aggregates surrounded by ill-defined fascicles of Schwann cells

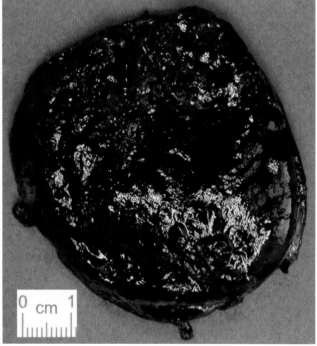

Fig. 1.78 Neuroblastoma. Neuroblastoma and ganglioneuroblastoma are derived from neuroblasts of the sympathetic nervous system. Their morphologic appearances represent a continuum of findings, with undifferentiated neuroblastoma at one end to ganglioneuroblastoma at the other end of the spectrum, a neoplasm that differs only minimally from ganglioneuroma. Neuroblastoma usually forms a solitary circumscribed ovoid or multinodular mass, which may be more than 10 cm in diameter. It may invade local structures or large veins. It is a soft, bulging, pink-white, plum-colored or tan tumor with varying degrees of hemorrhage, necrosis, cystic degeneration, and dystrophic calcification (*Image courtesy of* Paul Grabenstetter, MD)

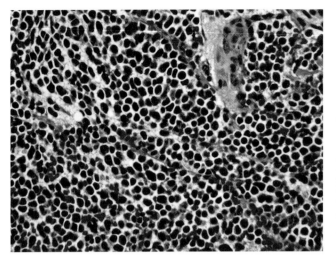

Fig. 1.79 Neuroblastoma. This tumor is undifferentiated, and composed of sheets of small blue cells with minimal cytoplasm, round and fairly uniform nuclei with dispersed nuclear chromatin and inconspicuous nucleoli, and indistinct cell borders. No neuropil is seen

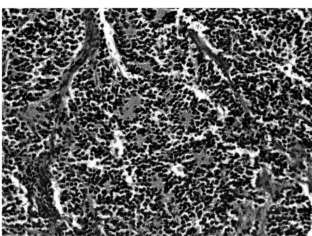

Fig. 1.82 Neuroblastoma. This tumor is poorly differentiated, and exhibits the presence of Homer Wright rosettes, composed of discrete clusters of neuronal processes surrounded by tumor cells

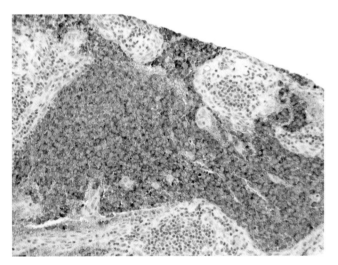

Fig. 1.80 Neuroblastoma. Tumor cells show positive immunostaining for neuron-specific enolase

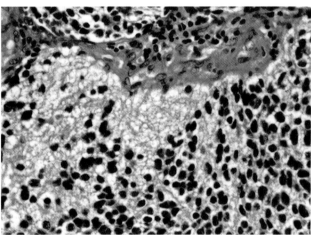

Fig. 1.83 Neuroblastoma. Neuronal processes impart a pale pink fibrillar background

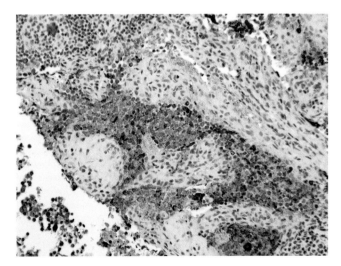

Fig. 1.81 Neuroblastoma. Tumor cells show positive immunostaining for chromogranin

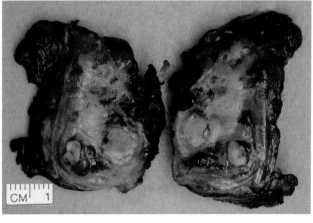

Fig. 1.84 Neuroblastoma. This tumor was excised following preoperative chemotherapy. Tumor is relatively small, and has areas of fibrosis and geographic necrosis (*Image courtesy of* Matthew Kuhn, MD)

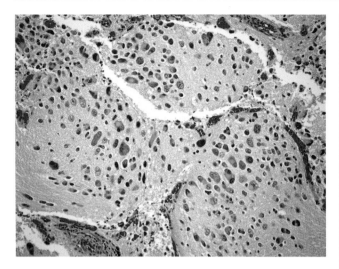

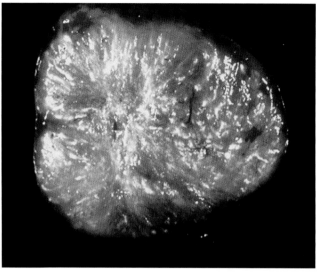

Fig. 1.85 Neuroblastoma. A section from the tumor shown in Fig. 1.84 shows features of differentiating neuroblastoma, in which more than 5% of the tumor shows evidence of ganglion cell differentiation. Tumor cells show nuclear enlargement, fairly abundant eosinophilic cytoplasm, and distinct cell borders. Nuclei are eccentrically located and have prominent nucleoli

Fig. 1.87 Ganglioneuroblastoma. Cut surface is bulging, with streaky necrosis and minimal hemorrhage (*see* MacLennan GT, Resnick MI, Bostwick DG 2003. With permission)

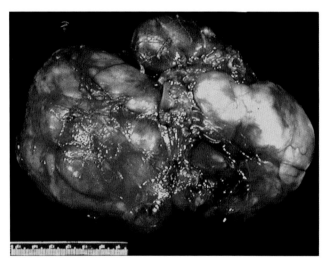

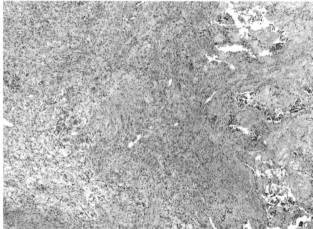

Fig. 1.86 Ganglioneuroblastoma. Tumor forms a very large multinodular mass that dwarfs the kidney, which is seen at the top of the image (*see* MacLennan GT, Resnick MI, Bostwick DG 2003. With permission)

Fig. 1.88 Ganglioneuroblastoma. The histologic appearance of the left half of this image is virtually indistinguishable from that of ganglioneuroma. However, at right are small aggregates of small dark blue cells that mimic a chronic inflammatory cell infiltrate

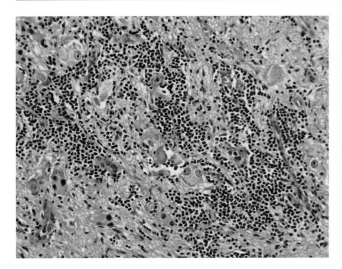

Fig. 1.89 Ganglioneuroblastoma. In this area of the tumor, there is an admixture of ganglion cells, Schwann cells and small dark blue cells of the type typically seen in neuroblastoma

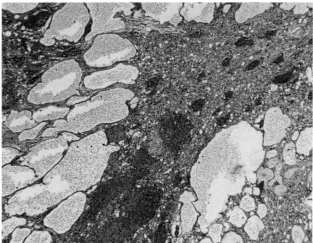

Fig. 1.91 Adenomatoid tumor of adrenal. At low power, tumor cells form solid nests or fenestrated channels and anastomosing tubules of varying size, set in a fibrous stroma

1.5 Other Adrenal Neoplasms

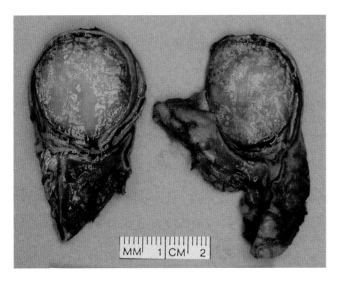

Fig. 1.90 Adenomatoid tumor of adrenal. This is a benign neoplasm of mesothelial origin, usually found incidentally, most often occurring in adults between 30 and 50 years of age. They are usually solid but rarely cystic and can measure up to 11 cm in diameter. Cut surface is pale and firm (*Image courtesy of* Paul Grabenstetter, MD)

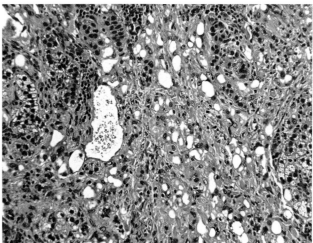

Fig. 1.92 Adenomatoid tumor of adrenal. Tumor cells range from plump epithelioid cells to flattened cells resembling endothelial cells. Many tumor cells exhibit prominent vacuolization, to an extent that may mimic a signet-ring appearance with apparent intracytoplasmic lumina. Tumor cells infiltrate between and around clusters of residual native adrenal cells, and sometimes involve adrenal capsule or peri-adrenal soft tissues. Tumor cells lack nuclear pleomorphism, necrosis, and mitotic activity

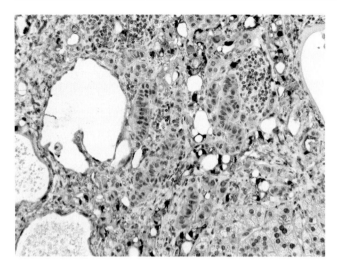

Fig. 1.93 Adenomatoid tumor of adrenal. Immunostain for calretinin highlights the tumor cells, consistent with their mesothelial derivation

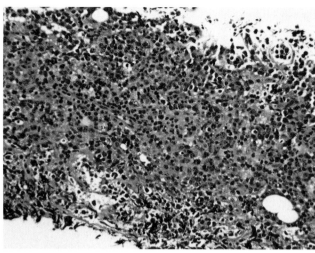

Fig. 1.96 Lymphoma of adrenal. Core needle biopsy of adrenal mass. Lesion proved to be diffuse large B-cell lymphoma

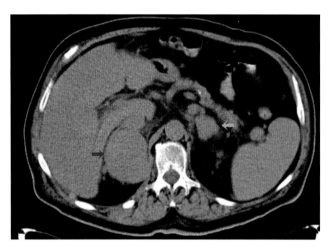

Fig. 1.94 Lymphoma of adrenal. Patient had marked enlargement of right (*red arrow*) and left (*green arrow*) adrenals on CT scan (*Image courtesy of* Nami Azar, MD)

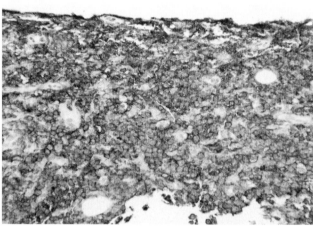

Fig. 1.97 Lymphoma of adrenal. Tumor cells of diffuse large B-cell lymphoma of adrenal show strong immunoreactivity to CD20

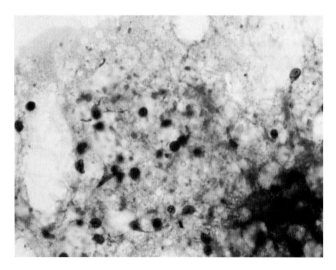

Fig. 1.95 Lymphoma of adrenal. Fine-needle aspiration biopsy of adrenal mass shows dyscohesive lymphoid cells

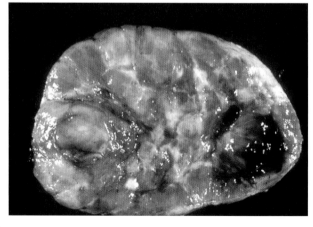

Fig. 1.98 Schwannoma of adrenal. Fewer than a dozen adrenal schwannomas have been reported. They are usually discovered incidentally, as in the case of this 50-year-old woman in whom a 10 cm adrenal mass weighing 990 g was found on CT scan performed for reasons unrelated to the adrenal mass. Schwannomas are typically tan or yellow, and often multinodular

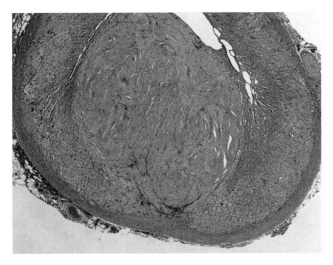

Fig. 1.99 Schwannoma of adrenal. Tumor is composed of spindle cells displaying fascicular growth, occupying the medullary aspect of the adrenal

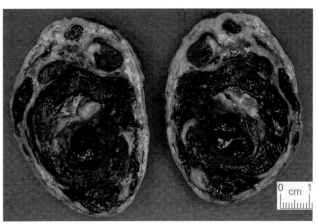

Fig. 1.101 Cavernous hemangioma and hematoma. As noted previously, the etiology of adrenal cysts and adrenal hematomas is often inapparent. In this case, an adrenal mass was noted incidentally on imaging studies, and after several months of observation the lesion was excised. It has the appearance of an organizing hematoma (*Image courtesy of* Erica Martin, MD)

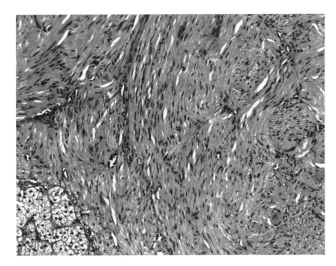

Fig. 1.100 Schwannoma of adrenal. This is a cellular schwannoma composed of intersecting fascicles of tumor cells with uniform spindled nuclei. Necrosis and mitotic figures are absent. Tumor cells showed strong diffusely positive immunostaining for S100 protein

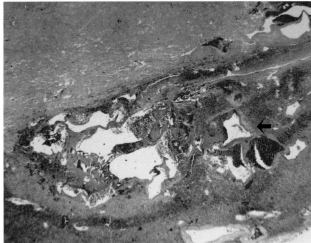

Fig. 1.102 Cavernous hemangioma and hematoma. At upper left is an organizing hematoma. *Arrow* indicates a vascular malformation

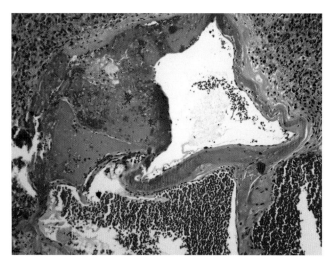

Fig. 1.103 Cavernous hemangioma and hematoma. Closer inspection of the region in Fig. 1.102 indicated by the *arrow* shows endothelial-lined vascular spaces consistent with cavernous hemangioma

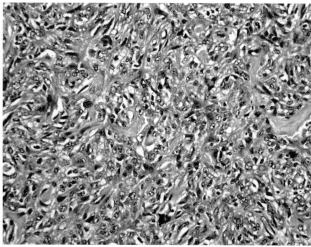

Fig. 1.105 Malignant solitary fibrous tumor of adrenal. Tumor was variably cellular, and showed pronounced cytologic atypia in areas of high cellularity, as shown in this image. Tumor cells showed no immunostaining for S100 protein, desmin, or pankeratin. Spindle cells with little nuclear atypia in hypocellular areas showed focal positivity for CD34

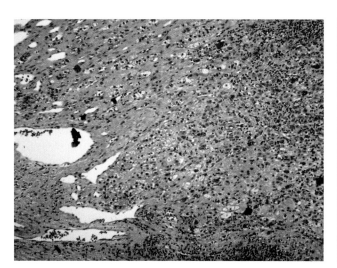

Fig. 1.104 Malignant solitary fibrous tumor of adrenal. Section from a 9 cm firm well circumscribed white adrenal mass in a 58-year-old male. The tumor (*right*), diffusely infiltrates the adrenal, which also exhibits an angiomatous proliferation (*left*). The cells lining the vascular spaces at left showed positive immunostaining for CD31. Tumor cells (*right*) showed no immunostaining for CD31

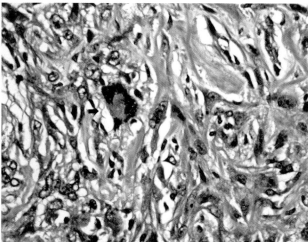

Fig. 1.106 Malignant solitary fibrous tumor of adrenal. Mitotic figures were readily evident throughout the tumor, and some had a bizarre appearance (*arrow*)

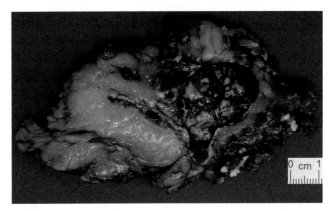

Fig. 1.107 Leiomyosarcoma arising in the adrenal, exhibiting a nodular whorled cut surface (*Image courtesy of* Marina Scarpelli, MD)

Fig. 1.110 Adrenal with metastatic cancer. This tumor was found in an adrenal gland removed as part of a radical nephrectomy procedure (Image courtesy of Christine Lemyre)

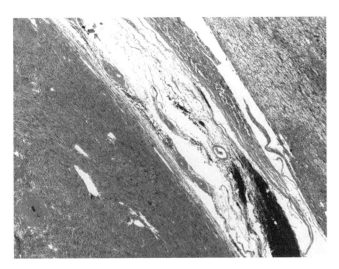

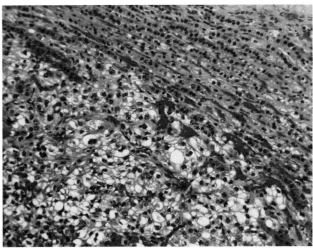

Fig. 1.108 Adrenal leiomyosarcoma, at lower left, showing cytologic atypia and focal necrosis (*Image courtesy of* Marina Scarpelli, MD)

Fig. 1.111 Adrenal with metastatic cancer. The tumor in Fig. 1.110 was metastatic renal cell carcinoma, clear cell type, high nuclear grade

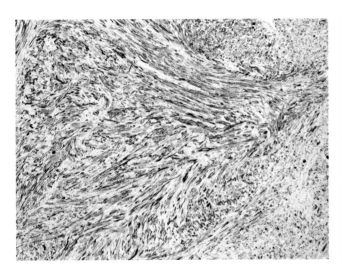

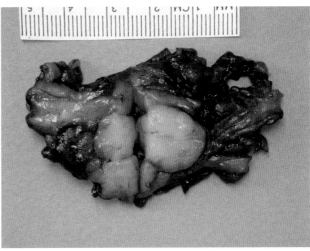

Fig. 1.109 Adrenal leiomyosarcoma. Tumor cells show positive immunostaining for desmin (*Image courtesy of* Marina Scarpelli, MD)

Fig. 1.112 Adrenal with metastatic cancer. In contrast to the primary tumor in Fig. 1.107, this adrenal leiomyosarcoma was a metastasis from a previously diagnosed lesion in another site

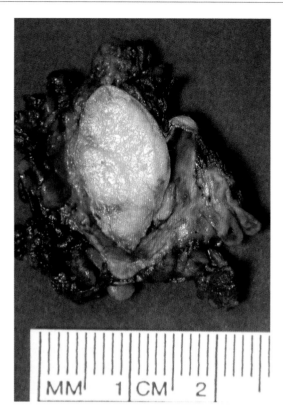

Fig. 1.113 Adrenal with metastatic cancer. Non-small cell lung cancer metastatic to adrenal several years after the initial diagnosis (*Image courtesy of* Richard Naturale, MD)

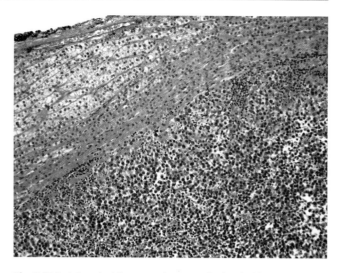

Fig. 1.115 Adrenal with metastatic cancer. Patient had been treated for testicular seminoma several years before discovery of this adrenal mass lesion on surveillance CT scan. Normal adrenal is shown at upper left. Tumor at lower right is morphologically typical of seminoma

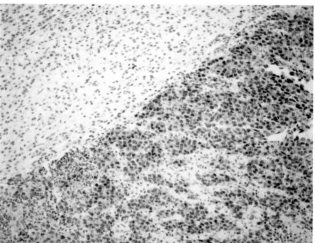

Fig. 1.116 Adrenal with metastatic cancer. The tumor cells of the metastatic cancer shown in Fig. 1.115, and occupying the lower right portion of the image, show positive immunostaining for OCT4, consistent with seminoma

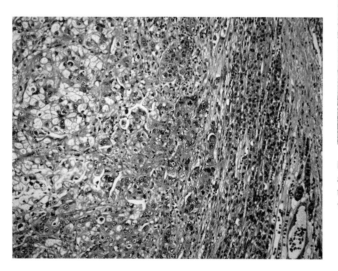

Fig. 1.114 Adrenal with metastatic cancer. Section of the adrenal mass shown in Fig. 1.113 shows findings consistent with metastasis of non-small cell lung cancer

The kidney is a paired bean-shaped organ located superiorly in the retroperitoneum, averaging 12 cm long, 6 cm wide, and 2.5 cm thick, and weighing between 115 and 170 g. It is contained within a thin fibrous capsule that ends at the renal sinus. Fat surrounds the cortical surface of the kidney and the blood vessels, nerves, and collecting structures at the hilum. The perirenal fat is enclosed within a thin but resilient translucent sheath known as Gerota's fascia. Each kidney is composed of 8–18 lobes, each of which constitutes a conical medullary pyramid capped by cortical tissue; downward extensions of cortical tissue between the pyramids are called columns of Bertin. The cortex is normally about 1 cm thick over the pyramids. Medullary rays of Ferrein, consisting of collecting ducts, straight segments of proximal and distal tubules, and vasa recta, extend from the cortex into the medulla. The inner medulla (papilla) drains through the orifices of the terminal collecting ducts (Bellini's ducts) into a minor calyx. Each kidney contains one to two million nephrons, which are the functional unit of the kidney. Each nephron includes a glomerulus, proximal tubule, distal tubule, connecting segment, and collecting duct, which actually is derived from the ureteric bud.

2.1 Normal Kidney

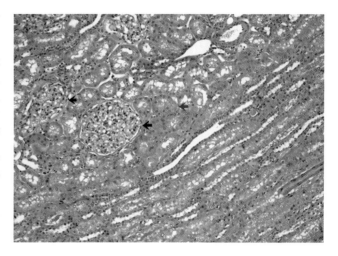

Fig. 2.1 Normal kidney. The section is from the corticomedullary junction, and demonstrates glomeruli (*black arrows*) surrounded by convoluted tubules (*blue arrows*), and long straight medullary rays of Ferrein (*green arrows*)

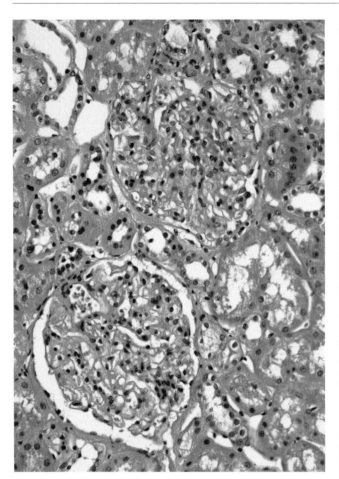

Fig. 2.2 Normal glomeruli, surrounded by cross sections of convoluted tubules

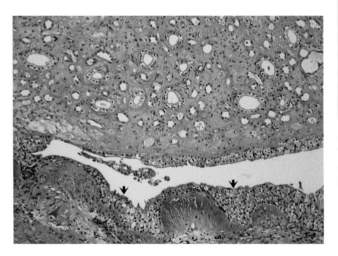

Fig. 2.3 Normal kidney. In the upper half is the tip of a papilla, with cross sections of collecting ducts. In the lower half is a minor calyx, lined by layers of urothelial cells (*black arrows*)

2.2 Congenital Malformations and Diseases

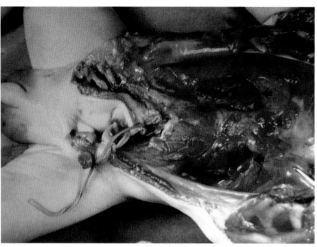

Fig. 2.4 Renal agenesis, bilateral. Potter's syndrome, as originally described, included bilateral renal agenesis, oligohydramnios and Potter's facies. Affected children are stillborn or die soon after birth of respiratory failure due to pulmonary hypoplasia. In this image, the two retroperitoneal structures are adrenal glands. No kidneys were present (*Image courtesy of* Beverly Dahms, MD)

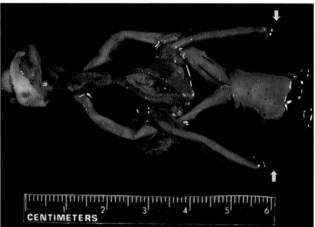

Fig. 2.5 Renal agenesis, bilateral. *Arrows* indicate the tips of two blind-ending ureters. The urachus and umbilical veins are patent and connected to the umbilicus at left. Umbilical arteries are still widely patent, as well (*Image courtesy of* Raymond Redline, MD)

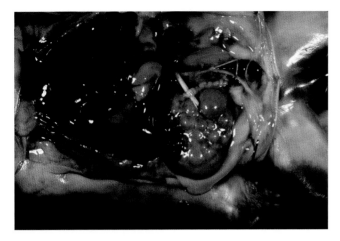

Fig. 2.6 Unilateral renal agenesis and contralateral multicystic dysplastic kidney. The left kidney is absent; left adrenal is visible in the retroperitoneum. The right kidney is present but distorted by multicystic dysplasia (*Image courtesy of* Raymond Redline, MD)

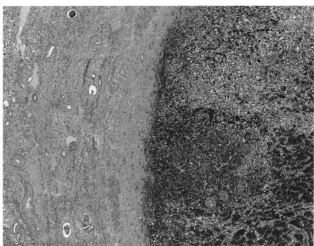

Fig. 2.8 Splenorenal fusion. At low power, the splenic tissue may mimic a vascular neoplasm

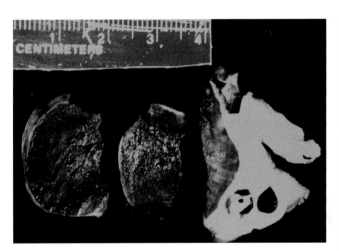

Fig. 2.7 Splenorenal fusion. In this condition, heterotopic splenic tissue is present within the renal capsule, usually due to the fusion of nephrogenic mesoderm and splenic anlage in the second month of gestation, but sometimes representing splenosis after splenectomy or trauma. The splenic tissue forms a beefy red well circumscribed mass within the renal capsule (*see* Tynski and MacLennan 2005. With permission)

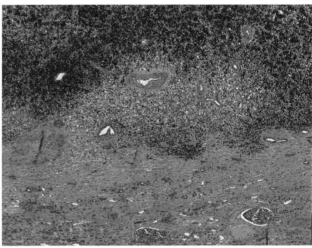

Fig. 2.9 Splenorenal fusion. On closer inspection, the splenic tissue shows its typical sinusoidal structures and scattered large blood vessels. Diagnosis in this case was made more difficult by the absence of typical lymphoid follicles in any of the submitted sections

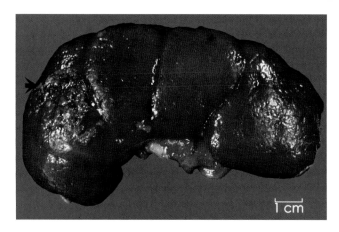

Fig. 2.10 Ectopic adrenal in kidney. The ectopic adrenal tissue is usually subcapsular and is most often in the upper pole. It may assume a plaque-like form (as in this image), but can also be wedge-shaped or spherical (*see* MacLennan GT, Resnick MI, Bostwick DG, 2003. With permission)

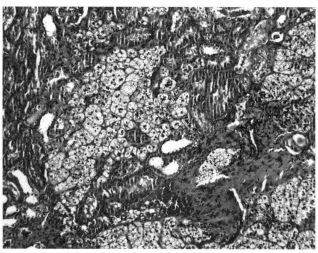

Fig. 2.12 Ectopic adrenal in kidney. Adrenal cortical tissue intermingles with normal renal tissue

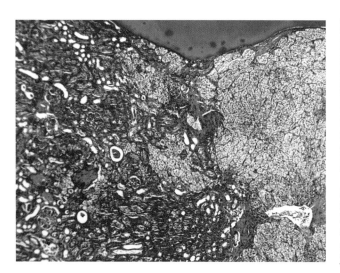

Fig. 2.11 Ectopic adrenal in kidney. The lack of circumscription imparts an infiltrative appearance. At times, this may be a diagnostic challenge; the level of difficulty is even more pronounced on intraoperative frozen sections

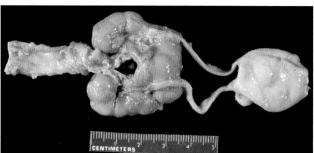

Fig. 2.13 Horseshoe kidney. This is the commonest form of renal fusion, comprising two distinct renal masses fused together in the midline by a broad isthmus connecting their inferior poles. The collecting systems face anteriorly, do not communicate with one another and frequently drain poorly because of anomalies of the ureteropelvic junction

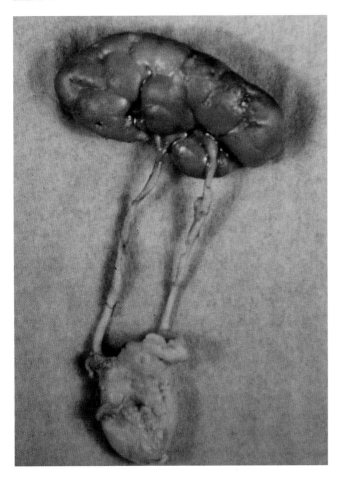

Fig. 2.14 Cake kidney. Similar to horseshoe kidney, but the fusion is more diffuse, rather than being localized to the inferior poles. Examples of inverted horseshoe kidneys, fused at the upper poles, have been reported

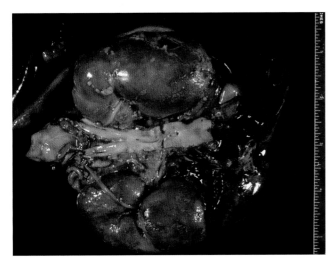

Fig. 2.15 Infantile autosomal recessive polycystic kidney disease. Both kidneys are massively enlarged, which can impede lung development and result in stillbirth or death in early neonatal life due to respiratory failure (*Image courtesy of* Raymond Redline, MD)

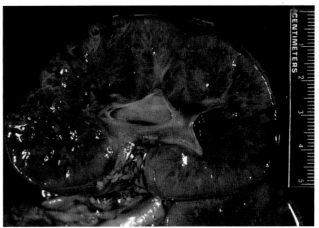

Fig. 2.16 Infantile autosomal recessive polycystic kidney disease. Kidneys retain their reniform shape, and collecting systems are normal. The cut surface has a spongy appearance due to the presence of innumerable small cystically dilated structures (*Image courtesy of* Raymond Redline, MD)

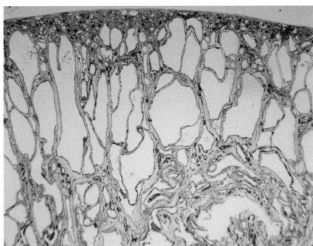

Fig. 2.17 Infantile autosomal recessive polycystic kidney disease. Normal cortical and medullary tissue is diffusely replaced by innumerable cystically dilated radially arranged collecting ducts

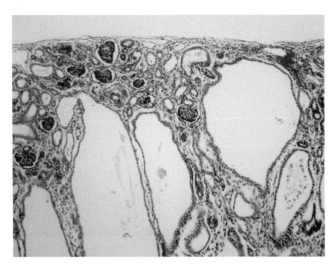

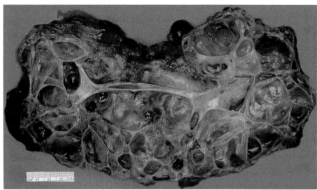

Fig. 2.20 Adult dominant polycystic kidney disease. Cut surface of one of the kidneys in Fig. 2.19 demonstrates the presence of innumerable cysts of variable size. The collecting system is normal. Despite distortion by the cysts, the kidneys retain a reniform shape (*Image courtesy of* Douglas Hartman, MD)

Fig. 2.18 Infantile autosomal recessive polycystic kidney disease. The cystically dilated collecting ducts are lined by small uniform cuboidal cells. A few normal looking residual glomeruli are present between the collecting ducts

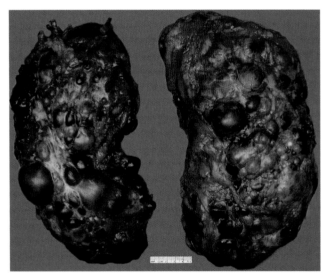

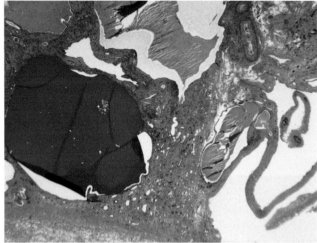

Fig. 2.21 Adult dominant polycystic kidney disease. Low power view shows cysts of varying sizes, lined by inconspicuous cuboidal epithelium; some contain proteinaceous fluid. There is obvious paucity of recognizable functional renal units

Fig. 2.19 Adult dominant polycystic kidney disease. This is the most common genetically transmitted disease and the most common cystic renal disease. When bilateral nephrectomy becomes necessary due to clinical considerations, the kidneys have often attained massive size, as in this case (*Image courtesy of* Douglas Hartman, MD)

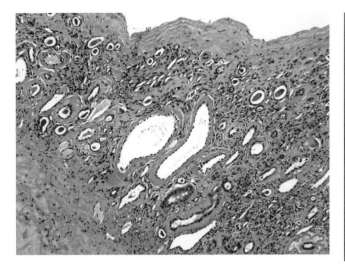

Fig. 2.22 Adult dominant polycystic kidney disease. The interstitium is fibrotic and contains an infiltrate of chronic inflammatory cells. Some tubules are atrophic; others are dilated and sclerotic

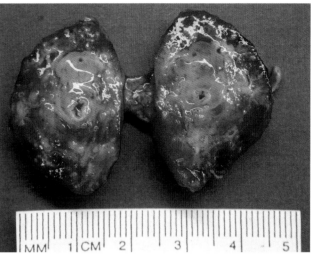

Fig. 2.24 Renal dysplasia: aplastic kidney. The term *dysplasia* connotes arrested organ development, with persistence of structures that never completely developed. Aplastic and multicystic dysplastic kidneys represent opposite ends of a spectrum, varying only in the degree of cyst formation. Aplastic dysplastic kidneys are extraordinarily small, as shown here, and exhibit very limited or absent cyst formation

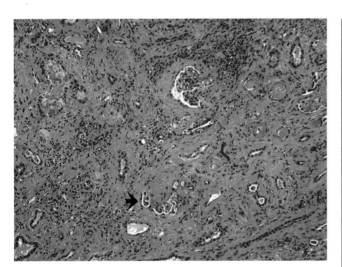

Fig. 2.23 Adult dominant polycystic kidney disease. One of the few remaining glomeruli is undergoing sclerosis (*arrow*)

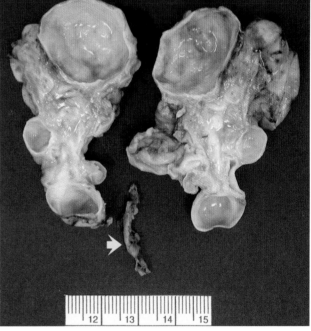

Fig. 2.25 Renal dysplasia: multicystic kidney. The extent of cyst formation is variable. In all instances, the ipsilateral ureter (*arrow*) is atretic or obstructed at the level of the ureteropelvic junction

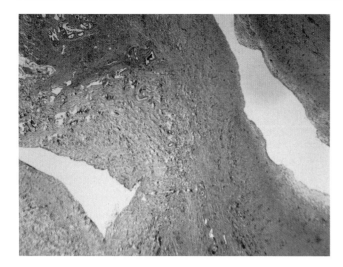

Fig. 2.26 Renal dysplasia. Microscopic findings vary widely. Cysts of variable size and number are commonly observed, lined by flat cuboidal cells and separated by fibrous stroma of variable prominence

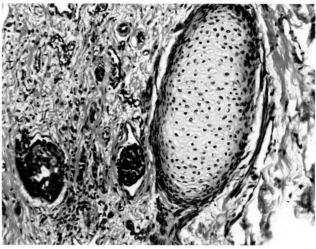

Fig. 2.28 Renal dysplasia. Poorly formed glomeruli are evident at left; islands of immature cartilage are often seen in dysplastic kidneys, possibly derived from renal blastema

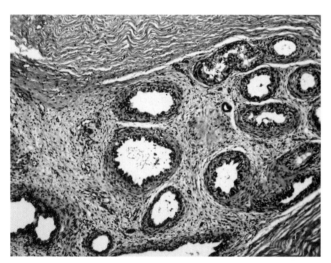

Fig. 2.27 Renal dysplasia. Collars of spindle cells surround dysplastic ducts lined by columnar epithelium. Dysplastic ducts are thought to be derived from the ampullary buds

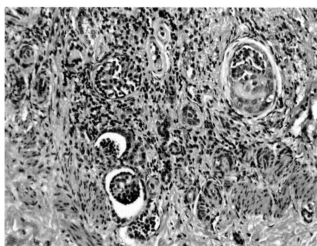

Fig. 2.29 Renal dysplasia. Poorly formed glomeruli and tubules

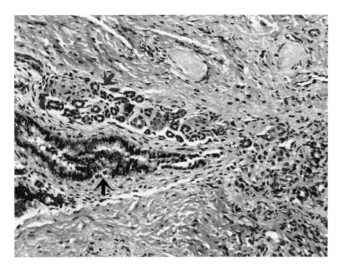

Fig. 2.30 Renal dysplasia. Poorly formed immature-appearing tubules (*blue arrow*) accompanied by a dysplastic ducts surrounded by spindle cells (*black arrow*)

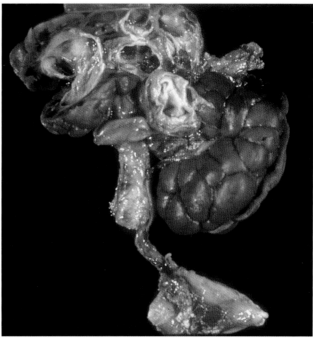

Fig. 2.32 Renal dysplasia in a horseshoe kidney. One of the renal units in the horseshoe kidney was obstructed and showed dysplastic changes

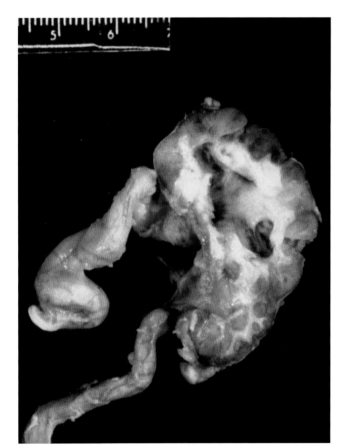

Fig. 2.31 Renal dysplasia: segmental dysplasia. Segmental dysplasia occurs in one segment (usually the upper pole) of a duplex kidney, and exhibits histologic changes similar to those noted in aplastic and multi-cystic kidneys. The affected segment is the one drained by a ureter, which is distally obstructed by ureterocele (as was the case in the image shown) or by ectopia of the ureteral orifice (*see* MacLennan GT, Resnick MI, Bostwick DG, 2003. With permission)

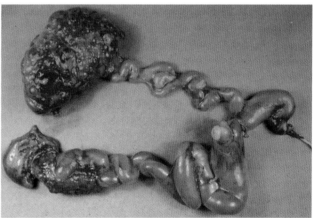

Fig. 2.33 Bilateral renal dysplasia. Lower urinary tract obstructions, such as congenital bladder neck obstruction, posterior urethral valves, and urethral stenosis and prune-belly syndrome (which was the etiology of the bilateral renal dysplasia in the image shown), can result in dysplasia that involves both kidneys

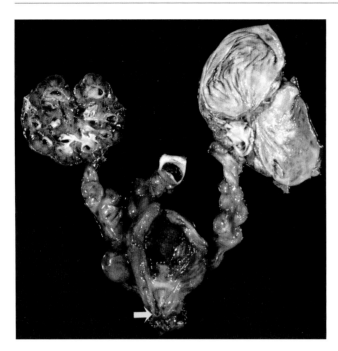

Fig. 2.34 Bilateral renal dysplasia. The renal changes were present at birth and were caused by posterior urethral valves (*arrow*) that had resulted in marked bladder outlet obstruction

2.3 Acquired Nonneoplastic Entities

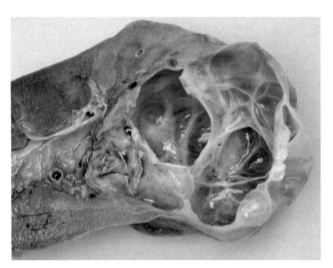

Fig. 2.35 Simple cortical cyst. Simple cortical cyst may be single, multiple, widespread or localized. It is usually located in the cortex, and is filled with clear serous fluid. The lesion shown was a conglomerate of closely situated simple cysts

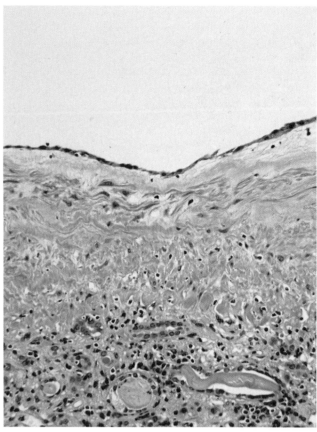

Fig. 2.36 Simple cortical cyst. The cyst is typically lined by flattened epithelium. Sometimes no lining epithelium is identified. The wall is often thick and fibrotic, and is occasionally calcified

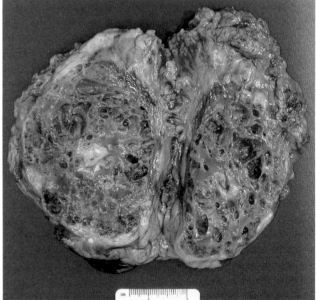

Fig. 2.37 Acquired cystic kidney disease (ACKD). Kidneys involved by ACKD contain multiple cysts ranging from 0.5 to 3.0 cm in diameter. The cysts are predominantly cortical in early stages, with involvement of the medulla as dialysis continues. Eventually all renal parenchyma is obliterated by cysts (*Image courtesy of* Peter Pavlidakey, MD)

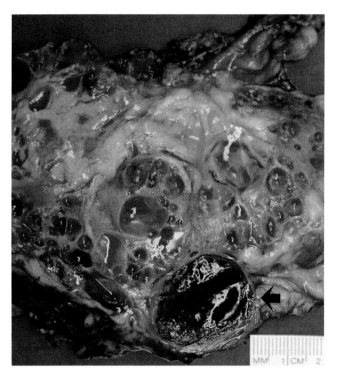

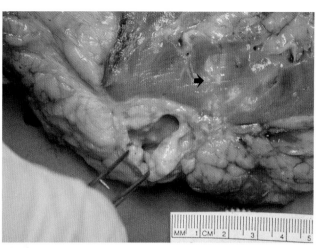

Fig. 2.40 Perirenal abscess, fungal. This fungal abscess developed in the left kidney of a 64-year-old man who was on immunosuppression after an orthotopic liver transplant. After prolonged efforts at conservative management, nephrectomy was performed. The abscess involves both renal parenchyma (*arrow*) and perirenal fat (*forceps*) (*Image courtesy of* Stacy Kim, MD)

Fig. 2.38 Acquired cystic kidney disease. Significant complications are associated with the development of ACKD, including local hemorrhage, infection, and the risk of acquiring renal cell carcinoma. The hematoma designated by the arrow developed in this patient on dialysis, and was radiologically indistinguishable from a solid neoplasm, prompting nephrectomy (*Image courtesy of* Richard Naturale, MD)

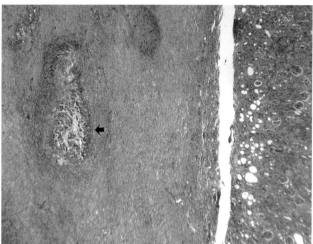

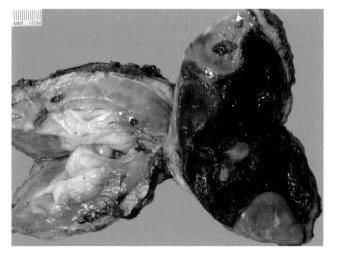

Fig. 2.41 Perirenal abscess, fungal. An abscess cavity is present within dense perirenal fibrous tissue (*arrow*)

Fig. 2.39 Perirenal abscess, bacterial. Perirenal abscess comprises necrotic renal or perirenal tissue and a collection of purulent material, enclosed within a fibrous wall, as exemplified by this image. This perirenal abscess complicated previous partial nephrectomy for infected calculi (*Image courtesy of* Felix Olobatuyi, MD)

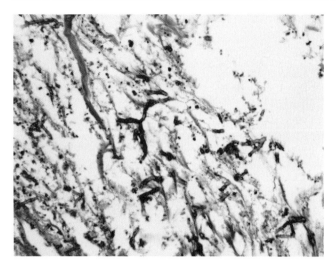

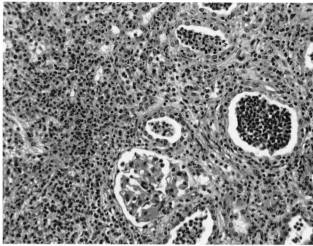

Fig. 2.42 Perirenal abscess, fungal. Fungal organisms consistent with *Aspergillus* species were readily visible within the abscess cavity shown in Fig. 2.40

Fig. 2.44 Acute pyelonephritis. Numerous neutrophils are present in the interstitium and within renal tubules

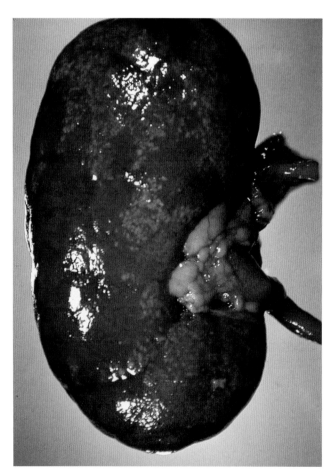

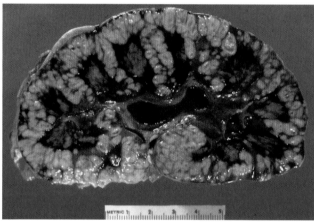

Fig. 2.45 Emphysematous pyelonephritis. This term is applied to gas bubble formation in the renal parenchyma or perirenal tissues; it is often accompanied by abscess and cortical infarcts. This is a kidney from a teenaged diabetic female who died of urosepsis. Tiny gas bubbles are visible within the purulent infiltrates in the renal cortex (*see* MacLennan GT, Resnick MI, Bostwick DG, 2003. With permission)

Fig. 2.43 Acute pyelonephritis. The affected kidney appears swollen and pale. Microabscesses may be visible in the papillae and the renal cortex. The kidney shown in this image was from a patient who died of urosepsis after a gynecologic surgical procedure during which the ureter was inadvertently ligated

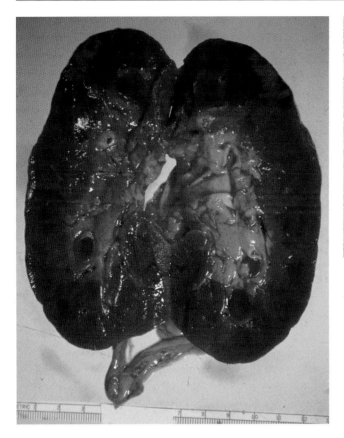

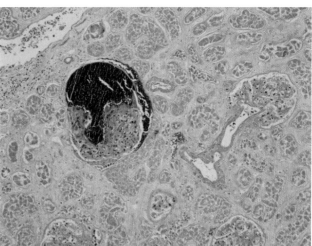

Fig. 2.48 Septic renal emboli. Bacterial overgrowth in and around a glomerulus of the patient described in Fig. 2.47

Fig. 2.46 Septic infarct of kidney. The pale and focally hemorrhagic region in the upper pole of this autopsy kidney represents a septic infarct, caused by vascular occlusion by a fragment of infected thrombus material, often secondary to bacterial endocarditis

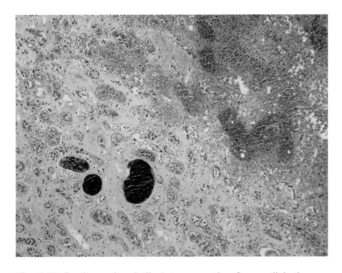

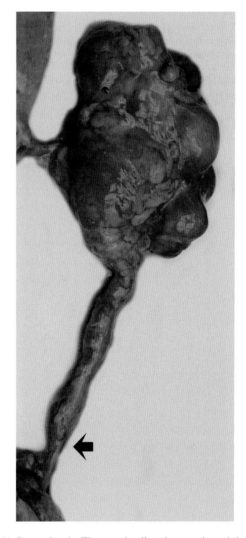

Fig. 2.47 Septic renal emboli. Autopsy section from a diabetic man who developed a mitral valve ring abscess that shed septic emboli infected with *Staphylococcus aureus* to brain, heart, kidneys, gastrointestinal tract, and kidneys. Bacterial overgrowth is evident in tubules and interstitium at upper right, and in several glomeruli at lower left

Fig. 2.49 Pyonephrosis. The term implies obstructed renal drainage – the collecting system is a contained abscess and a variable degree of renal parenchymal destruction is evident. Distension of the left renal unit is evident in this autopsy kidney; the caliber of the ureter changes abruptly at the level of the arrow (*Image courtesy of* Mark Costaldi, MD)

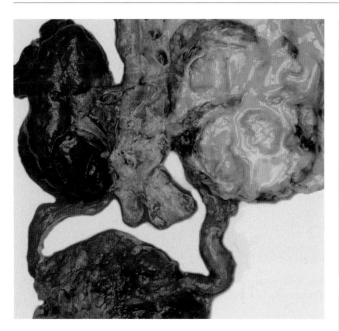

Fig. 2.50 Pyonephrosis. The collecting system of the kidney in Fig. 2.49 contained abundant purulent material. Only a thin rim of residual renal tissue was present. The ureter at the level of the abrupt caliber change showed fibrosis, calcification, and granulomatous inflammation. The etiology of the ureteral obstruction remained enigmatic (*Image courtesy of* Mark Costaldi, MD)

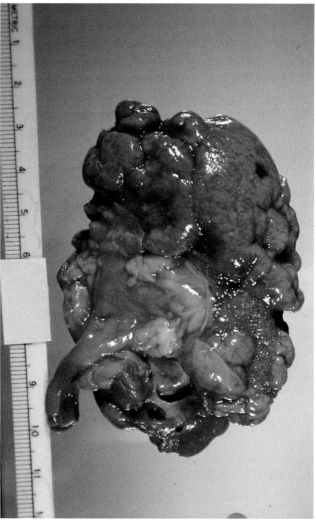

Fig. 2.51 Reflux nephropathy. This is a form of chronic pyelonephritis caused by reflux of urine from the urinary bladder into the upper collecting system, resulting in irregular cortical scarring. In the image shown, some portions of renal cortex are relatively preserved; in the scarred areas, there is virtually no residual cortex

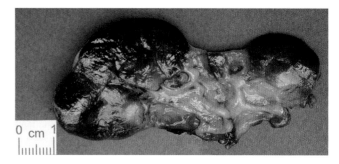

Fig. 2.52 Ask-Upmark kidney. Reflux nephropathy, usually in a child with hypertension, vesicoureteric reflux, and a small kidney with one or more circumferential saddle-shaped cortical scars, lacking inflammation, and sharply contrasting with essentially normal adjacent renal tissue, as shown here (*Image courtesy of* Philip Bomeisl, MD)

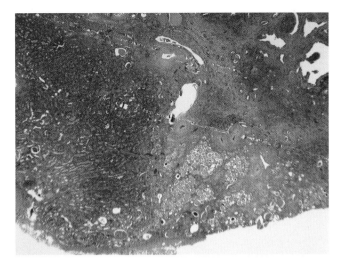

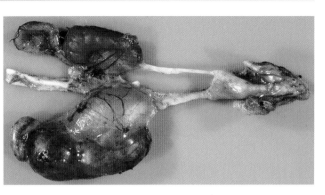

Fig. 2.55 Chronic obstructive pyelonephritis. The renal damage in a setting of obstructed renal drainage results from pressure-related atrophy and chronic infection. This image demonstrates bilateral congenital obstruction at the ureteropelvic junction. Both renal pelves are distended; distal ureters are of normal caliber

Fig. 2.53 Ask-Upmark kidney. There is an abrupt and distinct separation between relatively normal renal tissue on the left, and the area of scarring on the right. There is a scant inflammatory infiltrate in the cortical scar, but there is marked chronic inflammation in the collecting system tissue at upper right

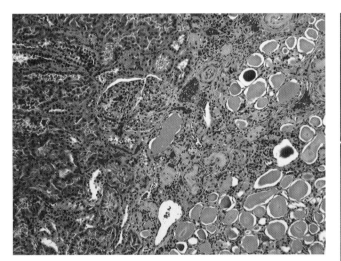

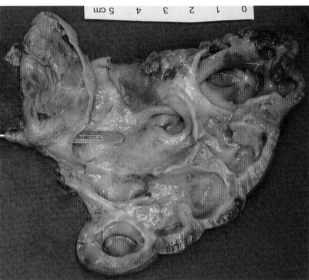

Fig. 2.54 Ask-Upmark kidney. The renal tissue on the left is essentially normal. On the right, in the area of scarring, glomeruli are absent, the interstitium shows fibrosis and is infiltrated by lymphocytes. The tubules appear atrophic and contain eosinophilic casts (thyroidization), and the blood vessels show intimal sclerosis

Fig. 2.56 Chronic obstructive pyelonephritis. Congenital ureteropelvic junction obstruction, with dilatation of renal pelvis and calyces, flattening or obliteration of papillae, and global thinning of renal cortex. Probe passes through the functionally obstructed ureteropelvic junction

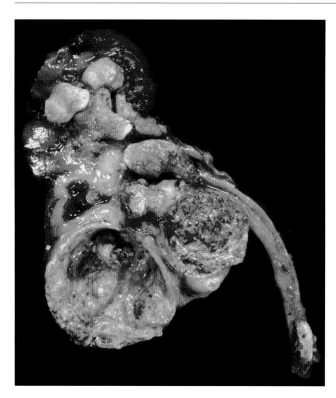

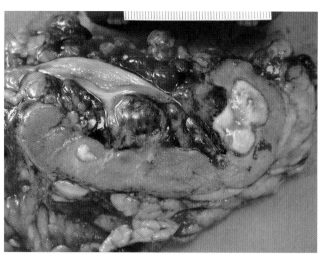

Fig. 2.59 Papillary necrosis. A line of demarcation develops between the viable kidney and the pale infarcted papillary tip. Two areas of papillary necrosis are evident. After the papilla sloughs, an irregular excavation remains (*Image courtesy of* Anaibelith Del Rio Perez, MD)

Fig. 2.57 Chronic obstructive pyelonephritis. Almost all of the renal parenchyma has been obliterated by impaired drainage due to the presence of infected staghorn calculi (*see* MacLennan et al. 2005. With permission)

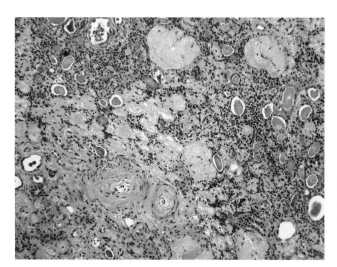

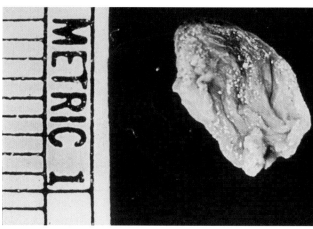

Fig. 2.58 Chronic obstructive pyelonephritis. The microscopic findings are similar to those noted in reflux nephropathy: the glomerular are sclerotic, the interstitium shows fibrosis and is infiltrated by lymphocytes, the tubules appear atrophic and contain eosinophilic casts (thyroidization), and the blood vessels show intimal sclerosis

Fig. 2.60 Papillary necrosis. This image shows a necrotic papilla that was withdrawn from the distal ureter using a stone basket. The initial clinical diagnosis in this diabetic patient was renal colic due to calculus (*see* MacLennan et al. 2005. With permission)

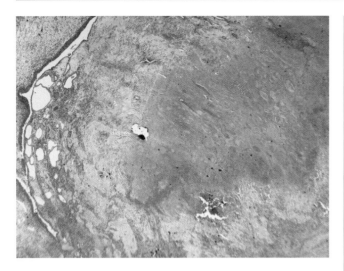

Fig. 2.61 Papillary necrosis. Most of this image demonstrates a papilla projecting into a calyx, visible at far left. The papilla shows an area of extensive infarction centrally

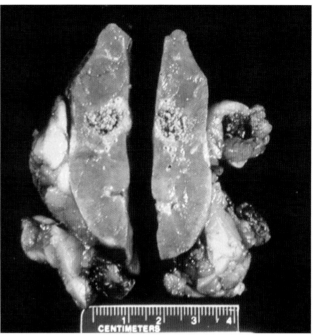

Fig. 2.63 Renal calculi mimicking neoplasm. Occasionally renal calculi, particularly if they are localized to a single calyx and accompanied by surrounding fibrosis, may not be readily distinguishable radiologically from a neoplasm with a necrotic center and a calcified fibrotic capsule, prompting excision, as in this case

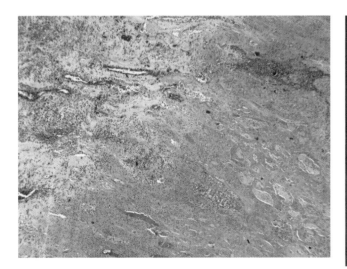

Fig. 2.62 Papillary necrosis. This image illustrates a line of demarcation between inflamed but viable papillary tissue at upper left, and a zone of infarcted and inflamed papilla at lower right

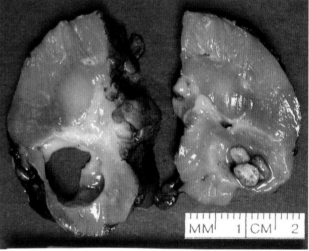

Fig. 2.64 Renal calculi mimicking neoplasm. Some renal calculi, such as uric acid calculi, contain no calcium, and hence are less readily identifiable as stone material. Others are predominantly matrix material, and only lightly calcified. This is another example of a partial nephrectomy necessitated by inconclusive radiologic findings, raising concern for the possibility of a necrotic calcified neoplasm

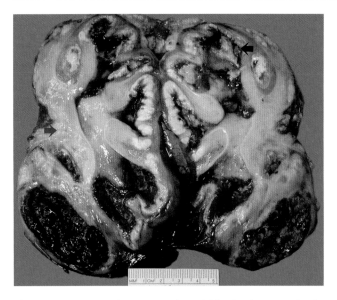

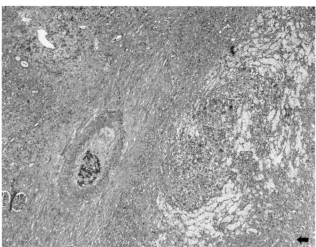

Fig. 2.67 Xanthogranulomatous pyelonephritis. The process has a zonal arrangement: necrotic debris and neutrophils centrally (*arrow at lower right*), surrounded by a zone of lipid-laden macrophages (which may be mistaken for tumor cells of clear cell carcinoma), plasma cells, eosinophils, and lymphocytes. There is usually a fibrous reparative reaction at the periphery of the inflammatory nodules, which may be difficult to distinguish from a spindle cell neoplasm

Fig. 2.65 Xanthogranulomatous pyelonephritis. Another example of a renal calculus-associated inflammatory process that may be difficult to distinguish radiologically from a renal neoplasm. The cut surface shows multiple gray-white to yellow nodules. The process may be diffuse, segmental, or focal. The papillae are blunted, and the renal pelvis commonly contains stones, often of the staghorn type (*black arrow*) and purulent material. The inflammatory process often extends into the perirenal and sinus fat (*blue arrow*) (*Image courtesy of* Douglas Hartman, MD)

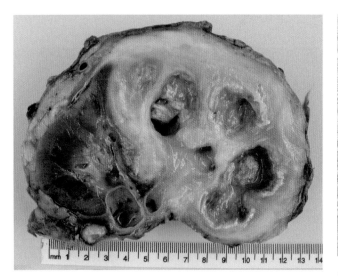

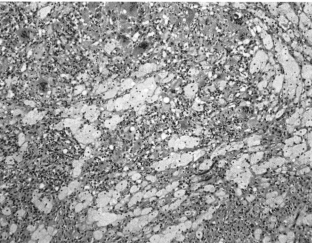

Fig. 2.66 Xanthogranulomatous pyelonephritis, segmental. Renal tissue at left is essentially normal. The tissue at right has been obliterated by chronic infection and obstruction. Calculi are present

Fig. 2.68 Xanthogranulomatous pyelonephritis. Multinucleated giant cells may also form part of the inflammatory cell population. The abundant large pale-staining cells are lipid-laden macrophages, which account for the yellow color of the cut surface of the nodules

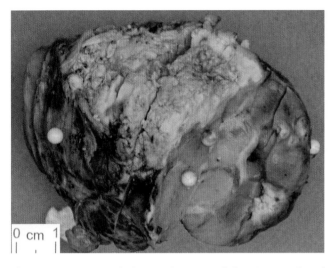

Fig. 2.69 Renal tuberculosis (*Mycobacterium chelonae*). An explanted transplant kidney that had become infected with *M. chelonae*, a rapidly growing mycobacterium most often found in skin, soft tissue, or postoperative wound infections. A perirenal abscess formed, necessitating removal (*Image courtesy of* Amber Petrolla, MD)

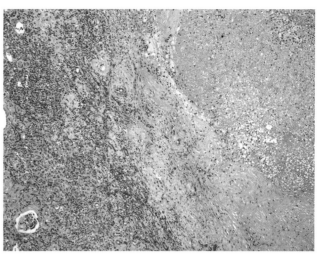

Fig. 2.71 Renal tuberculosis (*Mycobacterium chelonae*). Section from the kidney shown in Fig. 2.69. A fibrous-walled abscess cavity is shown at right. Prolonged antibiotic therapy preceded nephrectomy, and no viable organisms were demonstrable in the surgical specimen, although they were readily seen in the abscess cavity fluid preoperatively (*see* Figs. 2.72 and 2.73)

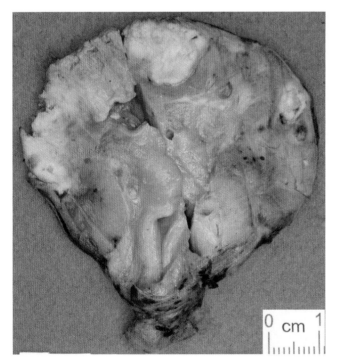

Fig. 2.70 Renal tuberculosis (*Mycobacterium chelonae*). Cross-section of the kidney shown in Fig. 2.69. Multiple areas of caseating necrosis are present (*Image courtesy of* Ambet Petrolla, MD)

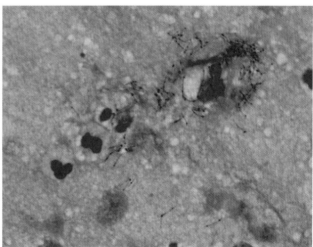

Fig. 2.72 Renal tuberculosis (*Mycobacterium chelonae*). Acid-fast stain demonstrating mycobacteria in fluid aspirated from perirenal abscess adjacent to kidney shown in Fig. 2.69

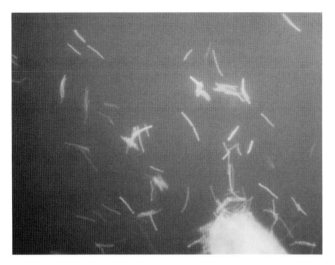

Fig. 2.73 Renal tuberculosis (*Mycobacterium chelonae*). Auramine-rhodamine stain highlighting mycobacteria in fluid aspirated from perirenal abscess adjacent to kidney shown in Fig. 2.69

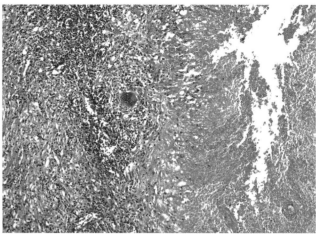

Fig. 2.75 Renal tuberculosis (*Mycobacterium tuberculosis*). Additional section from the lesion shown in Fig. 2.74. Central necrosis at right, and granulomatous inflammation and fibrosis at left. Multinucleated giant cells are present

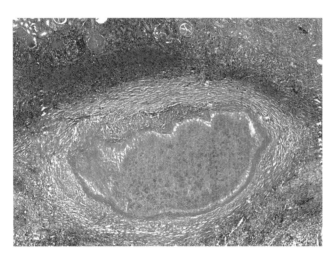

Fig. 2.74 Renal tuberculosis (*Mycobacterium tuberculosis*). This patient had a previous well-established history of pulmonary tuberculosis. Section from the patient's nephrectomy specimen shows a tuberculous granuloma, with central caseating necrosis and peripheral scarring

2.4 Benign Epithelial Tumors

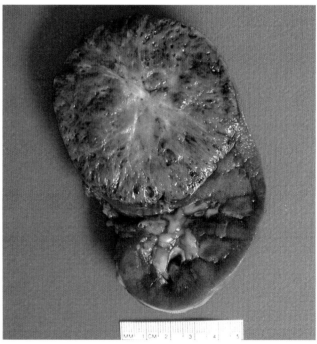

Fig. 2.76 Oncocytoma. Renal oncocytomas are usually solid and range from 0.3 to 26 cm in greatest dimension. They are typically mahogany brown and less often tan to pale yellow, and well circumscribed, with varying degrees of encapsulation. About one-third show central scarring; less often, one may observe hemorrhage, focal cystic degeneration, tumor extension into perirenal fat and, rarely, tumor growth into large blood vessels

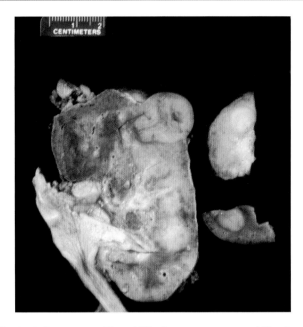

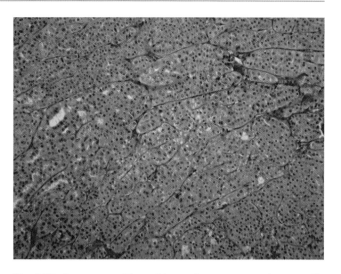

Fig. 2.77 Oncocytoma. Up to 13% of oncocytomas are multifocal, and up to 13% are bilateral. Other benign renal neoplasms are often present, including papillary adenomas and angiomyolipomas, and concurrent renal cell carcinoma has been observed in up to 32% of cases (*see* MacLennan GT and Cheng L, 2008. With permission)

Fig. 2.79 Oncocytoma. The architectural arrangement of tumor cells in oncocytoma may be described as nested or organoid (classic), tubulocystic, or mixed. In the classic form, tumor cells are arranged to form nests, islands, organoid clusters, cords, trabeculae, or confluent solid sheets of cells lacking stroma

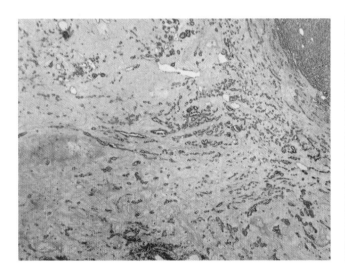

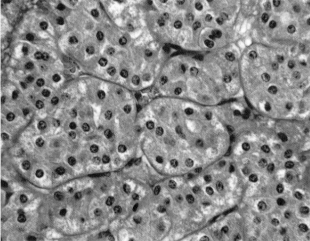

Fig. 2.78 Oncocytoma. Oncocytoma often exhibits areas where the tumor cells are embedded in a hypocellular hyalinized or myxoid stroma. Rarely, oncocytomas exhibit stromal calcifications, and osseous and myeloid metaplasia

Fig. 2.80 Oncocytoma. Oncocytoma is composed predominantly of round to polygonal cells with densely granular eosinophilic cytoplasm, round uniform nuclei with smoothly distributed chromatin, and a central nucleolus. Scattered binucleated cells are frequently present. Mitotic figures are absent or only rarely identified

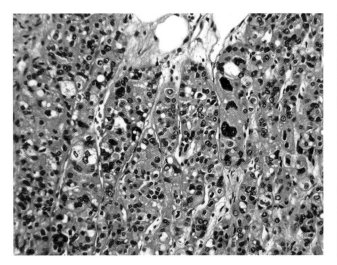

Fig. 2.81 Oncocytoma. A small population of cells with scant granular cytoplasm, dark hyperchromatic nuclei, and a high nuclear–cytoplasmic ratio may be present. Cells with pronounced nuclear atypia may be present; this is regarded as a degenerative change, provided that the rest of the findings in the tumor are consistent with oncocytoma

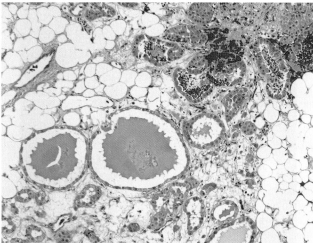

Fig. 2.83 Oncocytoma. Certain histologic findings, provided their extent is very limited, are considered compatible with a diagnosis of oncocytoma. Rare mitotic figures, hemorrhage, small foci of necrosis, focal nuclear pleomorphism, extension of tumor into perinephric fat (as shown in this image) or into adjacent renal parenchyma, small clusters of cells with clear cytoplasm embedded in hyalinized stroma, minute papillary projections into dilated tubules, and invasion of small, capillary-sized, or even venous-type vessels are considered permissible in an otherwise typical oncocytoma. Findings impermissible for a diagnosis of oncocytoma include areas of clear-cell or spindle-cell carcinoma, prominent papillary architecture, macroscopic or conspicuous microscopic necrosis, significant numbers of mitotic figures, and atypical mitotic figures

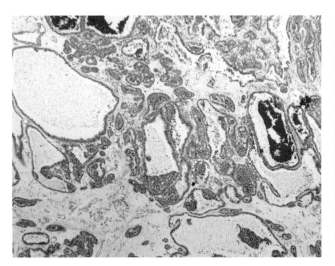

Fig. 2.82 Oncocytoma. Variably sized luminal structures lined by cells indistinguishable from cells of the classic pattern, as shown in this image, are often present; if extensive, this architecture is designated as the tubulocystic form of oncocytoma. The mixed form of oncocytoma includes both organoid and tubulocystic components

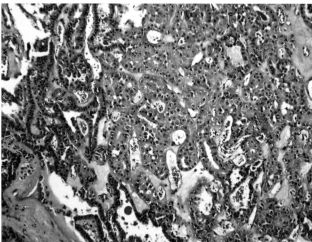

Fig. 2.84 Oncocytosis. Extreme examples of multifocality, with innumerable oncocytic neoplasms, are designated oncocytosis or oncocytomatosis. Some such cases contain "hybrid tumors," composed of both oncocytoma, as shown on the left, and chromophobe renal cell carcinoma, shown at right

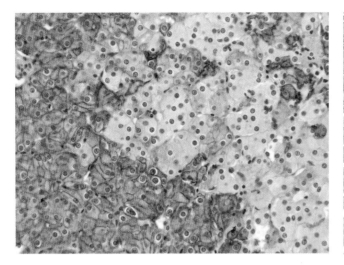

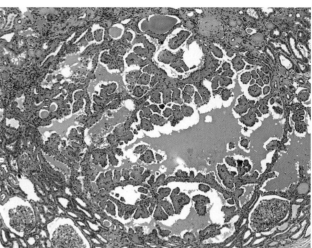

Fig. 2.85 Oncocytosis. Areas of this hybrid oncocytic neoplasm that showed features suggestive of chromophobe renal cell carcinoma showed positive immunostaining for cytokeratin 7; adjacent and intermingled cells more typical of oncocytoma showed little or no staining for this keratin marker

Fig. 2.87 Papillary adenoma. Although most have a seamless interface with the adjacent renal parenchyma, a thin fibrous pseudocapsule is apparent in some. In some cases, the tumor architecture is entirely papillary, as in this image

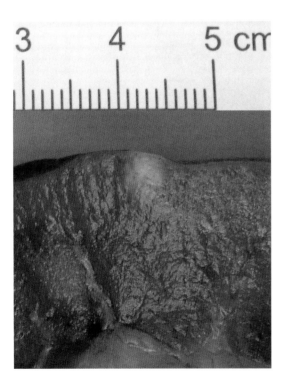

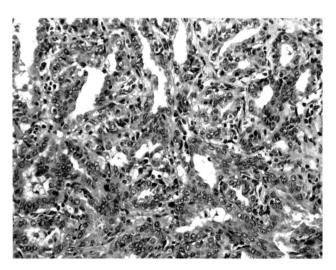

Fig. 2.88 Papillary adenoma. The tumor architecture may also be tubular, as in this image, or tubulopapillary. In most papillary adenomas, the tumor cells resemble those of type 1 papillary renal cell carcinoma, possessing nuclei that are round to oval and occasionally grooved, with stippled to clumped chromatin and inconspicuous nucleoli, lacking mitotic activity, and accompanied by scant cytoplasm that varies from pale to eosinophilic to basophilic

Fig. 2.86 Papillary adenoma. Papillary adenoma of the kidney is defined as a neoplasm having papillary or tubular architecture, low nuclear grade, a diameter less than or equal to 5 mm, and lacking histologic resemblance to clear cell, chromophobe, or collecting duct renal cell carcinoma. Papillary adenomas form well circumscribed gray white to tan nodules, frequently just below the renal capsule (*Image courtesy of* Michelle Stehura, MD)

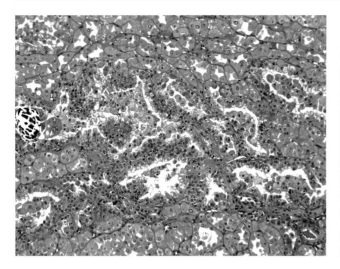

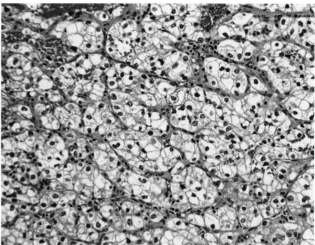

Fig. 2.89 Papillary adenoma. Infrequently, tumor cells resemble those of type 2 papillary renal cell carcinoma, exhibiting prominent nucleoli and voluminous eosinophilic cytoplasm. Psammoma bodies and foamy macrophages are sometimes seen within papillary adenomas

Fig. 2.91 Renal cell carcinoma, clear cell type. Classic clear cell carcinoma is composed of cells with distinct cell membranes and optically clear cytoplasm. Tumor cells are arranged in sheets, compact nests, alveolar, acinar, and microcystic, or even macrocystic structures, separated by an abundance of thin-walled blood vessels

2.5 Renal Cell Carcinoma

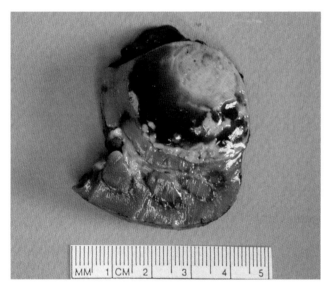

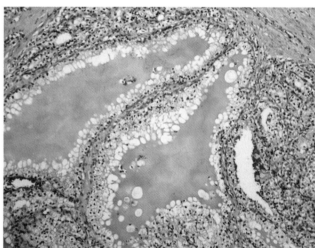

Fig. 2.92 Tubular structures vary in size. Microcysts contain eosinophilic fluid or extravasated red blood cells

Fig. 2.90 Renal cell carcinoma, clear cell type, Fuhrman nuclear grade 1. Clear cell carcinoma ranges in size from minuscule to tumors weighing several kilograms. It is typically unilateral and unicentric, and well demarcated from normal kidney by a fibrous pseudocapsule. The cut surface is usually variegated. Viable tumor is bright golden yellow, as shown here, due to various lipids within the tumor cells

2.6 Grading Renal Cell Carcinoma

One of the most important features of renal cell carcinoma for predicting outcome is the nuclear grade of the tumor. The nuclei of clear cell carcinoma show considerable variation in nuclear size, nuclear shape, and nucleolar prominence, and these features are assessed when assigning a nuclear grade to an individual tumor for prognostic purposes. The Fuhrman nuclear grading system is most commonly used in North America. The main grading parameters are nuclear size, nucleolar prominence, and nuclear shape

Fuhrman Nuclear Grading
I. Small round uniform nuclei, up to 10 µm, inconspicuous nucleoli
II. Nuclei slightly irregular, up to 15 µm, readily evident uniform nucleoli
III. Nuclei very irregular, up to 20 µm, large prominent nucleoli
IV. Nuclei bizarre, spindled or multilobated, larger than 20 µm, macronucleoli

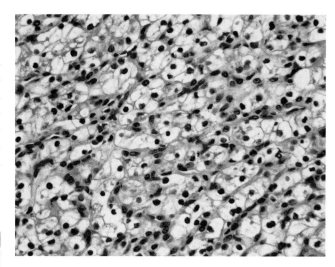

Fig. 2.93 Renal cell carcinoma, clear cell type, Fuhrman nuclear grade 1. In this image, the nuclei are only slightly larger than a red cell, and nucleoli are inapparent or inconspicuous, features consistent with Fuhrman grade 1

2.6.1 TNM Staging of Renal Cell Carcinoma

Tumor stage is a reflection of the extent of anatomic spread and involvement of disease, and is considered the most important factor in predicting the clinical behavior and outcome of renal cell carcinoma. Over the past several decades, the TNM (tumor, node, metastasis) system has been shown to be an excellent prognostic factor for patients with renal cell carcinoma

Primary Tumor – T Stage	
Tx	Primary tumor cannot be assessed
T0	No evidence of primary tumor
T1a	Confined to kidney, 4.0 cm or less
T1b	Confined to kidney, more than 4.0 cm but less than or equal to 7.0 cm
T2a	Confined to kidney, more than 7.0 cm but less than or equal to 10 cm
T2b	Confined to kidney, more than 10 cm
T3a	Tumor invades renal vein, or perinephric fat but not beyond Gerota's fascia
T3b	Tumor grossly extends into vena cava below the diaphragm
T3c	Tumor grossly extends into vena cava above the diaphragm or invades wall of vena cava
T4	Tumor invades beyond Gerota's fascia, or adrenal gland by contiguous extension (tumors involving ipsilateral adrenal but not by contiguous extension are regarded as M1)

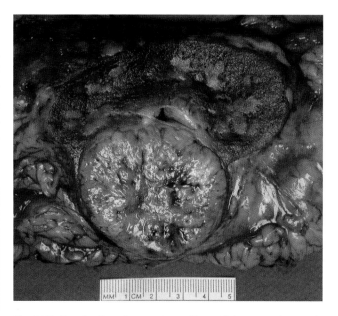

Fig. 2.94 Renal cell carcinoma, clear cell type, Fuhrman nuclear grade 2. Larger tumors and those of higher grade often show areas of gray-white fibrosis and recent or old hemorrhage. This tumor is stage T1b: it is between 4 and 7 cm and it protrudes into perirenal fat but does not infiltrate it (*Image courtesy of* Christine Lemyre)

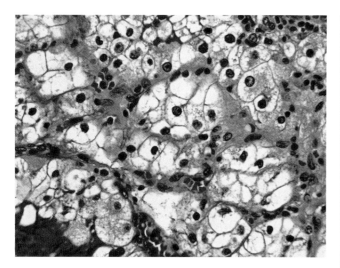

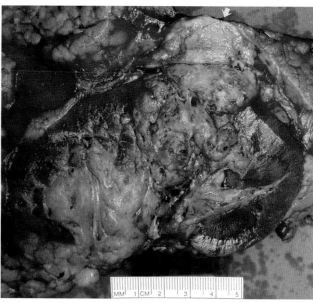

Fig. 2.95 Renal cell carcinoma, clear cell type, Fuhrman nuclear grade 2. Tumor cell nuclei are approximately twice the size of a red cell. Nucleoli are ready discernible in most nuclei, but are not particularly prominent. The outlines of some nuclei are a little irregular

Fig. 2.97 Renal cell carcinoma, clear cell type, Fuhrman nuclear grade 3. This tumor is stage T3a: it has infiltrated perirenal fat to the level of the black-inked Gerota's fascia (*arrow*), but not beyond it (*Image courtesy of* John Miedler, MD)

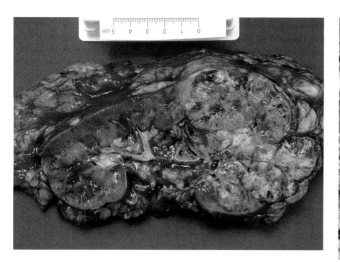

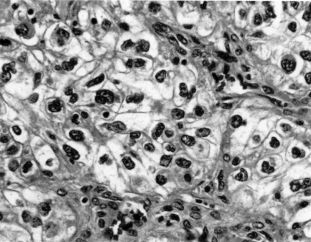

Fig. 2.96 Renal cell carcinoma, clear cell type, Fuhrman nuclear grade 3. Larger tumors often appear bosselated, and protrude from the cortical surface. This tumor is stage T2a: it is more than 7 cm but less than 10 cm, and it protrudes into perirenal fat but does not infiltrate it. T2b tumors are greater than 10 cm (*Image courtesy of* Anastasia Canacci, MD)

Fig. 2.98 Renal cell carcinoma, clear cell type, Fuhrman nuclear grade 3. Nuclei are at least three times larger than red cells, and they possess large prominent nucleoli. Nuclear outlines are quite irregular

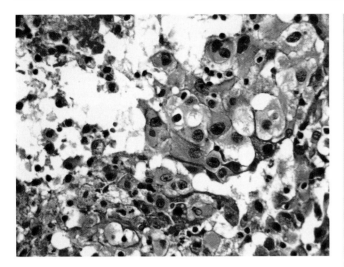

Fig. 2.99 Renal cell carcinoma, clear cell type, Fuhrman nuclear grade 3. Some clear cell carcinomas have components of cells with granular eosinophilic cytoplasm; such cells are more often seen in high-grade cancers, or near areas of hemorrhage or necrosis

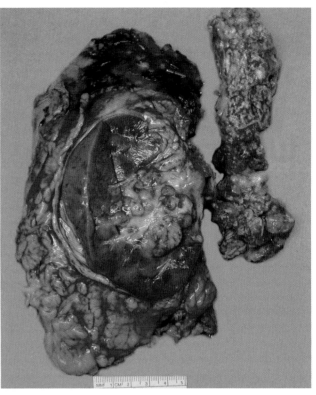

Fig. 2.101 Renal cell carcinoma, clear cell type, Fuhrman nuclear grade 4. This stage T3b high-grade clear cell carcinoma involved the renal vein, as well as the inferior vena cava below the diaphragm (*Image courtesy of* Michelle Stehura, MD)

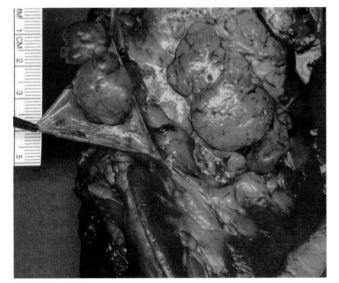

Fig. 2.100 Renal cell carcinoma, clear cell type, Fuhrman nuclear grade 3. Stage T3a tumor occupying the renal vein (*Image courtesy of* Li Yan Khor, MBBCh)

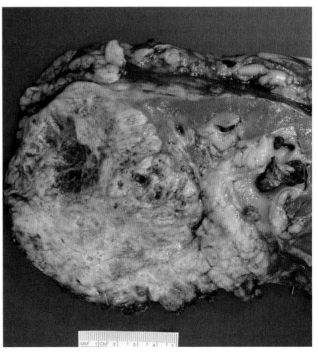

Fig. 2.102 Renal cell carcinoma, clear cell type, Fuhrman nuclear grade 4. Although most clear cell carcinomas have an expansile pushing growth pattern, some tumors irregularly infiltrate the adjacent renal parenchyma. This stage T4 tumor infiltrated sinus fat and extended through Gerota's fascia to involve skeletal muscle posteriorly

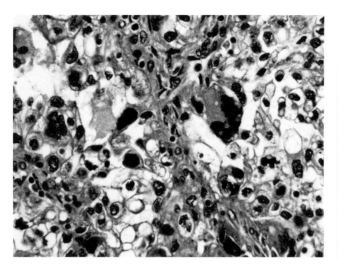

Fig. 2.103 Renal cell carcinoma, clear cell type, Fuhrman nuclear grade 4. Tumor cell nuclei are large and hyperchromatic. Some are spindled, some have prominent nucleoli, some are multilobed and some are simply bizarre in appearance

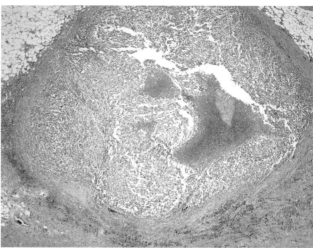

Fig. 2.105 Renal cell carcinoma, clear cell type, Fuhrman nuclear grade 4. Photomicrograph of one of the infiltrating nodules shown in Fig.2.104 confirms true invasion of fat with a fibroblastic and inflammatory response

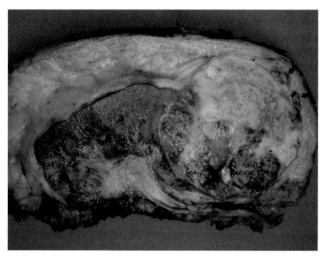

Fig. 2.104 Renal cell carcinoma, clear cell type, Fuhrman nuclear grade 4. In some cases it is difficult to ascertain whether a tumor is truly infiltrating perirenal fat, or simply displacing it by expansile growth. In this case, there appears to be true infiltration of fat (*arrows*) (*Image courtesy of* Hollie Reeves, MD)

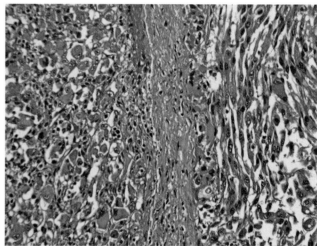

Fig. 2.106 Renal cell carcinoma, clear cell type, with sarcomatoid change. Sarcomatoid differentiation can be found in all of the major renal cell carcinoma subtypes. Fuhrman grade 4 clear cell carcinoma is at left; tumor cells have large bizarre nuclei and some have a rhabdoid appearance. At right, the tumor cells are spindled and resemble sarcoma

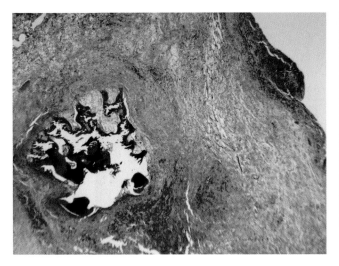

Fig. 2.107 Renal cell carcinoma, clear cell type, with unusual histologic findings. A small focus of clear cell carcinoma is present at upper right. Heterotopic bone formation is evident at left, in a background of inflammation and fibrosis

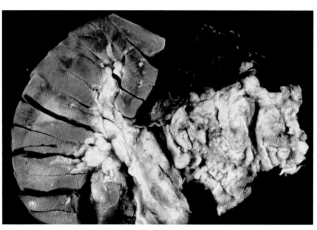

Fig. 2.109 Renal cell carcinoma, clear cell type, extrarenal. A bulky cancer, histologically classic clear cell renal cell carcinoma, was located in soft tissues adjacent to but entirely separate from an entirely normal kidney, which was extensively sampled but showed no evidence of a primary renal neoplasm. The opposite kidney was radiologically normal (*see* MacLennan GT and Cheng L, 2008. With permission)

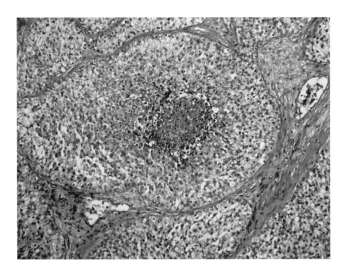

Fig. 2.108 Renal cell carcinoma, clear cell type, with unusual histologic findings. This clear cell carcinoma showed widespread comedo-type necrosis

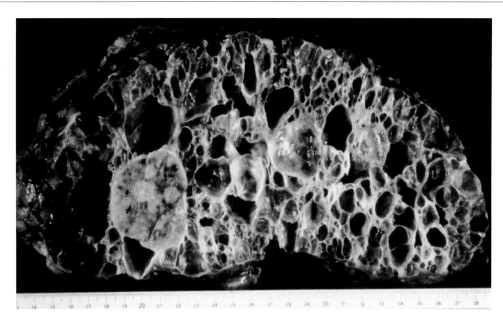

Fig. 2.110 Renal cell carcinoma in adult dominant polycystic kidney disease. More than 30 patients with autosomal dominant polycystic kidney disease have reportedly developed renal cell carcinoma, but there is no convincing evidence that autosomal dominant polycystic kidney disease confers a higher risk of renal cancer (*see* MacLennan GT, Resnick MI, Bostwick DG, 2003. With permission)

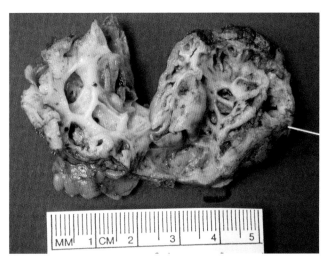

Fig. 2.111 Multilocular cystic renal cell carcinoma. Multilocular cystic renal cell carcinoma ranges from 0.5 to 13.0 cm in diameter. It is well circumscribed and usually unilateral and solitary. The cysts vary in size, contain clear or hemorrhagic fluid, and are separated by thin septa. No expansile tumor nodules are grossly visible (*Image courtesy of Shams Halat, MD*)

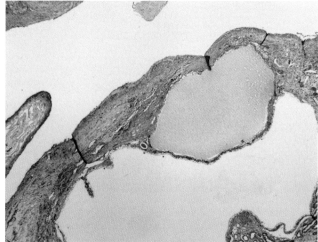

Fig. 2.112 Multilocular cystic renal cell carcinoma. By definition, it is entirely composed of cysts and septa with no expansile solid nodules; the septa should contain aggregates of epithelial cells with clear cytoplasm, cytologically indistinguishable from those of grade 1 renal cell carcinoma. Necrosis is absent. The cysts are lined by one or more layers of epithelial cells, occasionally forming minute papillary structures

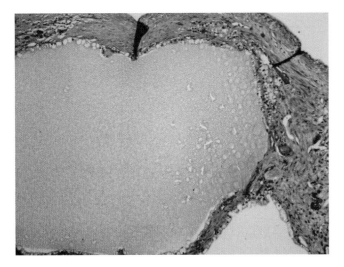

Fig. 2.113 Multilocular cystic renal cell carcinoma. The lining cells have variable amounts of clear or lightly eosinophilic cytoplasm. The cytologic characteristics of the lining epithelial cells are not part of the criteria for defining multilocular cystic renal cell carcinoma

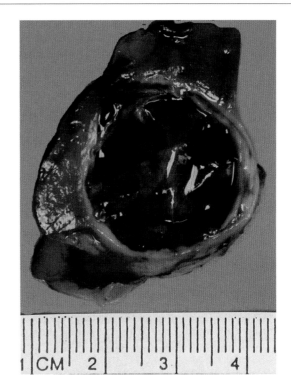

Fig. 2.115 Extensively cystic clear cell renal cell carcinoma. Grossly, this neoplasm had features suggestive of multilocular cystic renal cell carcinoma. Expansile nodules were not visible

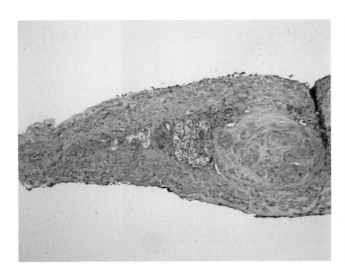

Fig. 2.114 Multilocular cystic renal cell carcinoma. The septa consist of fibrous tissue. In all cases there are clusters of epithelial cells with clear cytoplasm within the septa, typically with small dark nuclei. Confirmation of their epithelial nature with immunostains is sometimes necessary

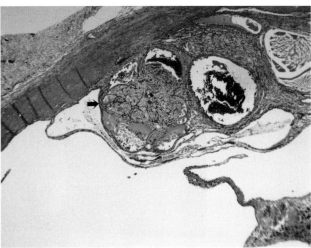

Fig. 2.116 Extensively cystic clear cell renal cell carcinoma. An expansile nodule of clear cell carcinoma is readily apparent. This feature excludes multilocular cystic renal cell carcinoma

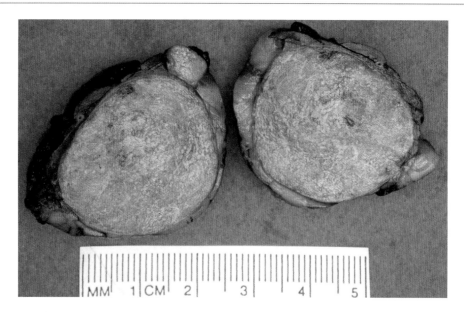

Fig. 2.117 Papillary renal cell carcinoma. Papillary renal cell carcinomas are typically well circumscribed. The cut surfaces vary from red-brown (if there is remote hemorrhage and hemosiderin accumulation) to yellow, if the stroma contains abundant stromal macrophages (*Image courtesy of* Anaibelith Del Rio Perez, MD)

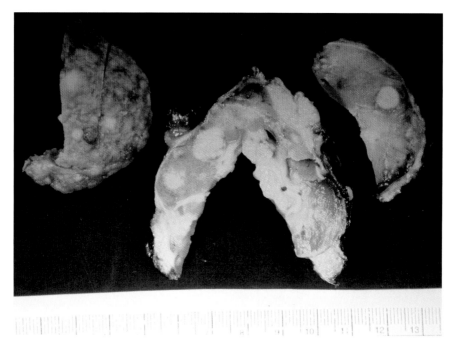

Fig. 2.118 Papillary renal cell carcinoma. Multifocality is noted in up to 8% of papillary renal cell carcinoma, and is pronounced when cancer develops in patients with hereditary papillary renal carcinoma, an example of which is illustrated here. Multiple papillary carcinomas of varying size are present

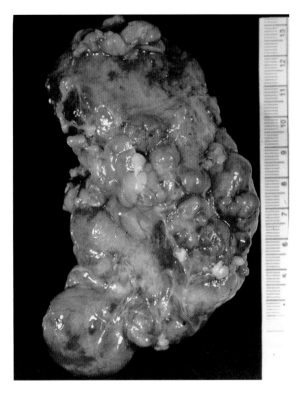

Fig. 2.119 Papillary renal cell carcinoma. The great majority of multifocal papillary renal cell carcinoma cases involve patients with no documented familial predisposition, as in this case. Multiple protruding papillary neoplasms are readily evident on the kidney surface

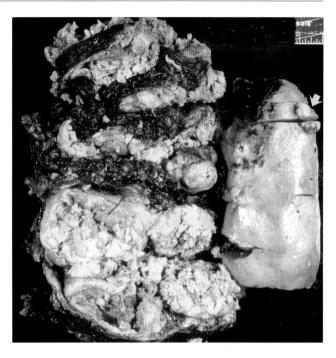

Fig. 2.121 Papillary renal cell carcinoma. A small and relatively inconspicuous papillary carcinoma (*arrow*) can form massive metastatic deposits, as shown here. The tumor mass at left is metastatic cancer in hilar soft tissues (*see* MacLennan GT and Cheng L, 2008. With permission)

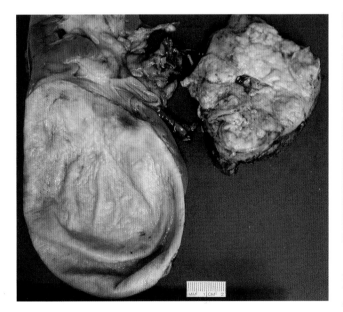

Fig. 2.120 Papillary renal cell carcinoma. A thick fibrous pseudocapsule is present in up to two thirds of cases, sometimes enclosing nothing more than old bloody necrotic material, as exemplified by this cystic tumor with only a small amount of mural sarcomatoid papillary carcinoma. The tumor mass at right is metastatic cancer in hilar soft tissues

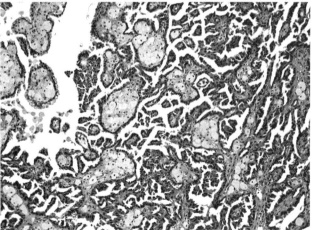

Fig. 2.122 Papillary renal cell carcinoma. Papillary renal cell carcinoma is composed of varying proportions of papillary and tubular structures, and some tumors consist only of cysts with a few papillary excrescences or with mural tumor. The stroma of the papillary structures commonly harbors variable numbers of macrophages. Papillae are lined by a single layer of tumor cells that may appear pseudostratified. The architectural arrangement of the papillary stalks varies. Classically, they form exquisite and readily recognizable papillae, as shown here

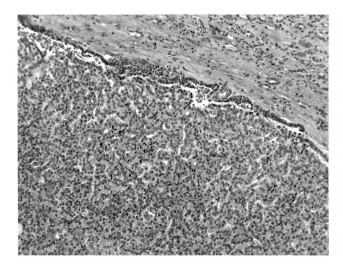

Fig. 2.123 Papillary renal cell carcinoma. Compact and tight packing of papillary structures in some tumors results in a solid appearance, as shown here

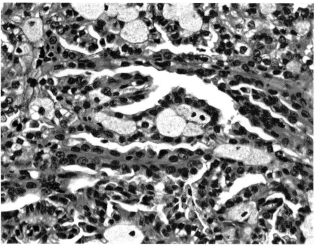

Fig. 2.125 Papillary renal cell carcinoma, type 1. Papillary renal cell carcinoma is subclassified into two morphologic variants. Tumor cells of type 1 are small and of low nuclear grade, with small round to ovoid nuclei with inconspicuous nucleoli, and with minimal pale or clear cytoplasm. The papillae of type 1 tumors are typically thin and delicate, often expanded by edema fluid and macrophages, and sometimes appear short or glomeruloid

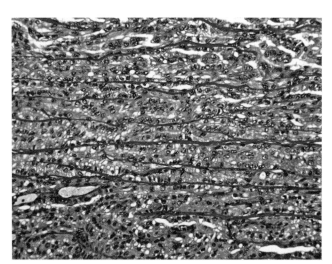

Fig. 2.124 Papillary renal cell carcinoma. In some tumors, the papillae are arranged in long parallel arrays, creating a trabecular appearance

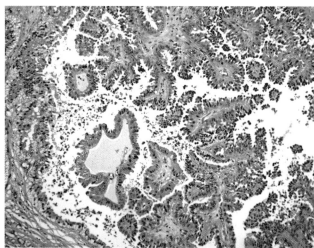

Fig. 2.126 Papillary renal cell carcinoma, type 2. Type 2 tumors are on average larger than type 1 tumors and of significantly higher nuclear grade. The fibrovascular cores of type 2 tumors tend to be dense and fibrous rather than thin and delicate. Macrophages are found near areas of necrosis, rather than within the stalks of the fibrovascular cores

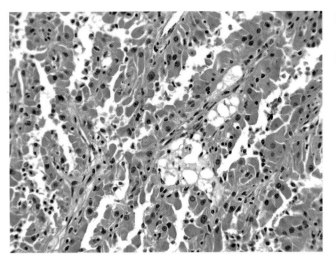

Fig. 2.127 Papillary renal cell carcinoma. Tumor cells in type 2 tumors exhibit large round or oval nuclei, prominent nucleoli, and varying degrees of nuclear pseudostratification. Their cytoplasm is usually abundant and eosinophilic

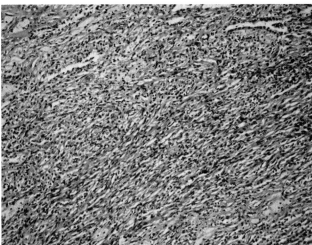

Fig. 2.129 Papillary renal cell carcinoma with low grade spindle cell foci. Infrequently, otherwise typical papillary carcinomas exhibit areas of low grade spindle cell morphology, comprising far more than half of the tumor. The spindle cells neither show significant mitotic activity or cytologic atypia, as would be expected if the spindle cell component were sarcomatoid, nor is there any mucin production, as would be expected in a mucinous tubular and spindle cell carcinoma

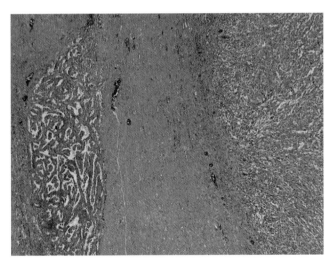

Fig. 2.128 Papillary renal cell carcinoma. Sarcomatoid morphology is noted in some papillary carcinomas, as shown on the right side of this image. Typical papillary carcinoma is seen at left

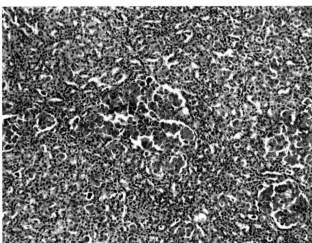

Fig. 2.130 Papillary renal cell carcinoma, mixed types. Some papillary tumors exhibit nuclear features typical of type 1, but cytoplasmic features typical of type 2, and some tumors consist of mixtures of cells of generally low nuclear grade but with substantial variations in cytoplasmic characteristics. This tumor contains both type 1 and type 2 cells

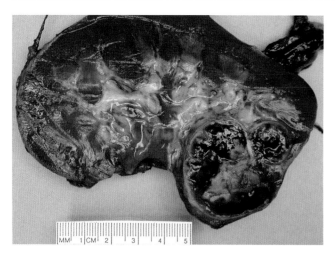

Fig. 2.131 Concurrent renal cell carcinomas. Reports of coexisting renal cell carcinomas of different types are infrequent. In this nephrectomy specimen, the larger mass was papillary carcinoma, and the smaller mass adjacent to it was clear cell carcinoma

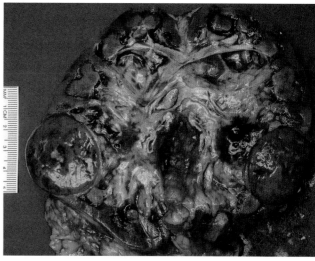

Fig. 2.133 Chromophobe renal cell carcinoma. This is an example of the eosinophilic variant of chromophobe carcinoma. It is mahogany brown, and resembles an oncocytoma, except that no central scar is present (*Image courtesy of* Mark Costaldi, MD)

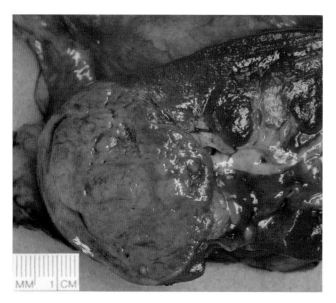

Fig. 2.132 Chromophobe renal cell carcinoma. Chromophobe renal cell carcinoma is usually solitary and well circumscribed. It varies from 1.5 to 25 cm in diameter. The cut surface is most often solid, homogeneous, and light brown, as shown here; less often the tumor is gray-tan, light pink, or yellow-white (*Image courtesy of* Felix Olobatuyi, MD)

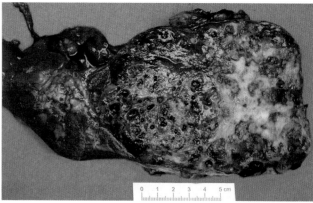

Fig. 2.134 Chromophobe renal cell carcinoma. This tumor is quite unusual in that it shows considerable cystic degeneration, areas of remote hemorrhage, and a prominent area of central scarring and necrosis. Hemorrhage and/or necrosis are unusual findings, and when present, are usually of limited extent (*Image courtesy of* Christine Lemyre)

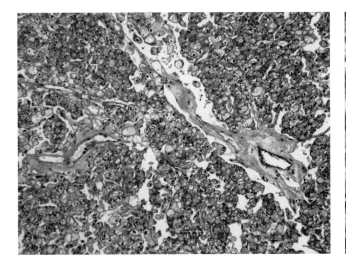

Fig. 2.135 Chromophobe renal cell carcinoma. The tumor cells of chromophobe carcinoma are usually arranged in solid sheets; in some cases, areas of tubulocystic architecture are present. Tumors are intersected randomly by delicate-to-broad fibrous septa containing blood vessels that are mainly of medium caliber, in contrast to the small sinusoidal vessels that are seen in clear cell carcinoma

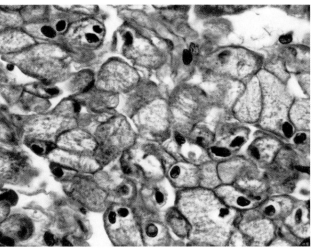

Fig. 2.137 Chromophobe renal cell carcinoma. Chromophobe cells are large polygonal cell with abundant nearly transparent and slightly flocculent cytoplasm and prominent, often "plant-like" cell membranes. They are frequently found adjacent to vascular channels

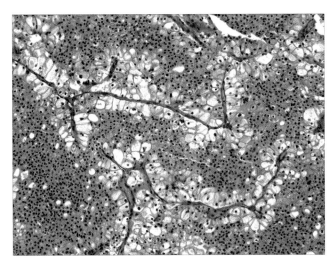

Fig. 2.136 Chromophobe renal cell carcinoma. Two types of tumor cells – chromophobe cells and granular eosinophilic cells – are usually present in varying proportions in the "typical" variant of chromophobe carcinoma

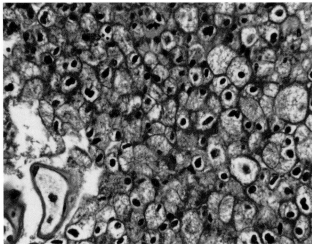

Fig. 2.138 Chromophobe renal cell carcinoma. Chromophobe cells are admixed with a second population of smaller cells with less abundant cytoplasm that is granular and eosinophilic. The nuclei of both cell types are hyperchromatic with irregular wrinkled "raisin-like" nuclear contours, and binucleation is often noted. Perinuclear halos are frequently present, and are more easily recognized in the smaller more eosinophilic cells

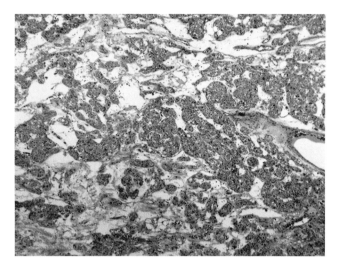

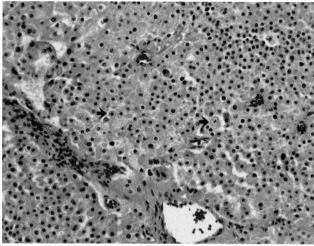

Fig. 2.139 Chromophobe renal cell carcinoma. The eosinophilic variant of chromophobe carcinoma is entirely composed of intensively eosinophilic cells with prominent cell membranes. This example of eosinophilic variant of chromophobe carcinoma shows the organoid architecture and the pale fibrous background often seen in oncocytomas

Fig. 2.141 Chromophobe renal cell carcinoma. Diagnosis of this eosinophilic variant of chromophobe carcinoma was facilitated by the presence of readily detected mitotic figures (*arrows*)

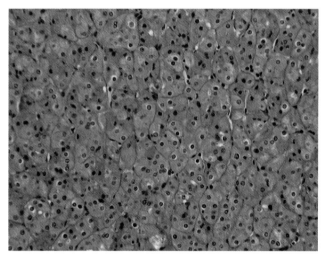

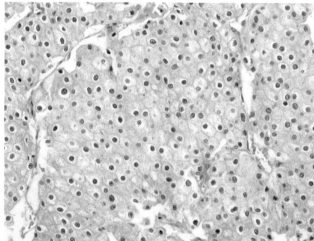

Fig. 2.140 Chromophobe renal cell carcinoma. Tumor cells of the eosinophilic variant of chromophobe carcinoma are morphologically similar to those of oncocytoma

Fig. 2.142 Chromophobe renal cell carcinoma. A diffuse cytoplasmic staining reaction with Hale's colloidal iron stain supports a diagnosis of chromophobe carcinoma; however, at least 11% of oncocytomas also show diffuse cytoplasmic staining for Hale's colloidal iron

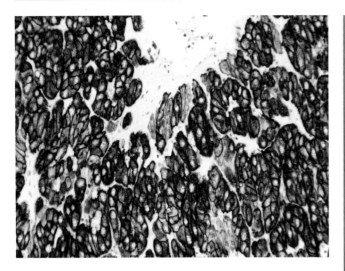

Fig. 2.143 Chromophobe renal cell carcinoma. Strong and diffusely positive immunostaining for cytokeratin 7 is characteristic of chromophobe carcinoma

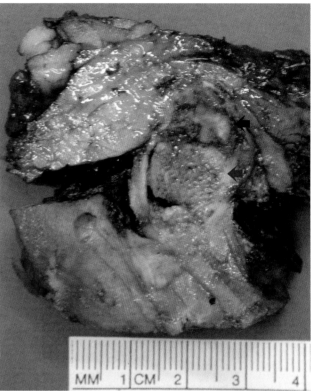

Fig. 2.145 Chromophobe carcinoma and concurrent papillary carcinoma. This is an unusual case in which a papillary carcinoma (*black arrow*) was situated immediately next to a chromophobe carcinoma (*blue arrow*) (*Image courtesy of* Amber Petrolla, MD)

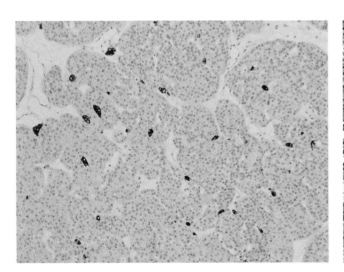

Fig. 2.144 Oncocytoma. In contrast to the findings in Fig. 2.143, this oncocytoma exhibits only scattered cells that show positive immunostaining for cytokeratin 7

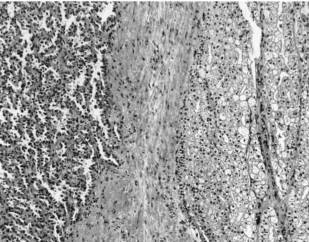

Fig. 2.146 Chromophobe carcinoma and concurrent papillary carcinoma. Papillary carcinoma is on the left; chromophobe carcinoma is on the right

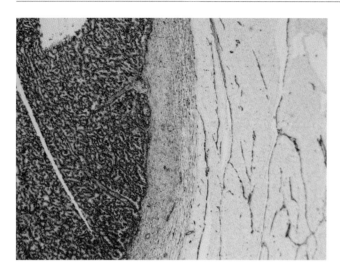

Fig. 2.147 Chromophobe carcinoma and concurrent papillary carcinoma. Papillary carcinoma, on the left, shows strong diffusely positive immunostaining for vimentin; chromophobe carcinoma, on the right, shows no immunostaining for vimentin, as expected

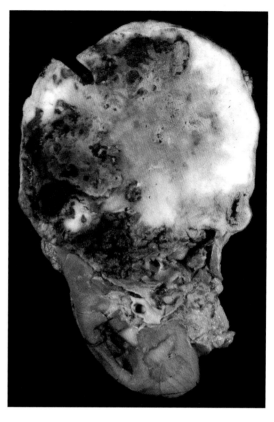

Fig. 2.149 Chromophobe renal cell carcinoma. Sarcomatoid differentiation is found in up to 9% of chromophobe carcinomas. The patient who underwent radical nephrectomy for this sarcomatoid chromophobe carcinoma died of cancer 6 months after surgery (*see* MacLennan GT and Cheng L, 2008. With permission)

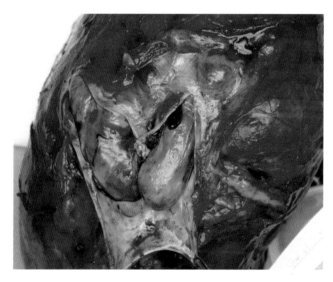

Fig. 2.148 Chromophobe renal cell carcinoma. Infrequently, chromophobe carcinoma exhibits aggressive features in the nephrectomy specimen. In this case, tumor is present in the renal vein (*Image courtesy of* Christine Lemyre)

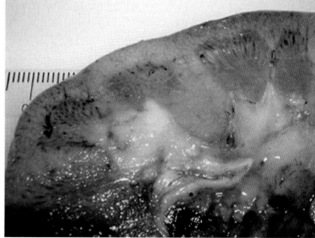

Fig. 2.150 Collecting duct carcinoma. Collecting duct carcinoma can originate anywhere in the parenchyma, but small cancers are often located centrally, as exemplified here. Tumor size varies from 1 to 16 cm in diameter. The cut surface of collecting duct carcinoma is typically gray-white and firm, sometimes with obvious necrosis, and with renal vein invasion in about 20% of cases (*see* MacLennan GT and Cheng L, 2008. With permission)

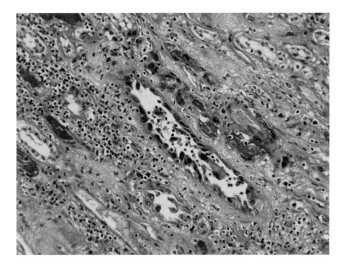

Fig. 2.151 Collecting duct carcinoma. The epithelium lining collecting ducts adjacent to or distant from the main tumor mass may show marked cytologic atypia or frank carcinoma in situ, as shown here. Intratubular extension of tumor may produce microscopic subcapsular deposits distant from the main tumor

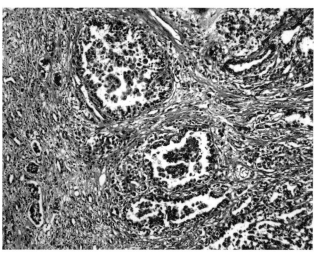

Fig. 2.153 Collecting duct carcinoma. Papillary and tubular structures in a desmoplastic and inflammatory background

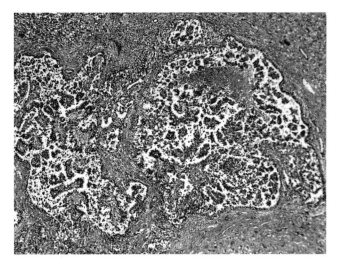

Fig. 2.152 Collecting duct carcinoma. Collecting duct carcinoma shows architectural complexity that can include papillary structures and solid cord-like areas. Some tumors have microcysts with intracystic papillary proliferations of high grade carcinoma

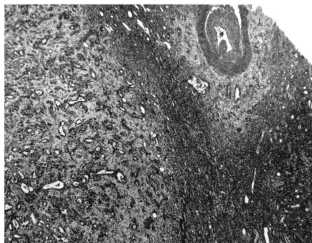

Fig. 2.154 Collecting duct carcinoma. The borders of the tumor are ill-defined with extensive infiltration of adjacent parenchyma and often a pronounced inflammatory infiltrate at the interface between tumor and normal parenchyma

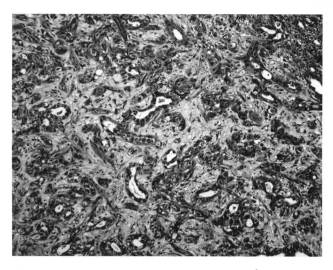

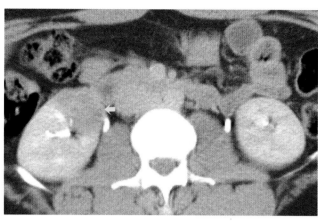

Fig. 2.157 Renal medullary carcinoma. This image is a CT scan of a 27-year-old black female with sickle cell trait and a 6-month history of intermittent hematuria. An ill-defined solid mass is present in one kidney (*arrow*) (*see* MacLennan GT and Cheng L, 2008. With permission)

Fig. 2.155 Collecting duct carcinoma. Pronounced stromal desmoplasia is a characteristic finding. Tubules lined by clearly malignant cells are present, sometimes forming complex interanastomosing structures. Tumor cells have varying amounts of eosinophilic cytoplasm and are usually of high nuclear grade, with nuclear pleomorphism and prominent nucleoli. Mucin is often demonstrable with mucicarmine, Alcian blue, or undigested periodic acid-Schiff stains, within tumor cell cytoplasm, at the luminal borders, or extracellularly. Sarcomatoid differentiation is seen in 16–36% of reported cases

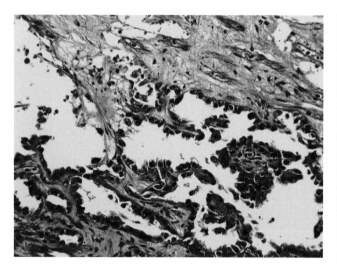

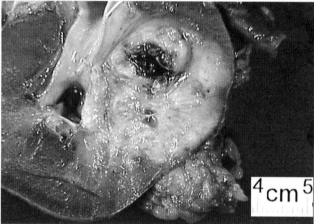

Fig. 2.158 Renal medullary carcinoma. Nephrectomy specimen of patient described in Fig. 2.157. These tumors typically occupy the renal medulla, as exemplified in this image, are poorly circumscribed, lobulated, firm to rubbery, tan to gray, with varying degrees of hemorrhage and necrosis, and range in size from 1.8 to 13 cm in diameter. Satellite nodules and extension into the perinephric and sinus fat are often seen (*see* MacLennan GT and Cheng L, 2008. With permission)

Fig. 2.156 Collecting duct carcinoma. Cells lining luminal structures may display a "hobnail" appearance, a finding that other types of renal cell carcinoma do not usually exhibit

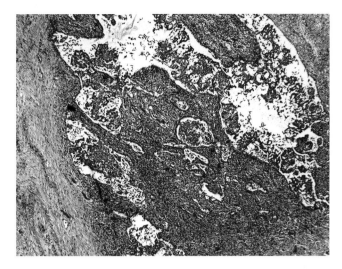

Fig. 2.159 Renal medullary carcinoma. The tumor exhibits a variety of morphologic patterns, including a reticular or microcystic growth pattern that resembles yolk sac tumor of the testis, areas that resemble adenoid cystic carcinoma, tubulopapillary formations, as shown here, or growth in diffuse sheets or solid nodules

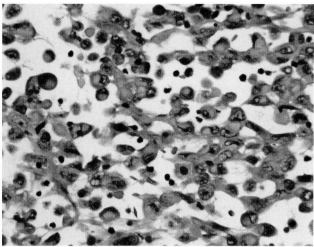

Fig. 2.161 Renal medullary carcinoma. Tumor cells are pleomorphic, with large nuclei, prominent nucleoli, and varying amounts of eosinophilic cytoplasm. Tumor cells may have a rhabdoid appearance, as exemplified here, or a squamoid appearance, particularly in areas of sheet-like growth

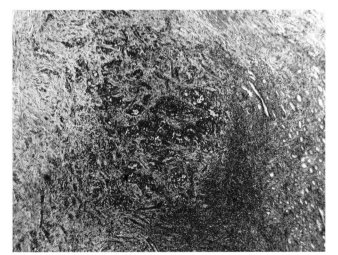

Fig. 2.160 Renal medullary carcinoma. The tumor incites a prominent desmoplastic stromal reaction, and there is often an intense inflammatory response at the interface between tumor and the adjacent renal parenchyma, findings that are remarkably similar to those of collecting duct carcinoma (compare with Fig. 2.154)

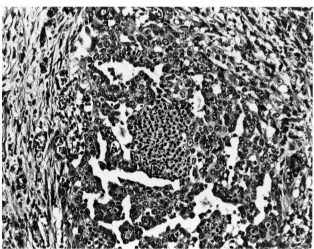

Fig. 2.162 Renal medullary carcinoma. Neutrophil aggregates may be noted within the tumor

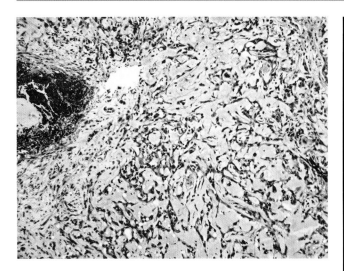

Fig. 2.163 Renal medullary carcinoma. Mucin production of variable extent is evident in the majority of renal medullary carcinomas

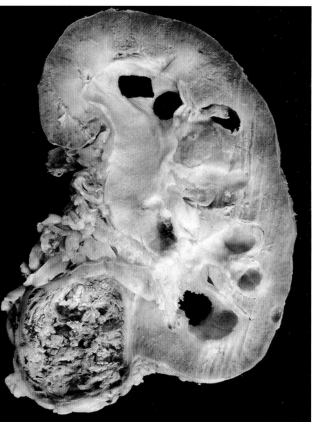

Fig. 2.165 Translocation carcinoma. PRCC-TFE3 carcinoma, shown here and defined by the t(X;1)(p11.2;q21) is typically yellow or gray, ranges in size from 3 to 14 cm in diameter, and has a fibrous pseudocapsule that has varying degrees of calcification in the majority of cases, sometimes substantial enough to impart an egg-shell consistency (*see* MacLennan GT and Cheng L, 2008. With permission)

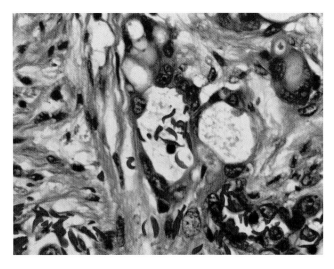

Fig. 2.164 Renal medullary carcinoma. In most histologic sections, sickled erythrocytes are identifiable

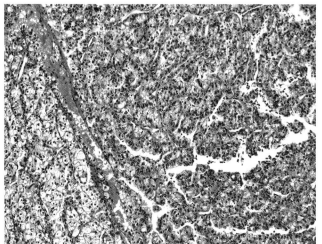

Fig. 2.166 Translocation carcinoma, PRCC-TFE3 type. Tumor cells are arranged in papillary formations and nests surrounded by thin-walled capillary vessels. The tumor cell nests, although usually solid, may be centrally dyscohesive, imparting an alveolar appearance, and a "bloody-gland" appearance is sometimes seen. Stromal macrophages and psammoma bodies, if present, are limited in number. Transitions between areas of nested (*left*) and papillary (*right*) architecture are usually sharply demarcated, as shown here

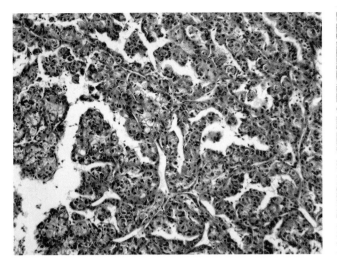

Fig. 2.167 Translocation carcinoma, PRCC-TFE3 type. Tumor cells are polygonal, with sharply outlined cell borders and abundant cytoplasm that varies from clear and finely granular to distinctly eosinophilic. Nuclei are wrinkled and irregular when viewed at high power. Areas of necrosis are seen in most cases, but mitotic figures are infrequent

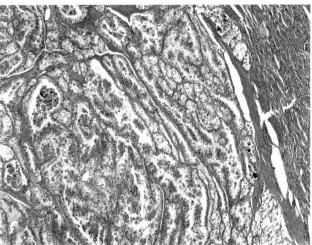

Fig. 2.169 Translocation carcinoma, ASPL-TFE3 type. ASPL-TFE3 carcinoma associated with the t(X;17)(p11.2;q25) exhibits nested and pseudopapillary growth patterns and conspicuous psammomatous calcifications. Foam cells and intracytoplasmic hemosiderin are not seen in the papillary structures

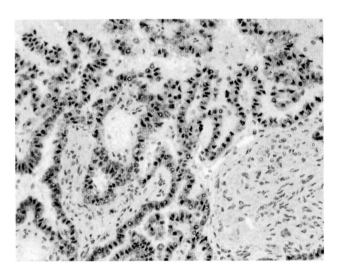

Fig. 2.168 Translocation carcinoma, PRCC-TFE3 type. The most distinctive, sensitive and specific immunohistochemical characteristic of these tumors is nuclear labeling for TFE3 protein, as shown here, using an antibody against a segment of the TFE3 gene that is retained in the gene fusions

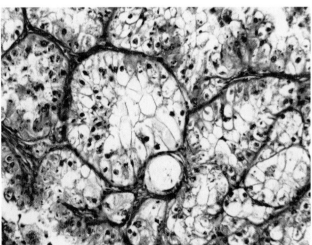

Fig. 2.170 Translocation carcinoma, ASPL-TFE3 type. Tumor cells appear epithelioid, with well-defined cell borders. The tumor cells possess voluminous cytoplasm that is predominantly clear, but may also be finely granular, eosinophilic, or densely granular. Nuclei have vesicular chromatin and a single prominent nucleolus

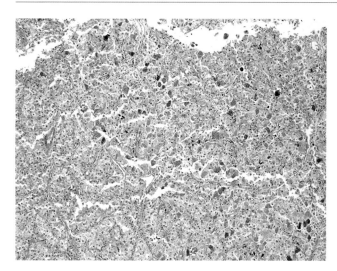

Fig. 2.171 Translocation carcinoma, melanotic. A rare renal tumor of childhood in which TFE3 gene fusions coexist with melanin production. This section of a 4 cm renal mass in a 14-year-old girl is composed of sheets and nests of cells with abundant cytoplasm, separated by delicate capillaries. Pigmentation is obvious in many cells, even at low power

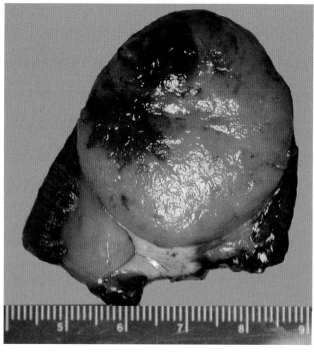

Fig. 2.173 Mucinous tubular and spindle cell carcinoma. Tumors are typically sharply circumscribed, gray-white, tan, or yellow, sometimes with minimal hemorrhage and/or necrosis; their cut surfaces are commonly bulging, shiny and mucoid, due to their content of mucin (*see* Yang et al. 2010. With permission)

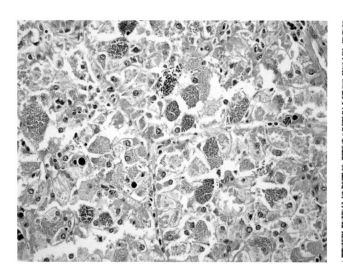

Fig. 2.172 Translocation carcinoma, melanotic. Tumor consists of polygonal epithelioid cells with fairly distinct cell borders and abundant clear to finely granular cytoplasm. Many cells contain brown-pigmented cytoplasmic granules. Tumor cells showed strongly positive immunostaining for TFE3 and HMB-45, and negative immunostaining for keratin AE1/AE3, epithelial membrane antigen, Melan A, microphthalmia transcription factor, and S-100 protein

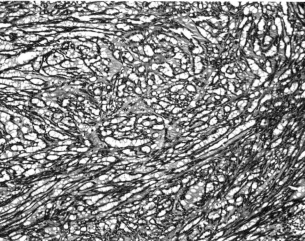

Fig. 2.174 Mucinous tubular and spindle cell carcinoma (MTSC). MTSC is composed of round, ovoid or elongated tightly packed tubules separated by abundant mucin that may have a "bubbly" appearance.

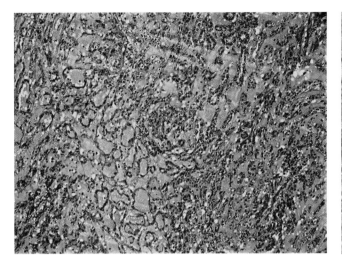

Fig. 2.175 Mucinous tubular and spindle cell carcinoma. Variably sized tubular structures are separated by basophilic extracellular mucin. Tubules are lined by uniform small cuboidal cells with minimal cytoplasm and round nuclei of low nuclear grade; nucleoli are absent or inconspicuous, and mitotic figures are rare

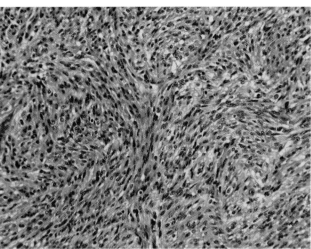

Fig. 2.177 Mucinous tubular and spindle cell carcinoma. Some tumors exhibit a component of spindled cells that may raise concern for sarcomatoid change, but necrosis, mitotic activity, and significant nuclear pleomorphism are absent

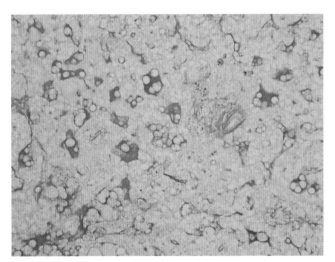

Fig. 2.176 Mucinous tubular and spindle cell carcinoma. Mucin within the tumor shows positive staining with Alcian blue

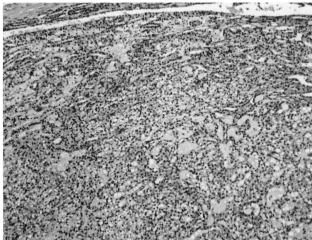

Fig. 2.178 Mucinous tubular and spindle cell carcinoma. The histologic spectrum includes cases in which the spindle cell component rivals or even exceeds the tubular component, as well as cases with relative paucity of mucinous matrix, aggregates of foamy macrophages, focal clear cell change in tubular cells, focal necrosis, oncocytic tubules, numerous small vacuoles, psammomatous calcification, or heterotopic bone formation. Rarely, neuroendocrine differentiation or true sarcomatoid differentiation is noted. In this case, mucin is noted at lower right, numerous macrophages are at upper left, and many of the tumor cells have clear cytoplasm

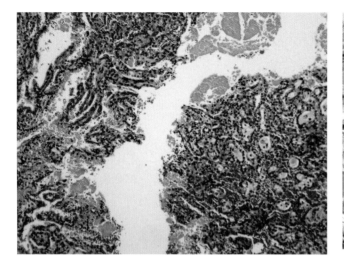

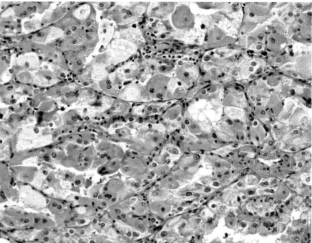

Fig. 2.179 Mucinous tubular and spindle cell carcinoma. Papillations or small components of well formed papillae are considered part of the spectrum of features that may be found in this tumor

Fig. 2.181 Postneuroblastoma renal cell carcinoma. Small foci of cells with abundant reticular cytoplasm are present, bearing some morphologic resemblance to chromophobe cells. Tumor cell nuclei are medium-sized and irregular, and many bear prominent nucleoli. Mitotic figures are infrequent. Diffuse parenchymal infiltration accompanied by desmoplasia is observed in some tumors

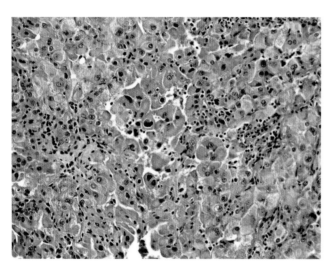

Fig. 2.180 Postneuroblastoma renal cell carcinoma. Postneuroblastoma renal cell carcinomas are composed of cells arranged in solid sheets or nests and in papillary arrangements. Occasionally, psammoma bodies are noted. Tumor cells have sharply defined cell membranes and abundant eosinophilic granular cytoplasm, giving it an "oncocytoid" appearance

2.7   Renal Cell Carcinoma, Unclassified

The following renal epithelial neoplasms are currently designated "renal cell carcinoma, unclassified." This is a diagnostic category for the designation of renal carcinomas that do not conform to any of the currently accepted categories of renal cell carcinoma, and therefore are not currently included in the 2004 WHO classification of renal neoplasms. Examples include tumors that are composites of recognized types, tumors composed of unrecognizable cell types, and renal carcinomas with entirely sarcomatoid morphology, lacking recognizable epithelial elements

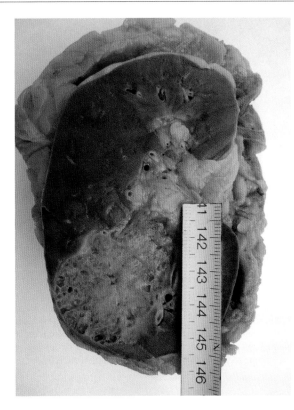

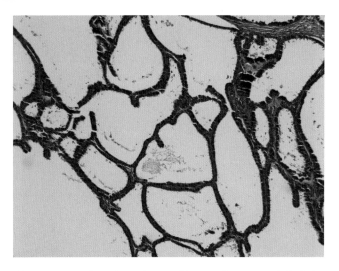

Fig. 2.184 Tubulocystic carcinoma. The tumor is composed of tubules and cystic structures of markedly variable size, separated by septa that are commonly very thin, delicate and "spider web-like"

Fig. 2.182 Tubulocystic carcinoma. Tubulocystic carcinoma is a well circumscribed tumor that ranges in size from 2 to 17 cm in diameter. On sectioning, it appears to be composed entirely of a myriad of small cysts, sometimes reminiscent of "bubble-wrap." Hemorrhage and necrosis are absent (*Image courtesy of* Jose I. Lopez, MD)

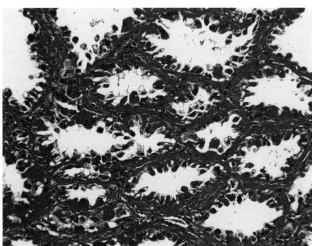

Fig. 2.185 Tubulocystic carcinoma. In some cases, septa between the tubules and cysts are thickened and fibrotic. Tubules are lined by a single layer of low cuboidal epithelial cells with modest to abundant amounts of eosinophilic cytoplasm, sometimes with a hobnail appearance, as shown here. Nuclei are round, with evenly dispersed chromatin, with conspicuous nucleoli in some cases. No necrosis is present, and mitotic figures are rarely identified

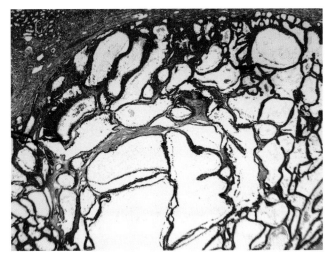

Fig. 2.183 Tubulocystic carcinoma. At very low power the appearance is that of variably sized cysts separated by thin septa, and is slightly reminiscent of a spider web or lace doily

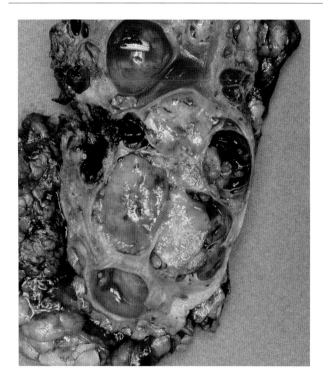

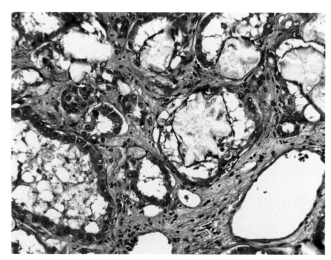

Fig. 2.188 Acquired cystic kidney disease (ACKD)-associated renal cell carcinoma. The tumor cells have modest amounts of granular eosinophilic cytoplasm, and large round to oval, mildly irregular nuclei with prominent nucleoli. About 80% of these tumors show abundant calcium oxalate crystals in stroma and in lumina. The crystals are unaccompanied by fibrosis, necrosis, increased mitoses or inflammation, and are unique to tumors arising in a background of ACKD

Fig. 2.186 End-stage renal disease (ESRD)-associated renal cell carcinoma. Kidneys with end-stage renal disease (ESRD), particularly those with acquired cystic kidney disease (ACKD), are prone to develop two types of renal cancer: ACKD-associated renal cell carcinoma (RCC), and clear cell papillary RCC of end-stage kidneys. This is an example of an ACKD-associated RCC

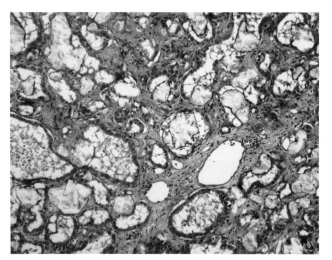

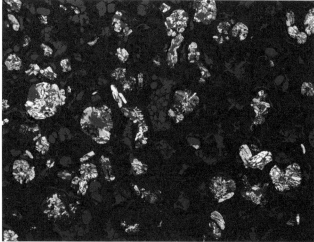

Fig. 2.187 Acquired cystic kidney disease (ACKD)-associated renal cell carcinoma. ACKD-associated renal cell carcinomas range from 1 to 8 cm, are often multifocal and bilateral, and generally well circumscribed, sometimes with focally calcified capsules. Foci of hemorrhage and necrosis are common. Tumor cells are arranged in solid sheet-like, papillary, acinar, cribriform, or tubulocystic patterns

Fig. 2.189 Acquired cystic kidney disease-associated renal cell carcinoma. The abundance of oxalate crystals within the tumor is even more striking under polarized light

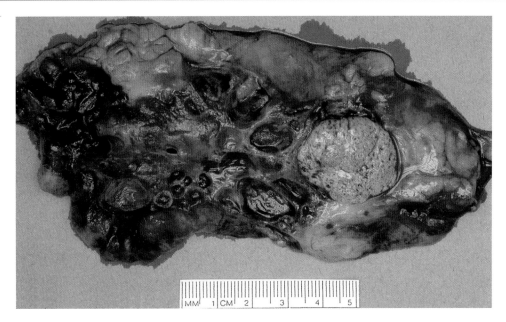

Fig. 2.190 Clear cell papillary RCC of end-stage kidneys. These distinctive tumors occur with almost equal frequency in ACKD and noncystic end-stage renal disease. They are well circumscribed and often cystic, with a thin fibrous capsule, and they lack hemorrhage or necrosis

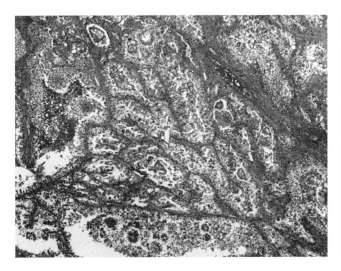

Fig. 2.191 Clear cell papillary renal cell carcinoma of end-stage kidneys. At low power, tumor architecture is predominantly papillary, but the tumor cells exhibit cytoplasmic clearing

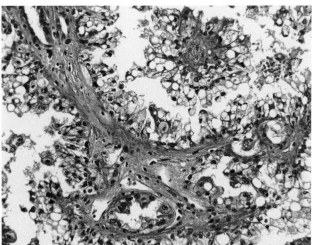

Fig. 2.192 Clear cell papillary renal cell carcinoma (RCC) of end-stage kidneys. The architecture is papillary, but the majority of tumor cells have clear cytoplasm. Typical sporadic papillary RCC and clear cell papillary RCC of end-stage kidneys both show positive immunostaining for cytokeratin 7; however, the former shows positive immunostaining for α-methylacyl-CoA racemase (AMACR), and the latter does not

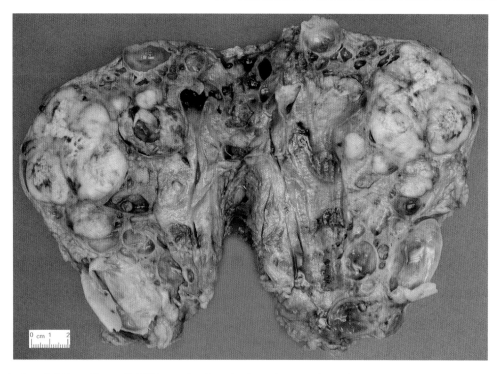

Fig. 2.193 Acquired cystic kidney disease (ACKD)-associated renal cell carcinoma (RCC) with sarcomatoid features. Sarcomatoid morphology is sometimes seen in end-stage renal disease-associated RCC, as exemplified in this case. A large multinodular and partially necrotic tumor is present in a background of ACKD (*Image courtesy of* Richard Naturale, MD)

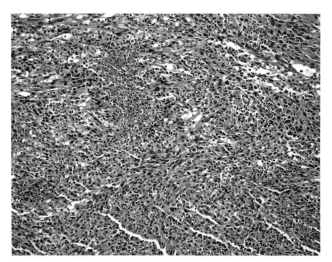

Fig. 2.194 Acquired cystic kidney disease-associated renal cell carcinoma with sarcomatoid features. Tumor cells have a spindled appearance, and the presence of abundant inflammatory cells raised the question of xanthogranulomatous pyelonephritis.

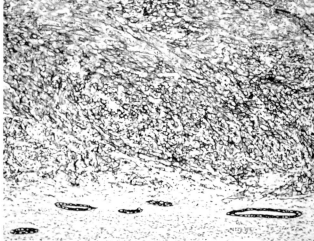

Fig. 2.195 Acquired cystic kidney disease-associated renal cell carcinoma with sarcomatoid features. Tumor cells showed strong diffusely positive immunostaining for keratin Cam 5.2.

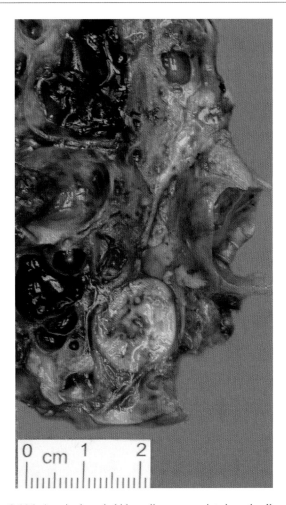

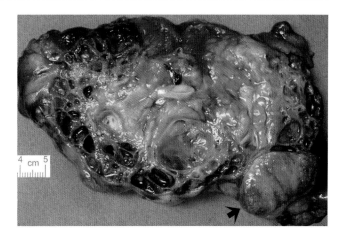

Fig. 2.198 End-stage renal disease-associated renal cell carcinoma. About 40% of renal neoplasms are well-recognized, conventional types of renal cell carcinoma. The shiny bulging tumor with a mucoid cut surface shown here (*arrow*), in a background of acquired cystic kidney disease, was a mucinous tubular and spindle cell carcinoma (*Image courtesy of* Anaibelith Del Rio Perez, MD)

Fig. 2.196 Acquired cystic kidney disease-associated renal carcinoma. This small tumor was noted distant from the large tumor mass shown in Fig. 2.193 (*Image courtesy of* Richard Naturale, MD)

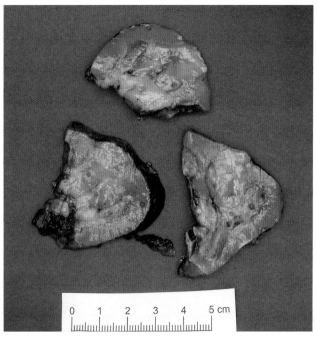

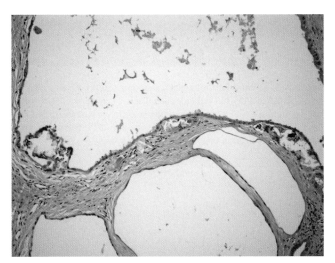

Fig. 2.199 Lipoid renal cell carcinoma. The unusual carcinoma illustrated here has a fatty appearance, grossly suggestive of angiomyolipoma (*Image courtesy of* Paul Grabenstetter, MD)

Fig. 2.197 Acquired cystic kidney disease (ACKD)-associated renal cell carcinoma. Sections from the separate small tumor demonstrated an ACKD-associated renal cell carcinoma, with the characteristic oxalate crystals

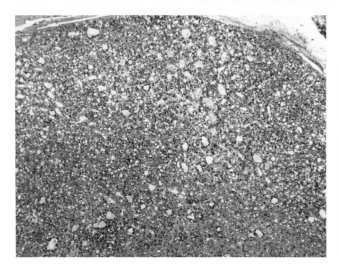

Fig. 2.200 Lipoid renal cell carcinoma. Section from the tumor shown in Fig. 2.199. At low power, at least part of the tumor is composed of cells similar to adipocytes. It does not resemble angiomyolipoma

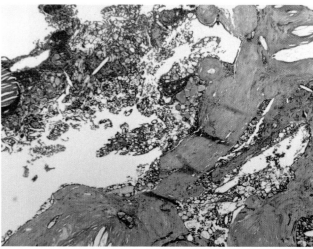

Fig. 2.202 Thyroid-like follicular carcinoma. Tumors range up to 4 cm in diameter and are encapsulated. Tumors appear to be composed entirely of microfollicles and macrofollicles containing inspissated colloid-like material

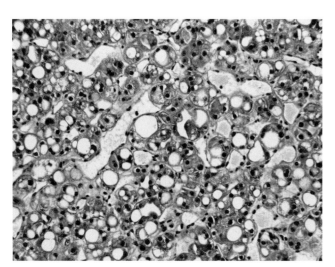

Fig. 2.201 Lipoid renal cell carcinoma. On closer inspection the tumor is composed of epithelial cells with extensively vacuolated cytoplasm. Tumor cells showed positive immunostaining for keratins AE1/AE3 and Cam 5.2, but did not stain for cytokeratin 7, HMB-45, Melan-A, S100 protein, 34βE12, or Ulex europaeus. It is possible that the tumor cells contained an overabundance of lipid material, which was removed by histologic processing

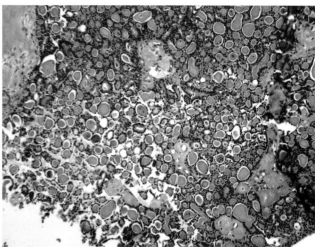

Fig. 2.203 Thyroid-like follicular carcinoma. Tumor bears a striking resemblance to a thyroid follicular neoplasm. These tumors show negative immunostaining for thyroglobulin and thyroid transcription factor-1. Immunostaining is prudent, because the differential diagnosis includes thyroid carcinoma metastatic to the kidney

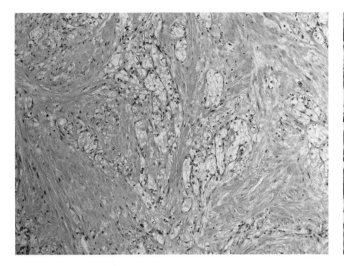

Fig. 2.204 Renal cell carcinoma with angioleiomyoma-like stroma. Only a few cases of this entity have been reported. The smooth muscle bundles are intimately admixed with clear cell carcinoma, usually of low grade. The smooth muscle component is believed to represent a prolific metaplastic stromal reaction induced by the carcinoma. Entities to be considered in the differential diagnosis include angiomyolipoma, leiomyoma and mixed epithelial and stromal tumor of kidney

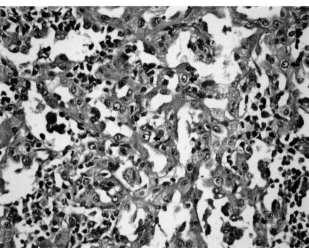

Fig. 2.206 Renal tumors in HLRCC syndrome. The hallmark of the renal cancers in this syndrome, regardless of their architecture, is the presence of large eosinophilic nucleoli with a clear perinuclear halo (*arrows*). This finding is virtually unique to HLRCC tumors

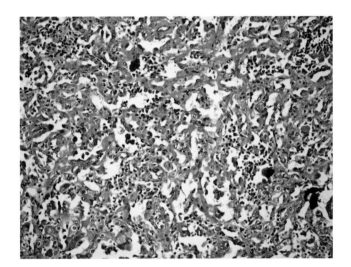

Fig. 2.205 Renal tumors in hereditary leiomyomatosis and renal cell carcinoma (HLRCC) syndrome. Patients with the inherited condition known as HLRCC syndrome have a high incidence of uterine and skin leiomyomas and renal cell carcinomas. The renal cancers exhibit a variety of architectural patterns: cystic, tubulopapillary, tubular, and solid. The example shown here was predominantly tubulopapillary, but had solid areas, as well

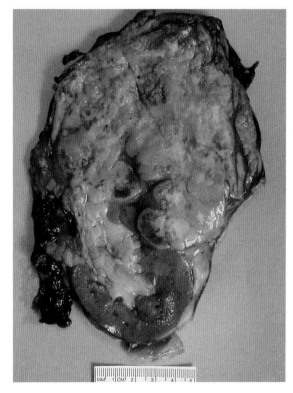

Fig. 2.207 Purely sarcomatoid carcinoma. This illustration shows a purely sarcomatoid renal carcinoma that infiltrated perirenal fat and was extensively present at the black-inked Gerota's fascia (*Image courtesy of* Shams Halat, MD)

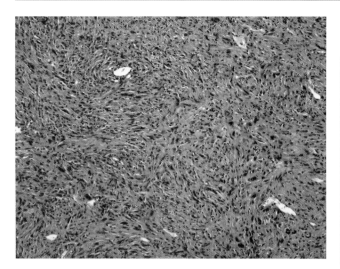

Fig. 2.208 Purely sarcomatoid carcinoma. Tumor is composed entirely of spindled and pleomorphic cells

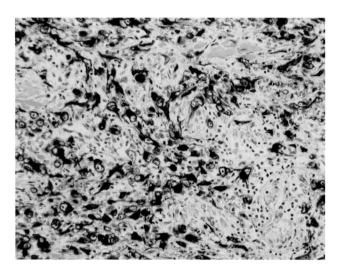

Fig. 2.209 Purely sarcomatoid carcinoma. Tumor cells show strong diffusely positive immunostaining for keratin Cam 5.2, confirming their epithelial differentiation

2.8 Metanephric Neoplasms

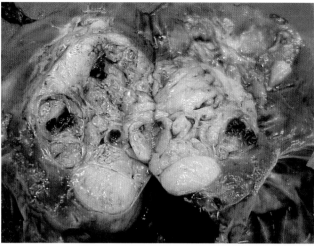

Fig. 2.210 Metanephric adenoma. Metanephric adenoma ranges from 0.3 to 20 cm in diameter and is typically unilateral and unifocal. It is either unencapsulated or invested with only a limited and discontinuous pseudocapsule. Tumors are tan to gray to yellow, and soft to firm. Most are solid, but some have areas of hemorrhage, necrosis, and cystic degeneration, as exemplified in this image. Calcifications are often noted within solid areas or within the walls of cystic structures (*Image courtesy of* Mark Barcelo, MD)

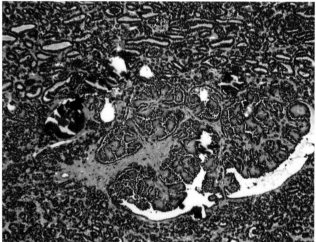

Fig. 2.211 Metanephric adenoma. Metanephric adenoma is composed of very small acini separated by variable amounts of acellular stroma consisting only of edema fluid or a smoothly hyalinized matrix, resulting in variation in the degree of acinar crowding. Tumor cells form variably sized tubules; papillary structures are commonly present. The great majority of tumors exhibit calcification, either as calcific deposits and foci of dystrophic calcification within areas of stromal hyalinization and scarring, or as psammoma bodies associated with papillary structures, as shown here

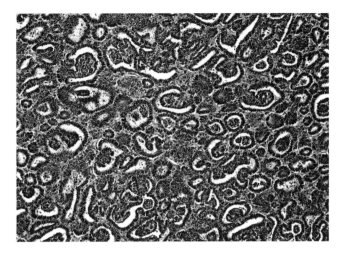

Fig. 2.212 Metanephric adenoma. Papillary structures, found in about half of cases, consist of polypoid fronds or short papillary infoldings within tubular or cystic spaces, producing a glomeruloid appearance. Infrequently, tumor cells form solid aggregates that resemble blastemal nodules of nephroblastoma

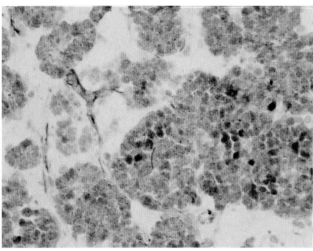

Fig. 2.214 Metanephric adenoma. Metanephric adenoma can be distinguished from epithelial-predominant Wilms tumor and the solid variant of papillary renal cell carcinoma with appropriate immunostains. Metanephric adenoma is typically immunopositive for WT1, shown here, and CD57, shown in Fig. 2.215

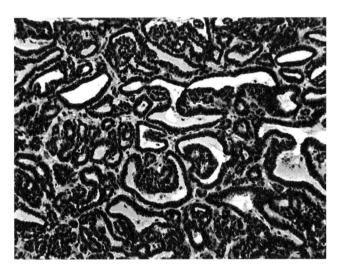

Fig. 2.213 Metanephric adenoma. Tumor cells of metanephric adenoma are closely spaced and often overlapping, and possess minimal pink or clear cytoplasm. Nuclei are slightly bigger than lymphocytes, irregularly rounded or ovoid, and sometimes display central folding. Nucleoli are absent or inconspicuous, and mitotic figures are rare or entirely absent

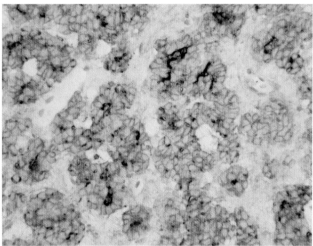

Fig. 2.215 Metanephric adenoma. Positive immunostaining for WT1 and CD57 (shown here), and negative immunostaining for α-methyla-cyl-CoA racemase (AMACR) and cytokeratin 7 (CK7) is the exact opposite of the immunoprofile of papillary renal cell carcinoma. Metanephric adenoma and nephroblastoma share immunopositivity for WT1 and immunonegativity for AMACR and CK7, but metanephric adenoma stains positively for CD57 and nephroblastomas shows negative immunostaining for CD57

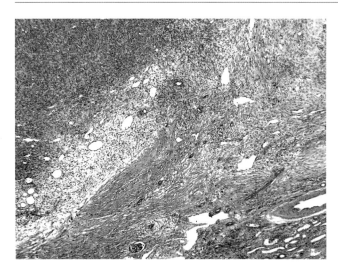

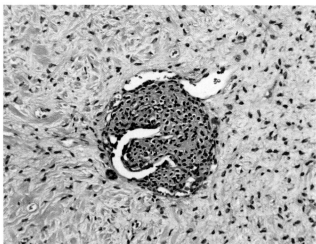

Fig. 2.216 Metanephric stromal tumor. Metanephric stromal tumor is typically a tan lobulated partially cystic fibrous tumor, often centered in the renal medulla, and usually unifocal. It is unencapsulated, and has an irregular margin that on close inspection subtly infiltrates the adjacent normal parenchyma, as illustrated here

Fig. 2.218 Metanephric stromal tumor. Tumor is composed of spindled and stellate cells with thin hyperchromatic nuclei and indistinct cytoplasmic extensions. Juxtaglomerular cell hyperplasia within entrapped glomeruli, as shown here, is observed in one-fourth of cases. Angiodysplasia in the form of epithelioid transformation of medial smooth muscle cells and myxoid change may be evident within entrapped arterioles

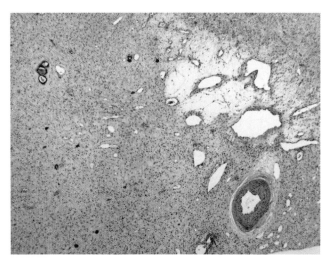

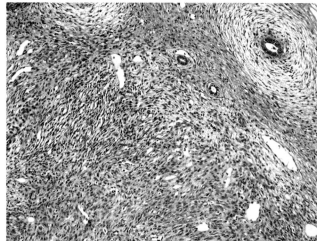

Fig. 2.217 Metanephric stromal tumor. Geographic differences in the degree of cellularity versus the degree of stromal myxoid change produces a vaguely nodular variation in tumor cellularity at low power

Fig. 2.219 Metanephric stromal tumor. The degree of cellularity is variable between different tumors (compare with Fig. 2.217). Tumor cells tend to surround native renal tubules and blood vessels, forming concentric "onionskin" rings or collarettes around these structures in a myxoid background (*upper right*). Heterologous stromal differentiation produces glial elements or cartilage in one-fifth of cases

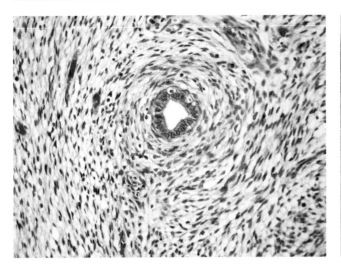

Fig. 2.220 Metanephric stromal tumor. High power view of a collarette of tumor cells around a native tubule

2.9 Nephroblastic Neoplasms

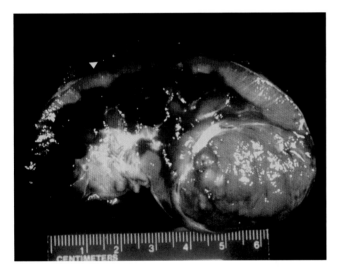

Fig. 2.221 Perilobar nephrogenic rests. Nephrogenic rests are putative precursors of nephroblastoma. There are two categories: perilobar nephrogenic rests (PLNR) and intralobar nephrogenic rests (ILNR). Perilobar nephrogenic rests involve only the periphery of a renal lobe. When a kidney is involved by a more or less continuous subcapsular band of nephrogenic rests, the condition is designated *diffuse hyperplastic perilobar nephroblastomatosis*, exemplified in this kidney from a patient who was found to have bilateral Wilms tumors, underwent chemotherapy, then underwent nephrectomy. *Arrow* indicates the region of diffuse hyperplastic perilobar nephroblastomatosis (*See* Bostwick and Cheng 2008. With permission)

Fig. 2.222 Perilobar nephrogenic rests. The rests are composed of blastema, embryonal epithelial cells and scant stroma, have an ovoid shape and a subcapsular location, and are sharply demarcated from the adjacent renal parenchyma. Hyperplastic perilobar nephrogenic rests (PLNRs) interface directly with adjacent normal renal tissue, lack the pseudocapsule that characterizes Wilms tumor, are strictly subcapsular, and tend to be ovoid, in contrast to the spherical expansile growth seen in Wilms tumor

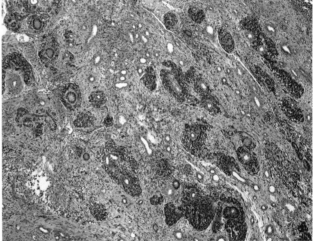

Fig. 2.223 Intralobar nephrogenic rests. Intralobar nephrogenic rests (ILNRs) can be situated anywhere in the renal lobe, in the renal sinus and even in the walls of the pelvicaliceal system. They lie between normal nephrons, forming an indistinct interdigitating interface with the adjacent normal tissue. ILNRs often contain stromal elements and epithelial tubules

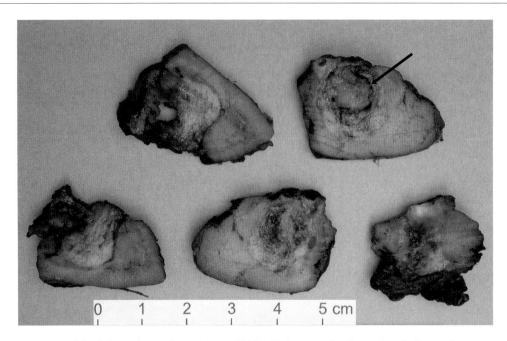

Fig. 2.224 Nephroblastoma arising in intralobar nephrogenic rests (ILNR). Patient was closely monitored after previous treatment for contralateral nephroblastoma, and developed a new lesion, which was excised by partial nephrectomy. The bulk of the lesion was ILNR, but the yellowish nodule (*arrow*) was a nephroblastoma (*Image courtesy of* Khaled Sarah, MD)

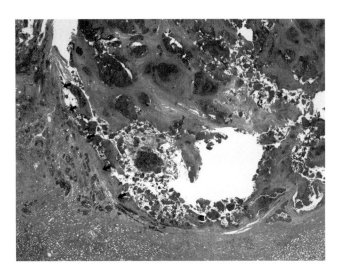

Fig. 2.225 Nephroblastoma arising in intralobar nephrogenic rests (ILNR). *Arrows* outline the sharply circumscribed fibrous boundary between ILNR at lower left, and a nephroblastoma that has arisen within this area of ILNR

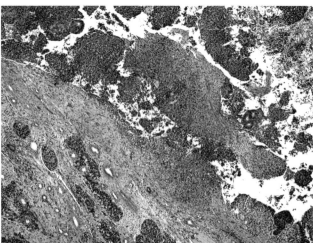

Fig. 2.226 Nephroblastoma arising in intralobar nephrogenic rests (ILNR). ILNR is at lower left. A classic triphasic nephroblastoma occupies the upper right aspect of the image

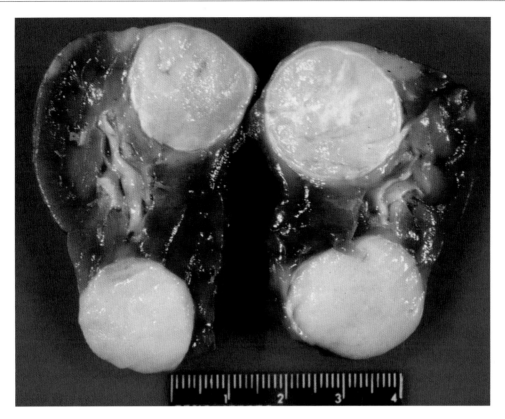

Fig. 2.227 Nephroblastoma. Although the great majority of nephroblastomas are solitary and unilateral, multiple tumors in a single kidney are found in 7% of cases, as shown here, and in 5% of cases, bilateral primary tumors are noted (*see* MacLennan GT and Cheng L, 2008. With permission)

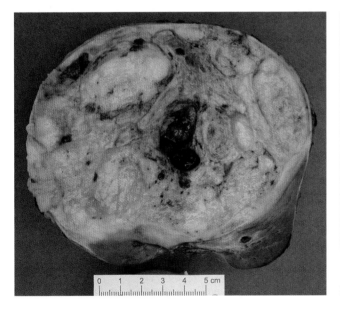

Fig. 2.228 Nephroblastoma, classic type. Nephroblastomas are usually sharply circumscribed and confined within a fibrous pseudocapsule, weighing up to 6 kg. Their color varies from pale gray to tan, and consistency varies from soft to firm. Hemorrhage, necrosis and cystic degeneration are commonly noted to a variable extent; rarely, protrusion of tumor into the renal pelvis results in a "botryoid" appearance

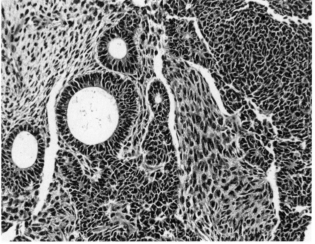

Fig. 2.229 Nephroblastoma, classic type. Most nephroblastomas are triphasic, containing variable proportions of blastema, epithelium and stroma, as shown in this image. Blastema is comprised of small, round, densely packed and overlapping cells with minimal cytoplasm and little evidence of differentiation. Their nuclei are round or polygonal, relatively uniform in size, and have evenly dispersed chromatin and small nucleoli. Abundant mitotic figures are usually present. Most nephroblastomas include an epithelial component in the form of tubular and occasionally glomeruloid structures. The stromal component typically is comprised of spindle cells in a myxoid background; it may show a wide range of differentiation patterns, including smooth muscle, fibrous tissue, cartilage, bone, adipose tissue, neuroglia, and mature ganglion cells

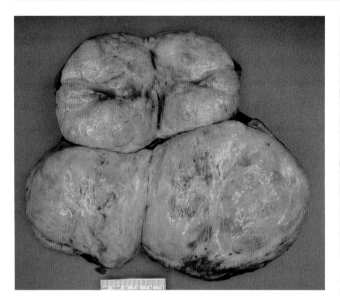

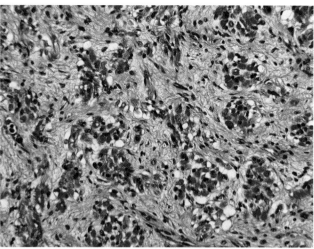

Fig. 2.232 Nephroblastoma, stroma-predominant. High power view showing skeletal muscle differentiation in the stroma

Fig. 2.230 Nephroblastoma, stroma-predominant. The gross appearance of this stroma-predominant nephroblastoma bears some resemblance to a leiomyoma (*Image courtesy of* Christina Wojewoda, MD)

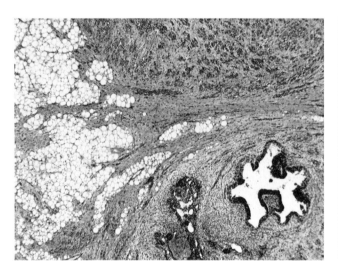

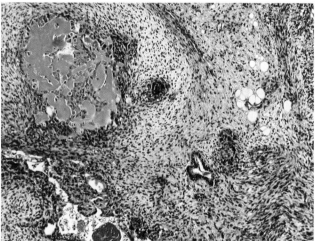

Fig. 2.231 Nephroblastoma, stroma-predominant. The stroma shows adipose (*left*) and skeletal muscle differentiation (*top*)

Fig. 2.233 Nephroblastoma, stroma-predominant. Tumor stroma shows osteoid (*left*), adipose tissue (*right*), and skeletal muscle differentiation (*lower right*)

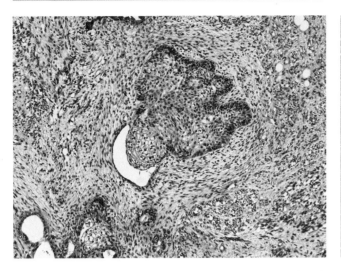

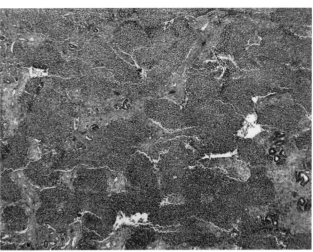

Fig. 2.234 Nephroblastoma, stroma-predominant. Squamous differentiation of the tubular epithelium is sometimes observed in nephroblastoma

Fig. 2.236 Nephroblastoma, blastema-predominant. About 75% of this tumor consisted of blastema. A few tubules are scattered through the rather scant stromal component

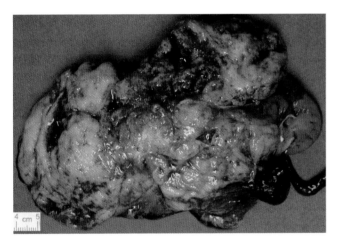

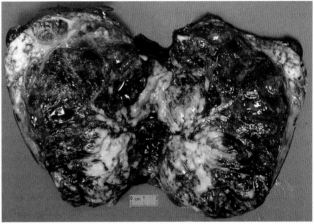

Fig. 2.235 Nephroblastoma, blastema-predominant. The gross consistency of the tumor was very soft (*Image courtesy of* Sean Fitzgerald, MD)

Fig. 2.237 Nephroblastoma, entirely blastemal (*Image courtesy of* Christina Wojewoda, MD)

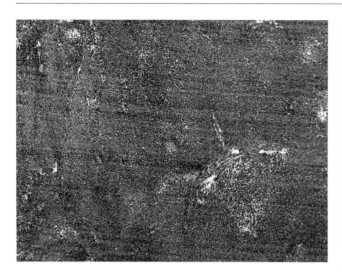

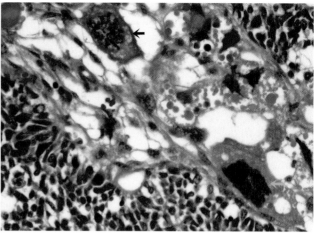

Fig. 2.238 Nephroblastoma, entirely blastemal. The tumor was composed only of blastemal elements; no tubular or stromal component were identified despite extensive sampling. Tumor cells showed positive immunostaining for WT1, CD56, vimentin, and bcl-2; immunostains for CD99, epithelial membrane antigen, keratin AE1/AE3, and for markers of muscle, lymphoid, and neuroendocrine differentiation were negative. Despite the absence of triphasic morphology, findings were regarded as consistent with nephroblastom

Fig. 2.240 Nephroblastoma, with nuclear anaplasia. A very large multipolar mitotic figure (*black arrow*) and a very large hyperchromatic nucleus (*green arrow*) are present (*see* MacLennan GT, Resnick MI, Bostwick DG, 2003. With permission)

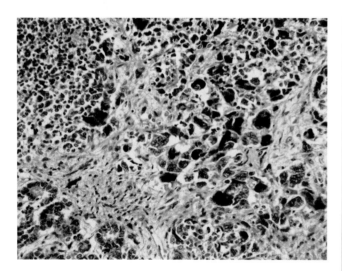

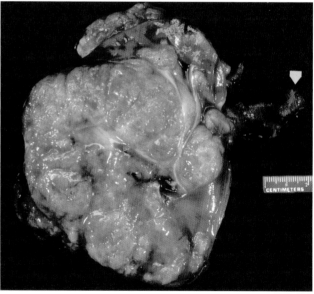

Fig. 2.239 Nephroblastoma, with nuclear anaplasia. Nuclear anaplasia, found in about 5% of nephroblastomas, means nuclear hyperchromasia and gigantism with multipolar mitotic figures. By definition, an anaplastic nucleus must be hyperchromatic and all its major dimensions must be at least three times larger than those of neighboring non-anaplastic nuclei. Each component of the abnormal metaphase of a multipolar polyploid mitotic figures must be as large as, or larger than, a normal metaphase. In this image, multiple very large hyperchromatic nuclei are readily apparent

Fig. 2.241 Nephroblastoma, high stage. Nephroblastomas, as they advance, typically extend locally into perirenal soft tissues, renal vein, and vena cava, and metastasize to regional lymph nodes, lungs and liver, and less frequently to spinal epidural space, central nervous system, and mediastinal lymph nodes after lung metastasis; they rarely metastasize to bone. The tumor shown here extensively infiltrates the sinus fat and fills the renal vein (*arrow*)

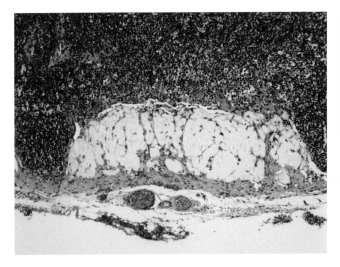

Fig. 2.242 Nephroblastoma. Lymph nodes in patients with nephroblastoma may be noted to contain amorphous proteinaceous material in the sinusoids, with or without apparent metastatic tumor. Although similar material may be found in the corresponding renal parenchyma, the presence of this amorphous material in lymph nodes is not, in itself, evidence of metastatic cancer

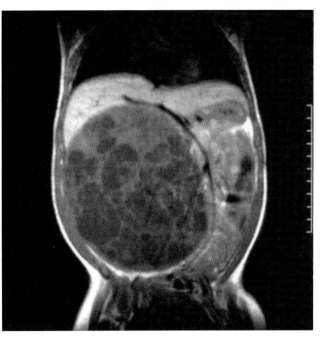

Fig. 2.244 Cystic partially differentiated nephroblastoma. MRI scan of the child in Fig. 2.243 shows a massive multicystic intraabdominal mass

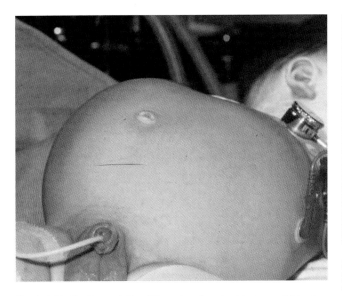

Fig. 2.243 Cystic partially differentiated nephroblastoma. Distortion of the abdominal contour by a mass was easily evident. Photo taken just before surgical excision (*Image courtesy of* Jonathan Ross, MD)

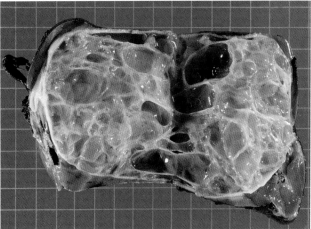

Fig. 2.245 Cystic partially differentiated nephroblastoma. Cystic partially differentiated nephroblastoma (CPDN) is a multilocular cystic Wilms tumor composed entirely of cysts separated by delicate septa, ranging up to 18 cm in diameter. They are typically well circumscribed, clearly demarcated from the adjacent normal kidney, entirely composed of cysts of variable size, and they lack expansile nodules of tumor (*Image courtesy of* David Grynspan, MD)

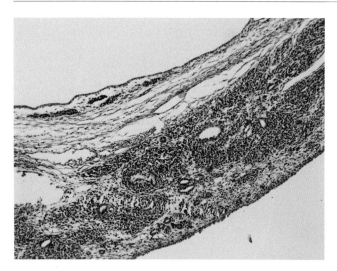

Fig. 2.246 Cystic partially differentiated nephroblastoma. The cysts are lined by flat, cuboidal or hobnail cells, and sometimes lack lining epithelium. The septa exhibit variable cellularity and may contain any of the following elements: blastema, nephroblastomatous epithelial elements in the form of luminal structures resembling tubules, ill-formed papillary structures resembling immature glomeruli, and undifferentiated and differentiated mesenchymal elements, most often in the form of skeletal muscle and myxoid mesenchyme, less often cartilage and fat

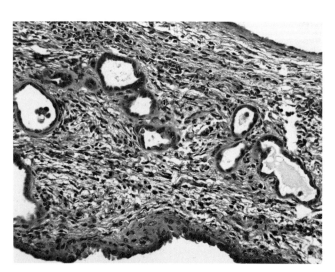

Fig. 2.247 Cystic partially differentiated nephroblastoma (CPDN). In some CPDNs, such as the one illustrated here, the septa harbor no nephroblastomatous elements, and such tumors have been designated "cystic nephroma," recognizing that these lesions are distinctly different on many levels from morphologically similar tumors, bearing the same name, that occur predominantly in adult females

2.10 Mesenchymal Renal Neoplasms Mainly Occurring in Children

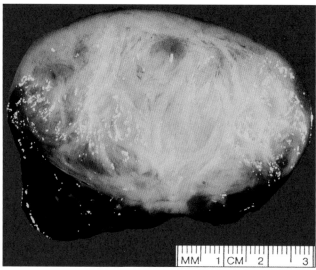

Fig. 2.248 Congenital mesoblastic nephroma (CMN). CMN takes two forms, designated classic and cellular. It is usually unilateral and solitary, and ranges from 0.8 to 14 cm in diameter. Classic CMN, illustrated here, accounts for about one quarter of cases. It is typically firm and may exhibit a whorled and myomatous texture; its interface with the adjacent normal kidney is not sharply demarcated (*see* MacLennan GT, Resnick MI, Bostwick DG, 2003. With permission)

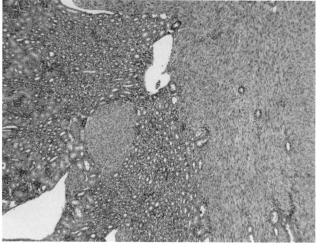

Fig. 2.249 Congenital mesoblastic nephroma (CMN). Classic CMN forms an irregular interface with the adjacent native renal parenchyma

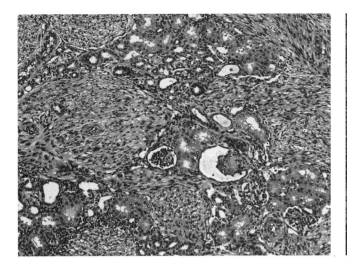

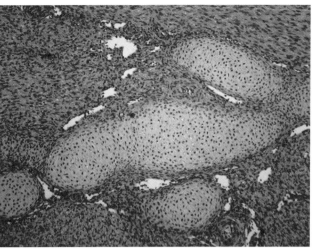

Fig. 2.250 Congenital mesoblastic nephroma (CMN). Classic CMN is composed of bland fibroblastic/myofibroblastic cells arranged in fascicles, with only rare mitotic figures and no necrosis. It subtly infiltrates adjacent tissue, encircling islands of native kidney at the interface between tumor and normal renal parenchyma. Long narrow tongues of tumor are often seen extending into perirenal soft tissue, particularly in the renal hilum

Fig. 2.251 Congenital mesoblastic nephroma (CMN). Classic CMN often exhibits islands of cartilaginous differentiation. These are considered to represent dysplastic changes in native renal parenchyma in response to the effect of tumor on normal renal development

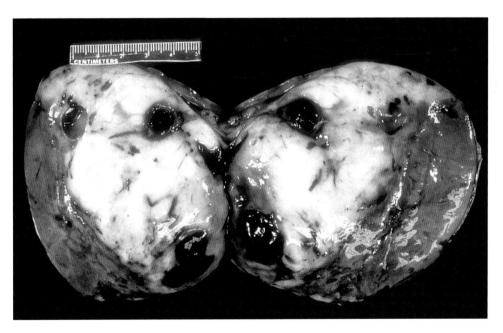

Fig. 2.252 Congenital mesoblastic nephroma (CMN). Cellular CMN accounts for about two thirds of case. In contrast to the classic form, cellular CMN is more often bulging and soft, with areas of hemorrhage, necrosis, and cystic degeneration, and its interface with the adjacent normal kidney is more sharply outlined (*see* MacLennan and Cheng 2008. With permission)

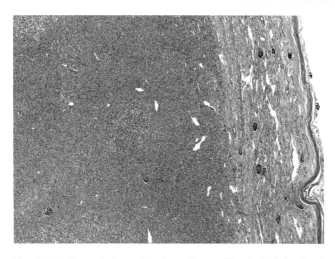

Fig. 2.253 Congenital mesoblastic nephroma (CMN). Cellular CMN is an expansile tumor that forms a "pushing" but unencapsulated border at its interface with normal kidney

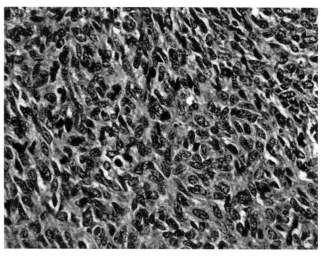

Fig. 2.255 Congenital mesoblastic nephroma (CMN). Section from a cellular CMN demonstrating numerous mitotic figures

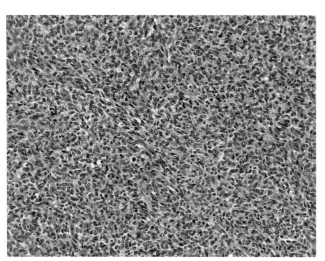

Fig. 2.254 Congenital mesoblastic nephroma. Cellular CMN is more densely cellular than classic CMN, and its architecture is more sheet-like than fascicular. It is composed of sheets of closely packed small cells that are usually quite uniform, with vesicular nuclei and minimal cytoplasm; some tumors exhibit plump and elongated tumor cells with slight to moderate nuclear pleomorphism

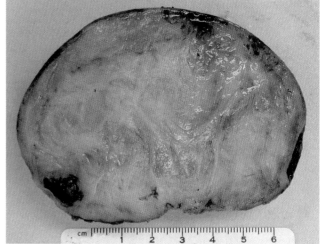

Fig. 2.256 Congenital mesoblastic nephroma (CMN). This neoplasm was a mixed CMN, composed of classic and cellular elements in variable proportions; it shows predominantly a whorled cut surface, but has areas that appear less firm

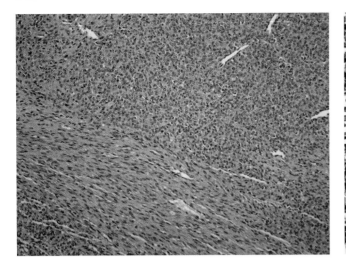

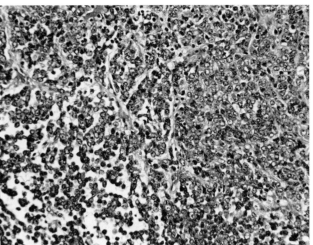

Fig. 2.257 Congenital mesoblastic nephroma (CMN). Section from a mixed CMN, showing classic morphology (*lower left*) and cellular morphology (*upper right*), quite sharply separated from one another. In mixed tumors, classic CMN is often seen at the periphery of a centrally expansile nodule of cellular CMN

Fig. 2.259 Rhabdoid tumor of kidney (RTK). RTK is composed of monotonous sheets of loosely cohesive cells

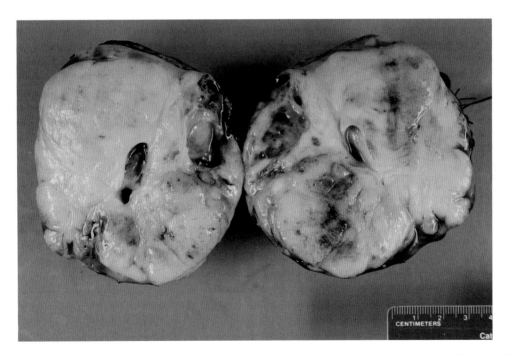

Fig. 2.258 Rhabdoid tumor of kidney (RTK). RTK is usually unicentric and unilateral, and usually weighs less than 500 g. As shown here, it is typically bulging, soft, and gray-white, sometimes with hemorrhage and/or necrosis, and forms an ill-defined interface with adjacent normal kidney

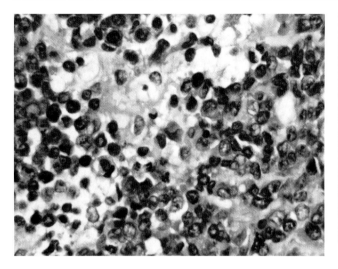

Fig. 2.260 Rhabdoid tumor of kidney (RTK). The tumor cells are large and polygonal, with vesicular nuclei, many of which have a single cherry-red nucleolus of variable prominence, and some exhibiting juxtanuclear, globular, eosinophilic cytoplasmic inclusions, composed ultrastructurally of whorled intermediate filaments. RTK infiltrates the adjacent renal parenchyma, and extensive vascular invasion is common

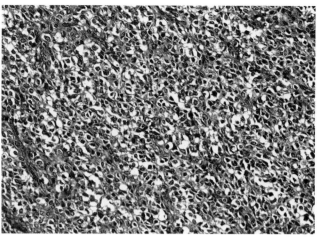

Fig. 2.262 Clear cell sarcoma of kidney (CCSK). Tumor cells are separated into cords or columns 4–10 cells in width by regularly spaced fibrovascular septa coursing through the tumor. The width of the fibrovascular septa varies considerably

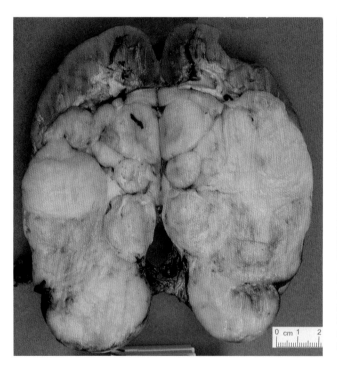

Fig. 2.261 Clear cell sarcoma of kidney (CCSK). CCSKs are large, well-circumscribed, and sharply demarcated unicentric masses ranging from 2.3 to 24 cm in diameter. Cut surfaces are gray-tan, soft, and mucoid, and cysts, hemorrhage and small foci of necrosis are commonly observed. Renal vein extension of tumor is present in 5% of cases; in 30% of cases lymph node metastases are found at the time of diagnosis (*Image courtesy of* Hollie Reeves, MD)

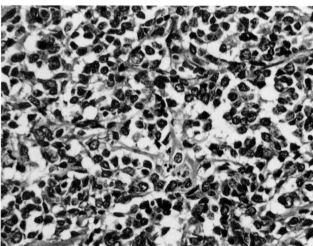

Fig. 2.263 Clear cell sarcoma of kidney (CCSK). Classically, tumor cells are plump and ovoid or spindled, with fairly uniform nuclei that are round to oval and often vesicular, with finely dispersed chromatin, inconspicuous nucleoli, and infrequent mitotic figures. Optically, clear material consisting of extracellular mucopolysaccharide matrix separates the tumor cells and imparts a clear cell appearance

2.11 Mesenchymal Renal Neoplasms Mainly Occurring in Adults

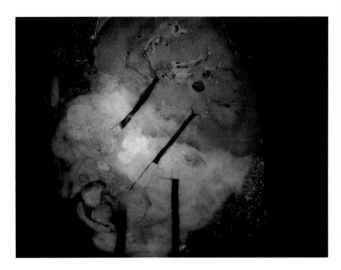

Fig. 2.264 Leiomyosarcoma. Tumors are solid and vary in size, but most are quite large – up to 23 cm in diameter. Necrosis is noted in up to 90% of cases, and cystic degeneration is common. Tumors are usually well-circumscribed, gray-white, and soft to firm; some have a whorled cut surface. The leiomyosarcoma illustrated here arose within an angiomyolipoma. The tumor is extensively necrotic and raggedly infiltrates the adjacent normal kidney (*see* MacLennan GT and Cheng L, 2008. With permission)

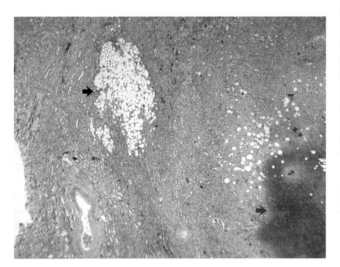

Fig. 2.265 Leiomyosarcoma, arising in angiomyolipoma. At low power, an angiomyolipoma is easily seen within renal parenchyma, at left (*black arrow*). A zone of necrosis is evident at lower right (*blue arrow*)

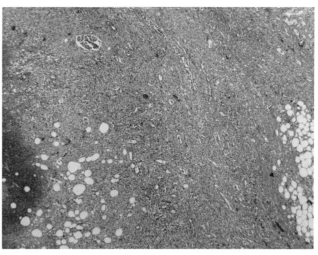

Fig. 2.266 Leiomyosarcoma, arising in angiomyolipoma. At low power, renal tubules and a glomerulus are admixed with adipocytes. Necrosis is seen at left

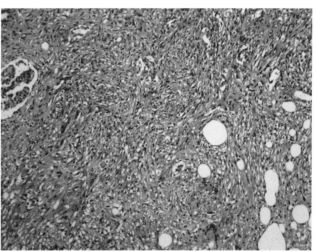

Fig. 2.267 Leiomyosarcoma, arising in angiomyolipoma. At higher power, native renal structures and adipocytes are readily seen. The renal interstitium is infiltrated and extensively replaced by a poorly differentiated malignant spindle cell neoplasm

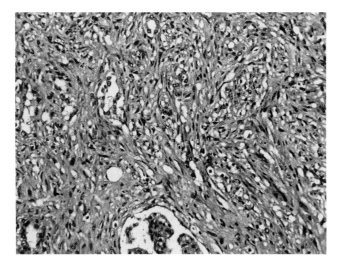

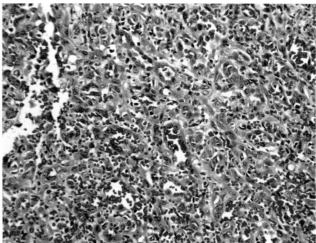

Fig. 2.268 Leiomyosarcoma, arising in angiomyolipoma. Pleomorphic malignant spindle cells replace the renal interstitium. The microscopic features of renal leiomyosarcoma are the same as those of leiomyosarcoma in other sites: eosinophilic cells with spindled nuclei, arranged haphazardly or in fascicles or plexiform structures. The degree of nuclear pleomorphism is variable, as are mitotic rates, which have a mean of 10.6 mitotic figures per ten high power fields

Fig. 2.270 Angiosarcoma. Tumors up to 23 cm in diameter have been reported. Tumors are hemorrhagic, yellow to gray-tan, soft, sometimes necrotic, with ill-defined borders and often grossly evident infiltration of adjacent structures. As illustrated here in a section of a tumor from a 48-year-old male, the tumor exhibits vasoformative architecture with channels resembling vascular spaces and sinusoids containing red blood cells, lined by epithelioid and spindled cells with eosinophilic cytoplasm, pleomorphic nuclei, and frequent mitotic figures

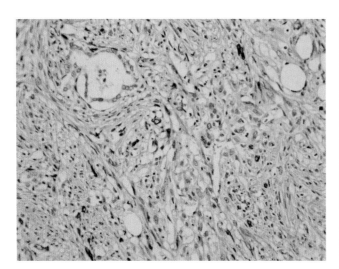

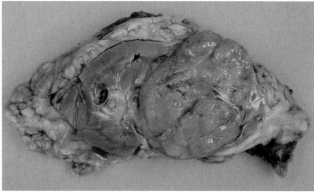

Fig. 2.271 Malignant fibrous histiocytoma (MFH). Most renal MFHs are large, up to 27 cm in diameter, and exhibit hemorrhage and necrosis. The case shown here is unusual in that it is relatively small, and shows neither hemorrhage nor necrosis; it was resected from a 61-year-old male

Fig. 2.269 Leiomyosarcoma, arising in angiomyolipoma. Tumor cells show positive immunostaining for muscle-specific actin

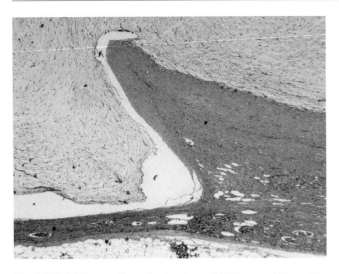

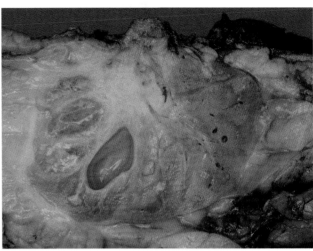

Fig. 2.272 Malignant fibrous histiocytoma (MFH), myxoid type. The majority of renal MFHs show a storiform-pleomorphic appearance typical of malignant fibrous histiocytoma in other sites. Sections from the tumor in Fig. 2.271 showed a variably cellular, prominently myxoid spindle cell neoplasm with a circumscribed and pushing border with adjacent kidney.

Fig. 2.274 Low-grade renal sarcoma, not further classified. This kidney from a 69-year-old female had an obvious inflammatory process that involved renal capsule, perirenal fat, and a portion of adjacent small bowel (*Image courtesy of* Carmen Kletecka, MD)

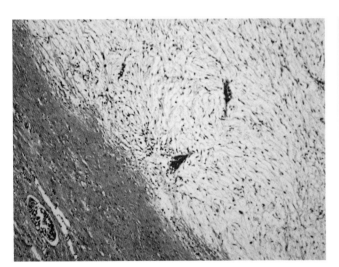

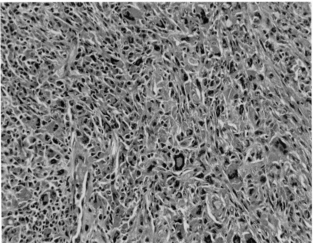

Fig. 2.273 Malignant fibrous histiocytoma (MFH), myxoid type. Tumor had a delicate vascular pattern and mild-to-moderate nuclear pleomorphism. Stains for c-kit, keratins AE1/AE3 and Cam 5.2, S-100 protein, and epithelial membrane antigen (EMA) were negative. Immunostain for CD34 was positive. Cytokeratin and EMA negativity argued against myxoid synovial sarcoma and sarcomatoid carcinoma; c-kit negativity argued against extragastrointestinal stromal tumor. CD34 positivity is often seen in solitary fibrous tumor, but the histology of this tumor excluded that diagnosis

Fig. 2.275 Low-grade renal sarcoma, not further classified. Much of the inflammatory component was consistent with xanthogranulomatous pyelonephritis. However, in addition to the inflammatory infiltrate, there was a substantial proliferation of mildly atypical spindle cells, exemplified in this image from the case shown in Fig. 2.274, that extended into the perirenal fat. The spindled cells lacked expression of keratins AE1/AE3 and Cam 5.2, S-100 protein, ALK1, CD34 or markers of melanocytic or muscle differentiation, arguing against sarcomatoid carcinoma, melanoma, myogenic sarcoma, solitary fibrous tumor, and inflammatory myofibroblastic tumor. Fluorescence in situ hybridization study for amplification in the MDM2 gene region were negative, arguing against well-differentiated liposarcoma. Findings were felt to fit best with a low grade mesenchymal neoplasm, not further classified

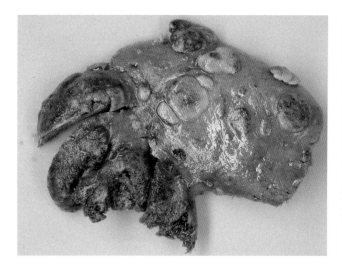

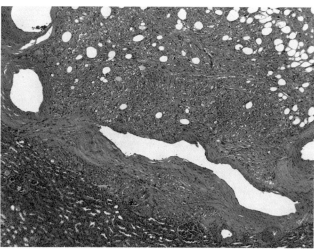

Fig. 2.276 Angiomyolipoma. Angiomyolipoma, the most common mesenchymal tumor of the kidney, is composed of varying quantities of myoid spindle cells, adipose cells, and dysmorphic blood vessels. Angiomyolipomas may be situated in the renal cortex, medulla, or capsule, and may be solitary or multiple, as in the case illustrated here

Fig. 2.278 Angiomyolipoma. The interface between angiomyolipoma and the adjacent renal parenchyma is sharp, with minimal intermingling of tumor and native renal tubules. Aggregates of thick-walled artery-like blood vessels are admixed with large mature fat cells and smooth muscle cells. The relative proportions of these components vary from tumor to tumor and even within different regions of the same tumor

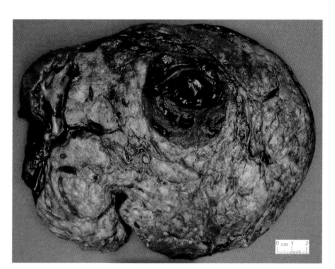

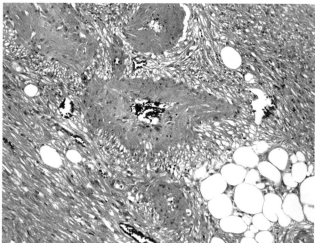

Fig. 2.277 Angiomyolipoma. Most angiomyolipomas removed surgically are greater than 4 cm in diameter, and can be as large as 30 cm in greatest dimension. They are typically smoothly rounded or ovoid and circumscribed but not encapsulated. They compress and distort the adjacent renal parenchyma but do not infiltrate it, although extension into perirenal fat or renal vein occurs, albeit infrequently. Depending upon the relative contents of smooth muscle and fat, tumor color varies from pink-tan or gray to yellow (*Image courtesy of* Anna Balog, MD)

Fig. 2.279 Angiomyolipoma. The blood vessels typically lack an elastica component. The smooth muscle cells may resemble normal smooth muscle cells or may assume a rounded epithelioid appearance. Focal areas of marked smooth muscle nuclear atypia are sometimes noted, with occasional mitotic figures. The smooth muscle cells tend to form a collar around the adventitia of the abnormal blood vessels and may assume a perpendicular orientation to the blood vessel lumen, creating a "hair on end" appearance, as shown here. Hemorrhage and areas of necrosis are often present

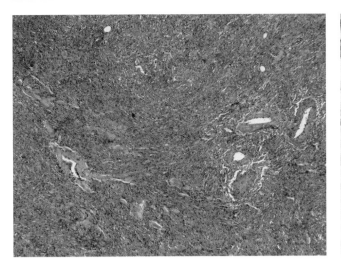

Fig. 2.280 Angiomyolipoma. Angiomyolipomas with classic morphology are not diagnostically challenging. Angiomyolipomas that are composed predominantly of smooth muscle, such as the case shown here, are less readily characterized, and in such circumstances, immunostains may be helpful

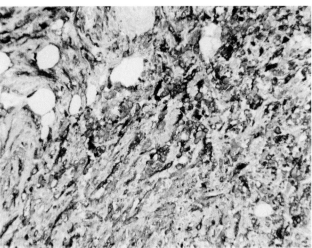

Fig. 2.282 Angiomyolipoma. Immunostain for Melan-A highlights the tumor cells strongly and diffusely

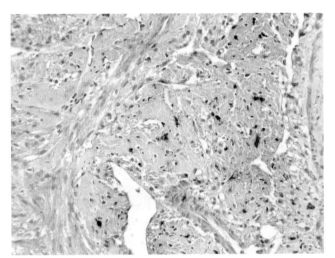

Fig. 2.281 Angiomyolipoma. The spindled and epithelioid smooth muscle cells of angiomyolipoma are immunoreactive to antibodies against a wide variety of markers; the combination of HMB-45 and Melan-A detects all classical renal angiomyolipomas. This image illustrates positive immunostaining in tumor cells for HMB-45

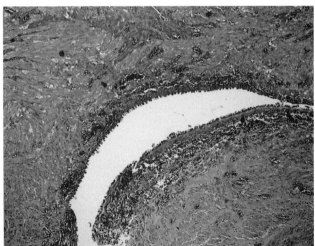

Fig. 2.283 Angiomyolipoma with epithelial cysts (AMLEC). Rarely, angiomyolipomas, usually muscle-predominant type, may be radiologically and grossly cystic. This is a section from an AMLEC. The tumor cells showed positive immunostaining for HMB-45, estrogen and progesterone receptors, desmin, and smooth muscle actin. The epithelial cells lining the cystic space are cuboidal to hobnail in appearance. The cysts are likely dilated entrapped native renal tubules

104

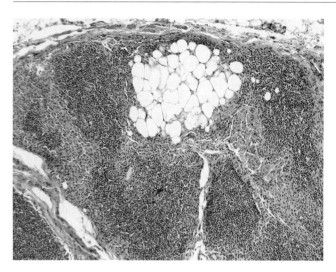

Fig. 2.284 Angiomyolipoma. Foci of angiomyolipoma are sometimes observed in regional lymph nodes, with no adverse patient outcomes, suggesting that the presence of angiomyolipoma in a lymph node, as illustrated here by the mature fat well within the confines of the lymph node, implies multicentricity of disease rather than metastasis

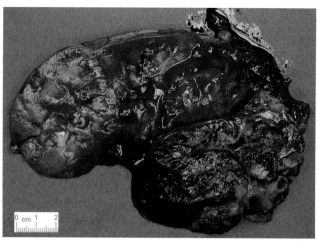

Fig. 2.286 Epithelioid angiomyolipoma (EAML). About 8% of renal angiomyolipomas are composed of an epithelioid component comprising more than 10% of the tumor, invoking a designation of "epithelioid angiomyolipoma." Only about 1% of renal angiomyolipomas are purely epithelioid. Renal EAMLs are often large, with a mean size of 8.6 cm, and are gray-tan, white or brown, often hemorrhagic, and sometimes partially necrotic (*Image courtesy of* Alan Siroy, MD)

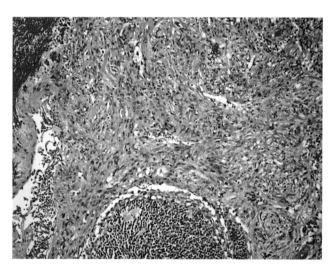

Fig. 2.285 Angiomyolipoma. This lymph node from a nephrectomy specimen containing renal angiomyolipoma contained abundant smooth muscle, consistent with multicentricity of angiomyolipoma characterized by smooth muscle proliferation, in contrast to the predominance of adipose tissue shown in Fig. 2.284

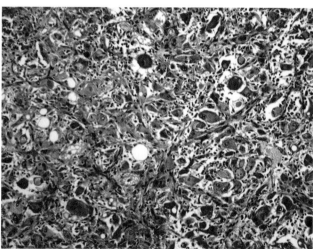

Fig. 2.287 Epithelioid angiomyolipoma (EAML). Tumors are composed of sheets of round to polygonal epithelioid cells with granular eosinophilic cytoplasm, admixed with variable amounts of the typical components of classic angiomyolipoma in most cases. The epithelioid cells show marked histologic variability: some have relatively small nuclei, small nucleoli, and limited amounts of cytoplasm, whereas others have large eccentrically placed vesicular nuclei, macronucleoli, and copious cytoplasm, and may resemble ganglion cells. Multinucleated giant cells with multiple peripheral nuclei are sometimes present. The extent of mitotic activity and necrosis is variable. Vascular invasion and invasion of perirenal soft tissues is sometimes observed

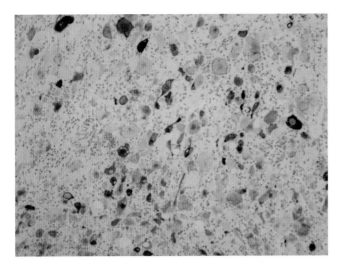

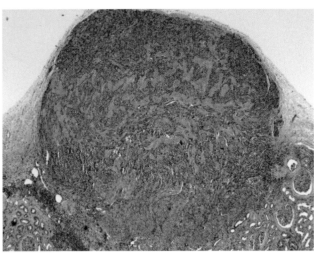

Fig. 2.288 Epithelioid angiomyolipoma (EAML). The epithelioid morphology in combination with cytological atypia, particularly when components of classic angiomyolipoma are absent, can be diagnostically challenging. Tumor cells of EAML show positive immunostaining for melanocytic markers such as HMB-45 and/or Melan-A (shown in this image), with variable expression of smooth muscle markers and negative immunostaining for epithelial markers and S-100 protein, which are usually positive in renal cell carcinoma and melanoma, respectively

Fig. 2.290 Leiomyoma. Small spindle cell neoplasm with areas of hyalinization

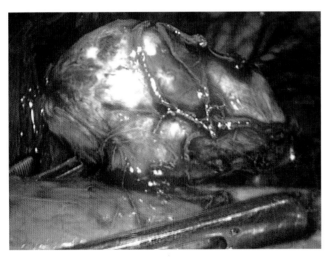

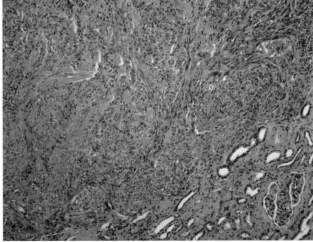

Fig. 2.289 Leiomyoma. The average size of renal leiomyomas is about 12 cm, and the largest reported renal leiomyoma was 57.5 cm in diameter and weighed 37 kg. They resemble leiomyomas in other locations: they are typically firm, bulging, and well-circumscribed, with a white whorled fibrous or trabeculated cut surface. This image is an intraoperative photo of a renal capsular leiomyoma removed laparoscopically (*see* Bostwick and Cheng 2008. With permission)

Fig. 2.291 Leiomyoma. Leiomyomas are composed of spindled cells usually arranged in small intersecting fascicles. Nuclear pleomorphism is minimal, and necrosis and mitotic figures are absent. Adipocytes and abnormal blood vessels are absent. Capsular leiomyomas often contain populations of cells strongly immunopositive for HMB-45, suggesting an undefined relationship with angiomyolipoma

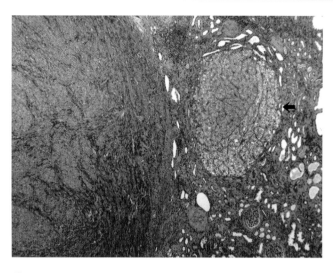

Fig. 2.292 Leiomyoma. An unexpected finding in this case of renal leiomyoma was a very small chromophobe renal cell carcinoma, at right (*arrow*)

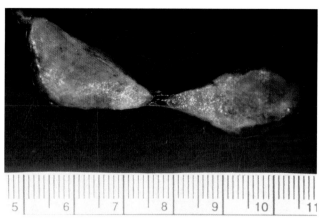

Fig. 2.294 Hemangioma. Hemangiomas involving the renal pelvis or a papilla may be very hard to identify grossly, appearing as a small mulberry-like lesion or a small red streak. Larger lesions often appear red or gray-tan, and spongy. The renal hilar mass described in Fig. 2.293 is shown here (*see* MacLennan GT and Cheng L, 2008. With permission)

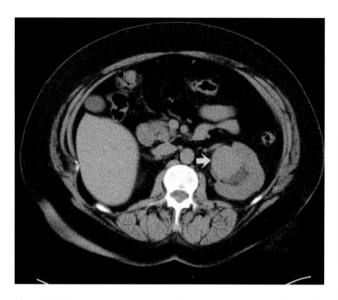

Fig. 2.293 Hemangioma. Most renal hemangiomas are only 1–2 cm in greatest dimension, but they may be as large as 18 cm. The commonest locations are the renal pelvis or renal pyramids, but hemangiomas also arise in the renal cortex, the renal capsule or within peripelvic blood vessels or soft tissues. *Arrow* indicates a solid mass lesion in the renal hilum. At surgery, it was peeled off the renal vein (*see* Bostwick and Cheng 2005. With permission)

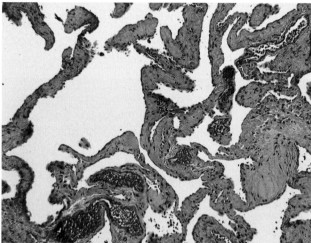

Fig. 2.295 Hemangioma. Lesions consist of irregular blood-filled vascular spaces lined by a single layer of endothelial cells that lack mitotic activity and nuclear pleomorphism. The lesion described in Figs. 2.293 and 2.294 was a cavernous hemangioma, shown here; capillary hemangiomas have also been reported

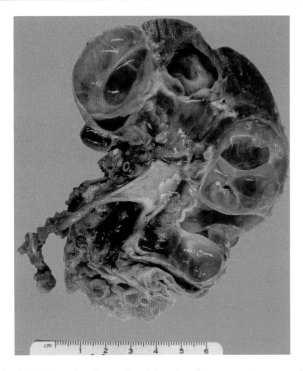

Fig. 2.296 Lymphangioma. Renal lymphangioma presents as a well-encapsulated multicystic mass that may be unilateral or bilateral, localized or diffuse. The cut surface is composed of innumerable fluid-filled cysts ranging from 0.1 to 2.0 cm in diameter, often mimicking a polycystic kidney disease or a multilocular renal cyst, as exemplified in this case

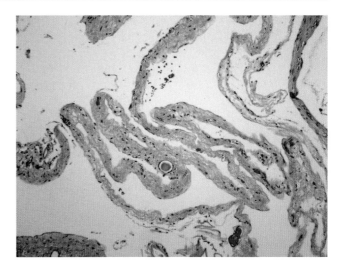

Fig. 2.298 Lymphangioma. The cysts are lined by flattened endothelial cells, and are separated by septal structures that may contain normal renal structures such as glomeruli, tubules, and blood vessels

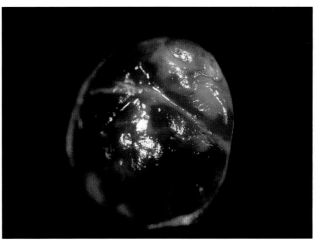

Fig. 2.299 Juxtaglomerular cell tumor. Juxtaglomerular cell tumors are usually well circumscribed, have a fibrous capsule of variable thickness, and are typically 2–4 cm in diameter, but can be much larger. They have a yellow to gray/tan and often hemorrhagic cut surface

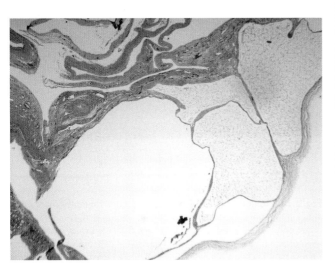

Fig. 2.297 Lymphangioma. At low power, lymphangioma consists of numerous thin-walled cysts separated by delicate fibrous septa

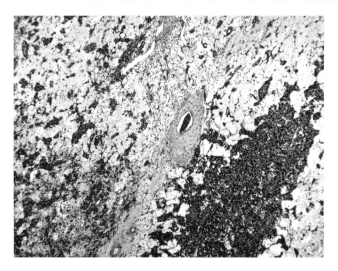

Fig. 2.300 Juxtaglomerular cell tumor. Tumor architecture is variable, and may be in the form of irregular trabeculae, papilla, organoid patterns, or solid compact sheets. The background stroma may be scant, abundant and hyalinized, or edematous, as in this image. Abundant thin-walled vessels are usually present, and most tumors demonstrate thick-walled blood vessels

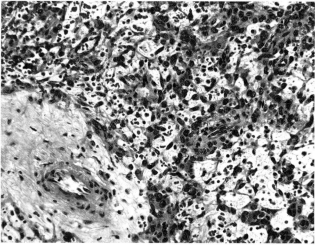

Fig. 2.302 Juxtaglomerular cell tumor. Features typical of this neoplasm include the large thick-walled blood vessel at left, the edematous stroma, the characteristic tumor cells, and a scant infiltrate of inflammatory cells

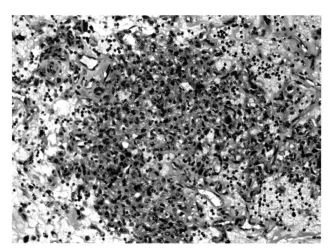

Fig. 2.301 Juxtaglomerular cell tumor. Juxtaglomerular cell tumors are composed of polygonal, round , or elongated spindle-shaped cells with slightly eosinophilic cytoplasm and centrally located nuclei. In most cases, some cells exhibit some degree of nuclear atypia. Mitotic figures are usually absent

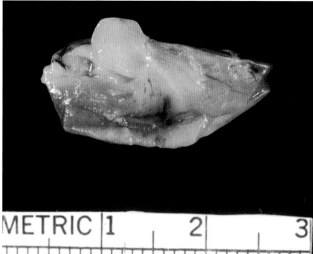

Fig. 2.303 Renomedullary interstitial cell tumor. Renomedullary interstitial cell tumors are small benign fibrous lesions in the renal medulla, commonly found incidentally. Most are 0.1–0.5 cm in diameter, as exemplified by the small gray-white interstitial cell tumor involving the tip of a papilla shown here, but rarely, they are large enough to obstruct renal pelvic outflow and cause pain (*see* MacLennan GT, Resnick MI, Bostwick DG, 2003. With permission)

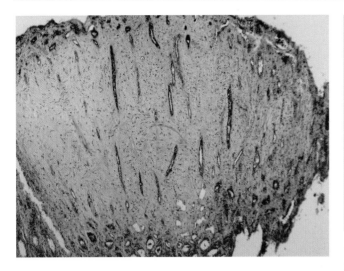

Fig. 2.304 Renomedullary interstitial cell tumor. The interstitium of this papilla is almost entirely occupied by small stellate or spindled cells set in a background of loose faintly basophilic stroma containing interlacing bundles of delicate fibers

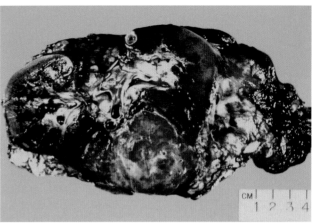

Fig. 2.306 Schwannoma. Schwannomas may originate in the renal parenchyma, the renal capsule, or the renal hilar soft tissues, and range from 4 to 16 cm in size. They are typically well circumscribed, tan to yellow, sometimes multinodular, and have a dense fibrous capsule (*see* MacLennan GT and Cheng L, 2008. With permission)

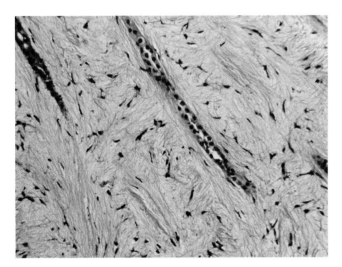

Fig. 2.305 Renomedullary interstitial cell tumor. A collecting duct is surrounded by spindled and stellate cells in a loose basophilic stroma

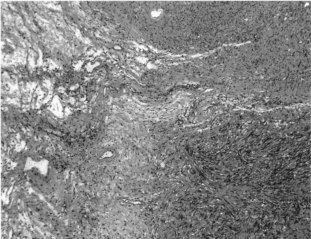

Fig. 2.307 Schwannoma. Schwannomas are classically characterized by a pattern of alternating Antoni A and Antoni B areas. The proportions of these elements vary, and the areas may subtly blend into one another. This image shows a rather cellular Antoni A area (*lower right*) and a relatively paucicellular Antoni B area (*left*). In the Antoni B area, spindle cells are arrayed haphazardly in a loosely textured matrix. Prominent blood vessels, characteristic of schwannoma, are readily seen in this area. Mitotic figures are absent or rare, and necrosis is absent

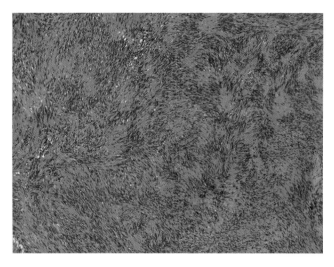

Fig. 2.308 Schwannoma. Antoni A areas consist of compact spindle cells with twisted nuclei, with characteristic palisading

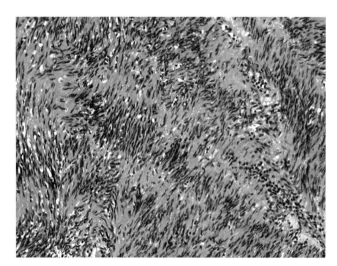

Fig. 2.309 Schwannoma. Approximately parallel rows of well-aligned palisaded tumor cells are separated by fibrillary cell processes, a formation designated as a Verocay body

Fig. 2.310 Schwannoma. Tumor cells show diffuse, strongly positive immunostaining for S-100 protein

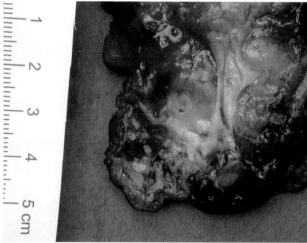

Fig. 2.311 Solitary fibrous tumor. Renal solitary fibrous tumors range from 2 to 25 cm in diameter, with a mean of 8.75 cm, and are typically well-circumscribed, pseudoencapsulated, lobulated, rubbery or firm masses that exhibit a homogeneous gray or tan-white, whorled cut surface, usually without necrosis, cyst formation, or hemorrhage

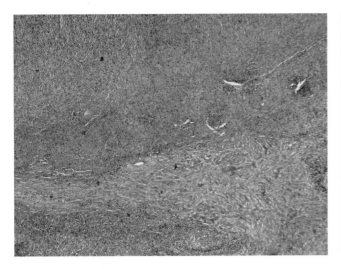

Fig. 2.312 Solitary fibrous tumor. Solitary fibrous tumors are composed of proliferations of spindle cells arranged in a patternless architecture, with areas of alternating hypocellularity and hypercellularity separated from one another by thick bands of hyalinized collagen

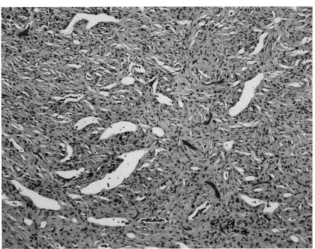

Fig. 2.314 Solitary fibrous tumor. Branching hemangiopericytoma-like blood vessels are often present

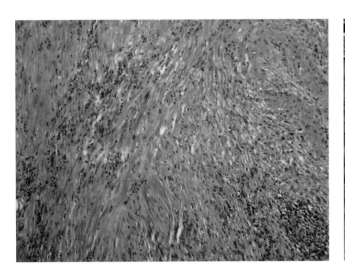

Fig. 2.313 Solitary fibrous tumor. Tumor cells possess minimal indistinct cytoplasm, and elongated nuclei with finely dispersed chromatin and only occasional nucleoli. Mitotic figures are absent or rare, and cellular atypia and necrosis are not observed in benign cases

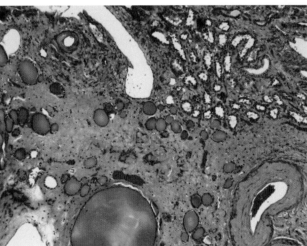

Fig. 2.315 Solitary fibrous tumor. The tumor infiltrates subtly around native renal structures, causing thyroidization of tubules

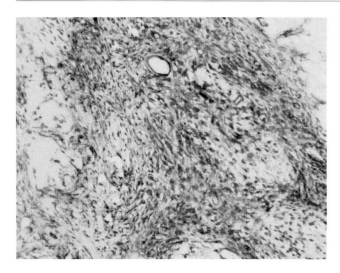

Fig. 2.316 Solitary fibrous tumor. Tumor cells show positive immunostaining for CD34, a finding that is considered characteristic and indispensible in making the diagnosis

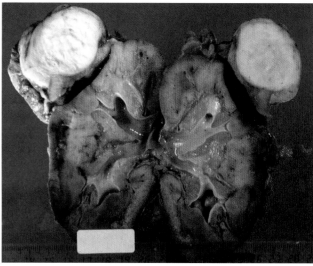

Fig. 2.318 Inflammatory myofibroblastic tumor (IMT). The tumor is white and fibrous, predominantly intrarenal, and well circumscribed, without hemorrhage or necrosis. Some IMTs have a myxoid or gelatinous cut surface (*Image courtesy of* Antonio Lopez-Beltran, MD)

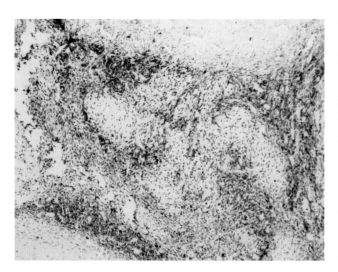

Fig. 2.317 Solitary fibrous tumor. Tumor cells show positive immunostaining for bcl-2, a finding observed in 70% of solitary fibrous tumors. Immunostains for S100 protein, cytokeratins, and/or desmin are usually negative or only weakly positive in a few cells

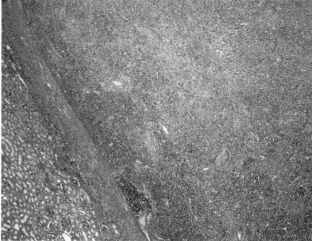

Fig. 2.319 Inflammatory myofibroblastic tumor (IMT). Three histologic patterns are described. One pattern is characterized by loosely organized spindle cells admixed with inflammatory cells and small blood vessels in an inflammatory background. In a second pattern, exemplified by this section from a perirenal IMT, spindle cells are much more abundant, and are admixed with collagen and inflammatory cells. The third type consists of hypocellular fibrous tissue with dense keloid-like fibrosis and relatively few inflammatory cells

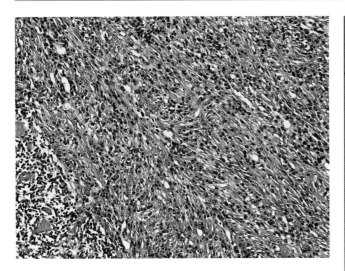

Fig. 2.320 Inflammatory myofibroblastic tumor. Tumor is an intimate admixture of spindle cells, lymphocytes, and plasma cells. The spindle cells in these lesions show myofibroblastic differentiation, and are usually anaplastic lymphoma kinase-1 negative

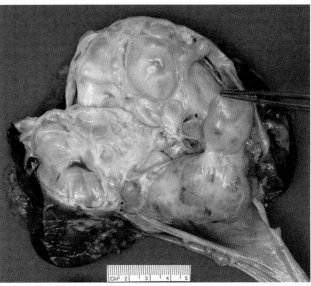

Fig. 2.322 Cystic nephroma. In some cases, cystic nephroma protrudes into the renal pelvis, as exemplified in this image

2.12 Mixed Mesenchymal and Epithelial Tumors

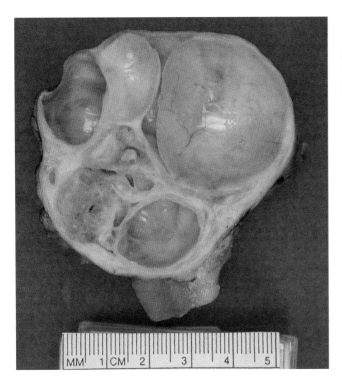

Fig. 2.321 Cystic nephroma. Cystic nephromas are well-circumscribed, usually unilateral but rarely bilateral, and range in size from 1.4 to 13 cm in diameter. They are composed of variably sized multilocular cysts containing serous fluid. No solid areas are discernible. Most tumors involve the renal cortex, as did the tumor shown in this image

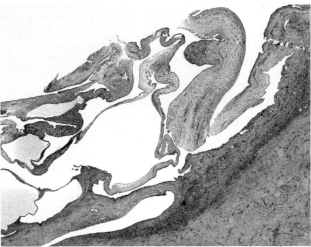

Fig. 2.323 Cystic nephroma. Cysts are encompassed by septa of variable thickness, which correspond to the outlines of the cysts; expansile nodules are absent. The stroma of the septa is composed of spindle cells in a collagenous background

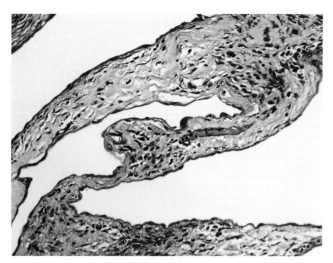

Fig. 2.324 Cystic nephroma. The cyst lining consists of epithelial cells that are flattened, cuboidal, or hobnail in appearance. Some lining cells may possess clear cytoplasm. Mitotic figures are not seen

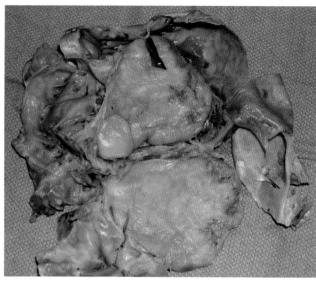

Fig. 2.326 Cystic nephroma with secondary sarcoma. There are at least eight reports of sarcoma arising in a background of cystic nephroma in adults. This image shows a solid neoplasm in a background of a cystic lesion in a middle-aged woman (*see* MacLennan GT and Cheng L, 2008. With permission)

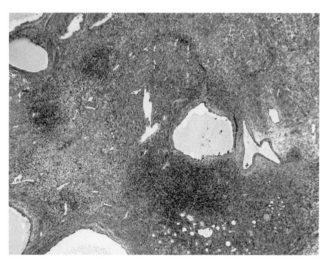

Fig. 2.325 Cystic nephroma. In some areas, stromal cell nuclei are very closely packed, imparting an ovarian stroma-like appearance. Acellular structures somewhat reminiscent of corpora albicantia/corpora fibrosa of the ovary are often seen. Small tubular structures may be present in septal stroma, but the septal stroma does not contain aggregates of clear cells, which would raise concern for multilocular cystic renal cell carcinoma, nor does it contain skeletal muscle, fat, smooth muscle, blastema, or other immature elements, which would raise concern for Wilms tumor

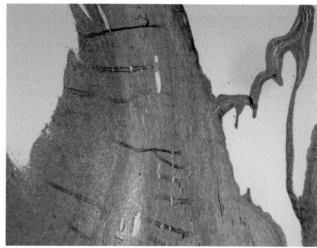

Fig. 2.327 Cystic nephroma with secondary sarcoma. Findings at right are consistent with cystic nephroma. At left is a densely cellular spindle cell neoplasm

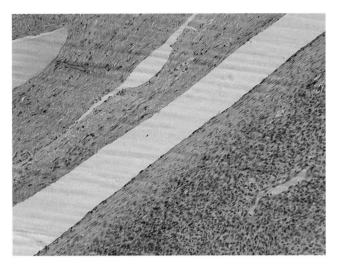

Fig. 2.328 Cystic nephroma with secondary sarcoma. The spindle cell neoplasm (*lower right*) was diagnosed as sarcoma, not otherwise specified, following extensive immunohistochemical and molecular studies

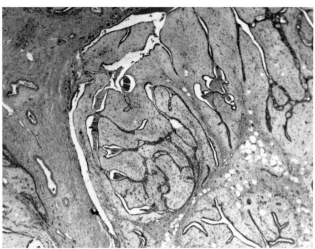

Fig. 2.330 Mixed epithelial and stromal tumor of kidney (MESTK). MESTK is biphasic, with spindle cell and epithelial components, both of which show a myriad of morphologic findings. The epithelial component consists of variably sized glands that may be uniformly dispersed or closely aggregated; in some tumors, tubular structures show complex branching or phyllodes-like structures, as shown here. Adipocytes may be present, as shown at lower right

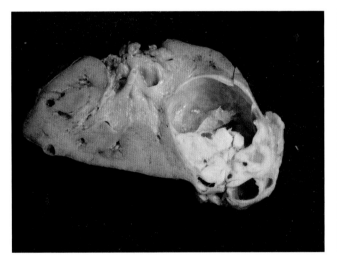

Fig. 2.329 Mixed epithelial and stromal tumor of kidney (MESTK). MESTK is typically single, unilateral, and well-circumscribed, ranging from 2 to 16 cm in diameter, and sometimes protrudes into the collecting system. Tumors typically have both solid and cystic components; the cysts may be clustered or dispersed, and the solid areas may be fleshy, or firm and rubbery (*see* MacLennan GT and Cheng L, 2008. With permission)

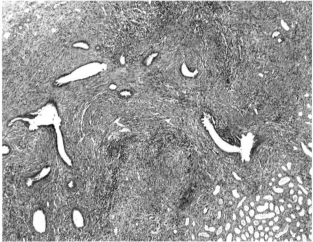

Fig. 2.331 Mixed epithelial and stromal tumor of kidney (MESTK). Glandular epithelial cells may be low cuboidal, columnar, or hobnail type, with variable amounts of clear, foamy, eosinophilic, or amphophilic cytoplasm. Neither the spindle cell nor the epithelial components show significant cytologic atypia or mitotic activity

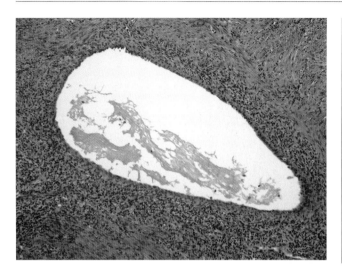

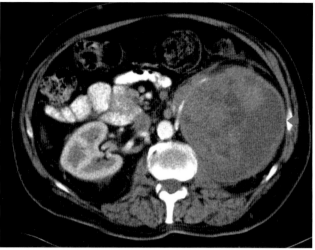

Fig. 2.332 Mixed epithelial and stromal tumor of kidney (MESTK). The spindle cell component may be hypocellular with extensive collagenization or with myxoid change, or cellular and arranged in fascicles resembling smooth muscle or in a woven pattern resembling ovarian stroma, or densely cellular, resembling fibrosarcoma or synovial sarcoma. It may show alternating zones of hypocellularity and hypercellularity with fibrocytic cells in a keloid-like background resembling solitary fibrous tumor. Often spindle cells show condensation around cystic areas, as illustrated in this image

Fig. 2.333 Synovial sarcoma. Renal synovial sarcoma is often quite large, ranging from 5 to 20 cm in diameter, as can be appreciated from this CT scan of an elderly man whose tumor (*arrow*) was biopsied but was deemed inoperable (*Image courtesy of* Nami Azar, MD)

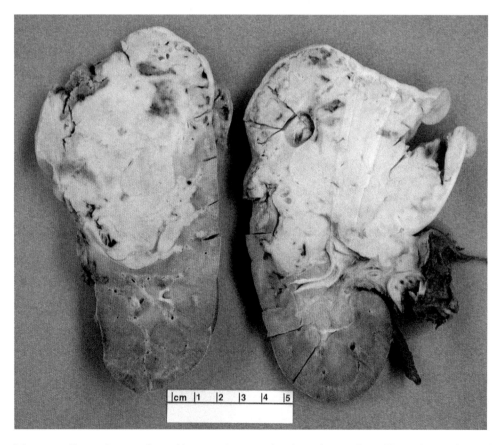

Fig. 2.334 Synovial sarcoma. Tumors have a soft or rubbery consistency and variegated cut surfaces. Hemorrhage and necrosis are usually evident, and most contain smooth-walled cysts. Tumor extension into large vessels is sometimes noted

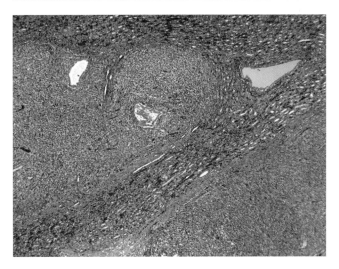

Fig. 2.335 Synovial sarcoma. Renal synovial sarcoma is composed of monomorphic plump spindle cells growing in solid sheets or in short intersecting fascicles that infiltrate native renal parenchyma, encircling normal structures

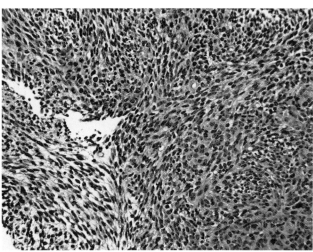

Fig. 2.337 Synovial sarcoma. The spindle cells are usually quite uniform in size, with ovoid nuclei and indistinct cell borders; rare cases with rhabdoid cell morphology have been reported. Mitotic figures are abundant. Tumor cellularity may be quite variable: hypocellular myxoid, edematous, or sclerotic areas may intermingle with densely populated regions

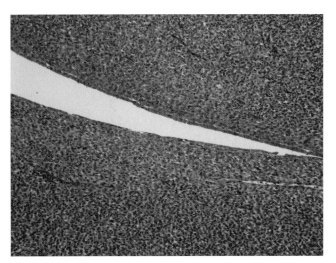

Fig. 2.336 Synovial sarcoma. Cysts of variable size are usually present, lined by mitotically inactive epithelium with abundant eosinophilic cytoplasm. The cysts are thought to represent entrapped and cystically dilated native renal tubules

2.13 Neuroendocrine Tumors

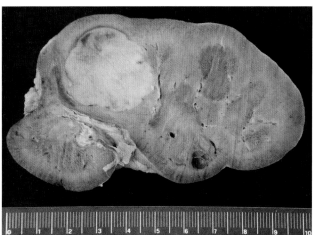

Fig. 2.338 Carcinoid tumor. Primary renal carcinoid tumor ranges in size from 1.5 to 30 cm in diameter. Tumors are yellow-white to red-tan, and most are solid, as shown here, but about one third are partially or predominantly cystic. About half are confined to the kidney, but one third involve perirenal fat, and about 10% invade the renal vein (*see* MacLennan GT and Cheng L, 2008. With permission)

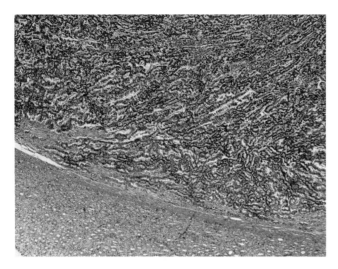

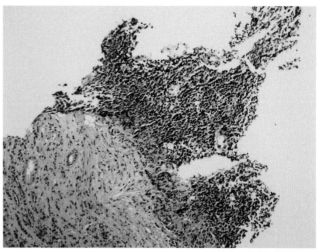

Fig. 2.339 Carcinoid tumor. At low power, the tumor has a sharply circumscribed interface with native kidney

Fig. 2.341 Small cell carcinoma. The majority of renal small cell carcinomas probably originate in the urothelium of the renal pelvis or calyces. The great majority of tumors are between 10 and 18.5 cm in diameter. They are typically solid, poorly circumscribed, gray-yellow, and extensively necrotic and hemorrhagic. Histologically, immunohistochemically and ultrastructurally, they resemble small cell carcinomas that arise elsewhere

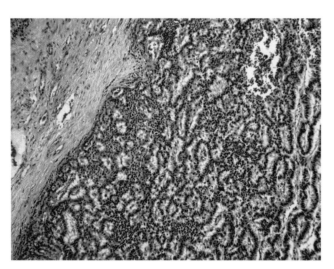

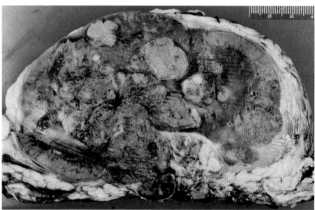

Fig. 2.342 Primitive neuroectodermal tumor (PNET). Renal PNETs are typically large, often greater than 10 cm in diameter. They are poorly circumscribed gray-tan to white tumors that extensively obliterate native renal parenchyma. Hemorrhage, necrosis, and renal vein invasion are commonly present (*Image courtesy of* Zhanyong Bing, MD)

Fig. 2.340 Carcinoid tumor. The morphology of renal carcinoid tumor is the same as that of carcinoid tumors that arise elsewhere. Most display a mixed growth pattern, with cells arranged in solid nests, ribbons, rosette-like structures, or tubular structures. Mitotic figures are infrequent

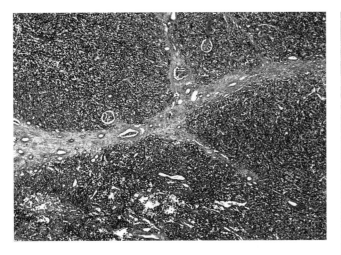

Fig. 2.343 Primitive neuroectodermal tumor (PNET). PNET consists of sheets of monotonous small round blue cells with high nuclear to cytoplasmic ratios. Tumor cells freely infiltrate adjacent renal parenchyma, sometimes leaving native structures intact

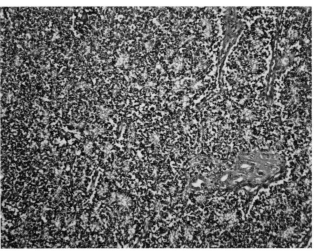

Fig. 2.345 Primitive neuroectodermal tumor. Pseudorosette formation may be present, as shown here

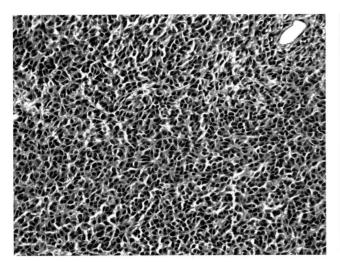

Fig. 2.344 Primitive neuroectodermal tumor. Nuclei are round and hyperchromatic, with dispersed chromatin and absent or inconspicuous nucleoli. Mitotic figures are readily apparent, and may be numerous. Cell overlapping is not prominent

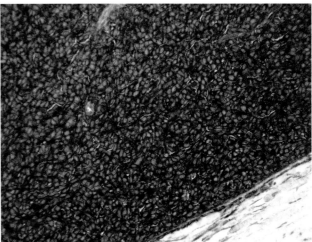

Fig. 2.346 Primitive neuroectodermal tumor. Tumor cells show strong, diffusely positive immunostaining for CD99

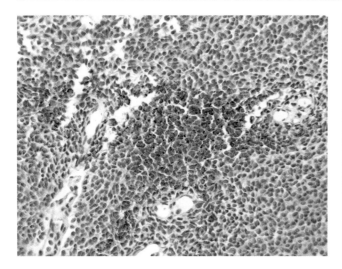

Fig. 2.347 Primitive neuroectodermal tumor. Tumor cells shows scattered positive immunostaining for FLI-1

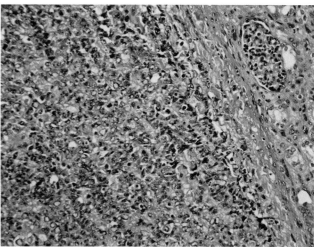

Fig. 2.349 Neuroblastoma, intrarenal. On closer inspection, the tumor shown in Fig. 2.348 is an undifferentiated neoplasm, consistent with neuroblastoma, based on positive immunostaining for neuron-specific enolase, synaptophysin, chromogranin, and PGP9.5, and negative immunostaining for CD45RB, vimentin, desmin, EMA, CD99, MYF-4, and cytokeratin

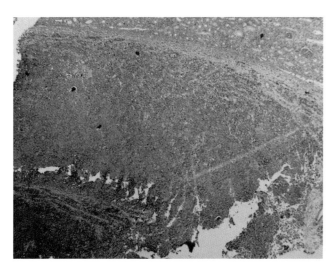

Fig. 2.348 Neuroblastoma, intrarenal. It is unclear whether neuroblastoma is ever primary in the kidney; secondary renal involvement by adrenal or retroperitoneal neuroblastoma is fairly common. This sections is from a renal mass in an 11-month-old male suspected of having nephroblastoma. A small round blue cell tumor was present in kidney, pancreas, and numerous retroperitoneal lymph nodes. Adrenal gland was normal

2.14 Hematopoietic and Lymphoid Tumors

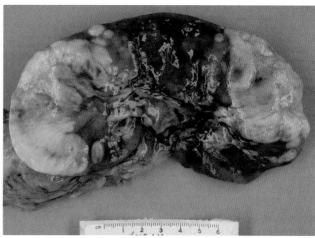

Fig. 2.350 Lymphoma. Renal lymphoma takes the form of single or multiple pale tan, pink, or gray-white nodules that may be friable, soft and fleshy, firm, or rock hard, with varying degrees of necrosis and/or hemorrhage. Tumors often obliterate substantial portions of the renal parenchyma. Infiltration of perirenal soft tissues, adrenal, and/or renal hilar vessels is often noted

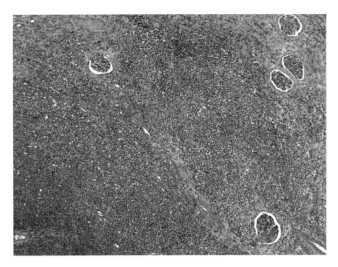

Fig. 2.351 Lymphoma. Lymphoma obliterates the underlying parenchyma except at the interface between tumor and normal kidney, where the lymphoma cells infiltrate in an interstitial pattern, sparing tubules and glomeruli, as shown here

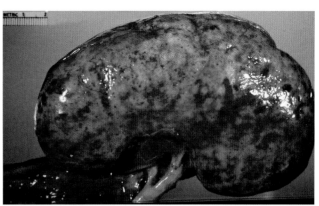

Fig. 2.353 Leukemia. Autopsy photo, from a patient who died of eosinophilic leukemia. Kidney is hyperemic, ecchymotic, and swollen (*see* Bostwick and Cheng 2008. With permission)

2.15 Metastatic Neoplasms in Kidney

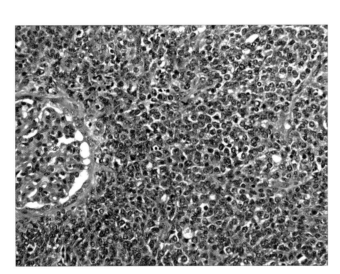

Fig. 2.352 Lymphoma. Virtually all histologic lymphoma subtypes reportedly involve the kidney. Diffuse large B-cell lymphoma (shown here) and its variants account for the majority of renal lymphomas

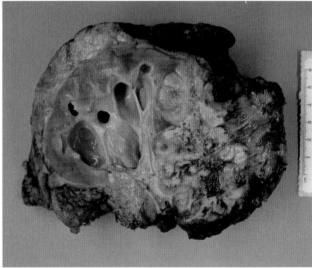

Fig. 2.354 Metastasis to kidney. Melanoma of skin, and cancers of lung, breast, opposite kidney, gastrointestinal tract, ovary, and testis (as in this case of metastatic seminoma) are the commonest primary sites. In patients with prior cancers, renal metastases outnumber new renal cell carcinomas by a ratio of about 4:1

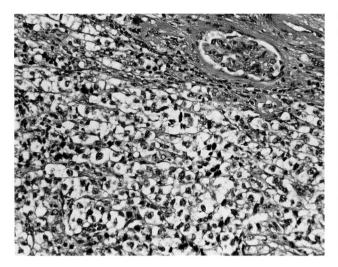

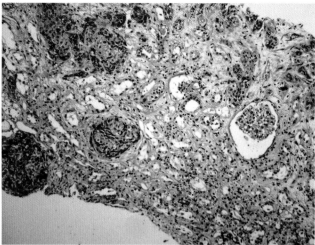

Fig. 2.355 Metastasis to kidney. Section of the metastatic seminoma illustrated in Fig. 2.354

Fig. 2.357 Metastasis to kidney. In some cases, metastases are confined to the glomeruli, and, rarely, this may result in renal insufficiency. Section from a renal biopsy of a 68-year-old man who presented with hematuria and renal failure. Diagnosis was acute glomerulonephritis until this biopsy showed extensive glomerular metastases from the patient's previously unknown lung cancer

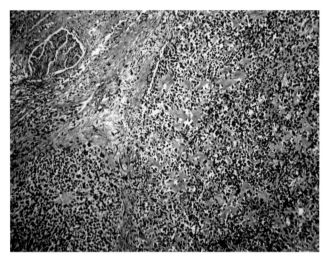

Fig. 2.356 Metastasis to kidney. Section from a nephrectomy specimen containing metastatic osteosarcoma, in a 25-year-old man treated for osteosarcoma 7 years previously

The renal pelvis and ureter are conduits composed of interlacing bundles of spirally oriented smooth muscle, lined by urothelium. Their function depends upon the presence of intrinsically normal musculature and proper spatial orientation relative to the bladder. Surgical correction of malformations may involve excision of an intrinsically defective segment of the collecting system (as in ureteral diverticulum, congenital ureteropelvic junction obstruction, ureterocele, and primary megaureter), or the reconstitution of proper anatomy (as in correction of ureteral reflux, ureteral ectopia, or paraureteral diverticulum). The status of the musculature of an excised segment of the drainage system is of prime importance; the overlying mucosa is generally normal.

3.1 Malformations, Congenital and Acquired

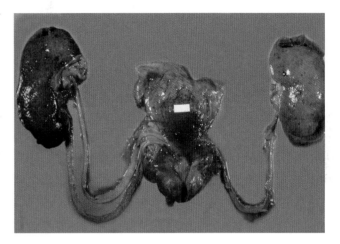

Fig. 3.1 Ureteral duplication. Two complete ureters (*right*) each drain separate portions of the kidney, and each has its own ureteral orifice in the bladder. In a setting of complete duplication, the orifice of the upper pole ureter is often ectopically placed, closer to the bladder neck, or outside the bladder proper (e.g., in the urethra or even in the vagina). This may result in obstructive changes in the renal segment drained by the anomalous ureter (*see* Fig. 2.31)

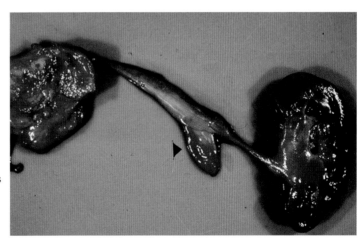

Fig. 3.2 Incomplete bifid ureter with a blind end. The ureteral outpouching (*arrow*) is most likely a portion of a bifid ureter that failed to connect to the renal parenchyma. Alternatively, it may represent a true congenital ureteral diverticulum, but this is less likely. Both entities are characterized by a complete wall, including urothelium, lamina propria, and muscularis propria (*see* MacLennan GT, Resnick MI, Bostwick DG, 2003. With permission)

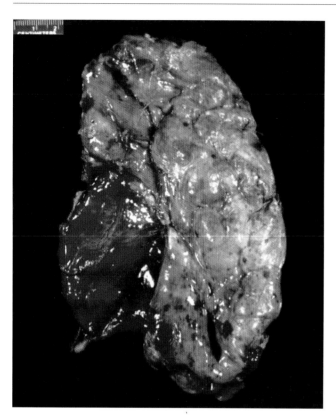

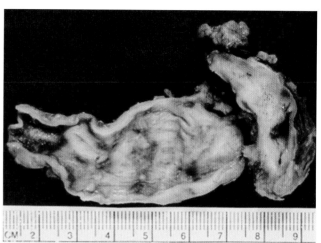

Fig. 3.5 Megaureter. Primary megaureter is a rare condition characterized either by functional intrinsic obstruction of the distal ureter, or by congenital deficiency of the musculature of the proximal ureter. Secondary ureteral dilatation may be due to vesicoureteric reflux, or to longstanding distal mechanical obstructions, such as ectopic orifice, stone, neoplasm, or ureterocele, shown here. The distal ureter (*left*) is markedly dilated. A decompressed ureterocele is at right

Fig. 3.3 Congenital ureteropelvic junction obstruction. External view of a kidney with longstanding obstruction at the ureteropelvic junction. The renal pelvis is markedly distended. The renal cortex is scarred and thin. Because attempts at repair and renal conservation are usually made, the fact that the kidney was removed implies that it was virtually nonfunctioning (*see* MacLennan GT, Resnick MI, Bostwick DG, 2003. With permission)

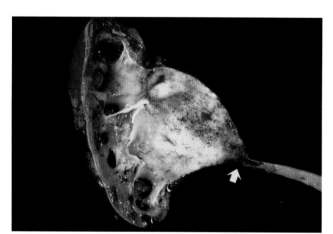

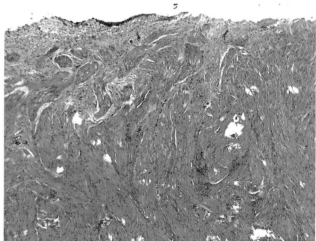

Fig. 3.4 Congenital ureteropelvic junction obstruction. *Arrow* indicates the region of obstruction. The renal pelvis and calyces are dilated; renal cortex is markedly thinned. The microscopic findings in this condition vary: the muscle layers in the area of the ureteropelvic junction may be normal, attenuated, disorganized, or predominantly longitudinal. In a minority of cases, the obstruction is extrinsic to the collecting system, and due to impingement of polar vessels associated with renal malrotation (*see* MacLennan GT, Resnick MI, Bostwick DG, 2003. With permission)

Fig. 3.6 Megaureter. There is marked hyperplasia of the ureteral smooth muscle

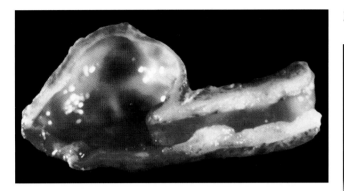

Fig. 3.7 Ureterocele. This is a congenital anomaly characterized by an abnormally small ureteral orifice. The distal ureter becomes dilated and balloons into the bladder lumen, sometimes becoming large enough to undermine the trigone and protrude into the urethra. The great majority involve the upper pole ureter of a duplex collecting system, and the renal unit drained by the affected ureter shows segmental dysplasia in nearly three-quarters of cases (*see* Bostwick and Cheng 2008. With permission)

3.2 Acquired Nonneoplastic Disorders

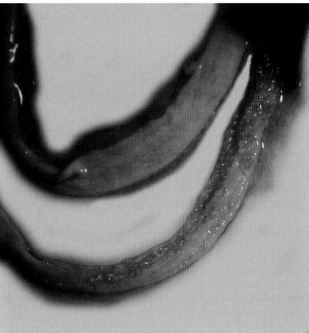

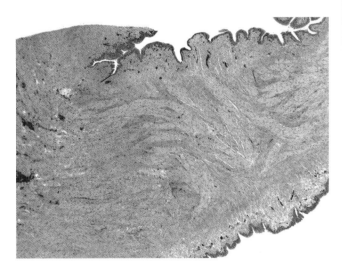

Fig. 3.8 Ureterocele. The musculature of the wall of a ureterocele may be relatively abundant, as in this case. The ureteral lumen is at top center; the bladder lumen is at bottom right

Fig. 3.10 Ureteritis cystica and glandularis. The presence of foreign bodies such as renal calculi or indwelling ureteral stents is sometimes associated with pyelitis or ureteritis cystica, or pyelitis or ureteritis glandularis, depending upon the location of the small fluid-filled mucosal vesicles, exemplified in the lower ureter in this image, and whether they are lined by urothelium or columnar cells

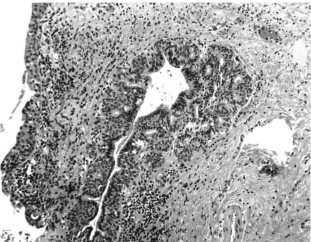

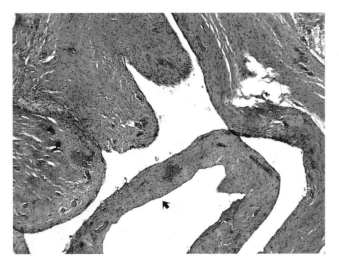

Fig. 3.9 Ureterocele. In this case, the wall of the ureterocele (*arrow*) is essentially devoid of muscle

Fig. 3.11 Ureteritis cystica and glandularis. In the lamina propria are clusters of cells, many of which have a central lumen lined by columnar cells. The columnar cells are accompanied by normal urothelial cells in some of the nests

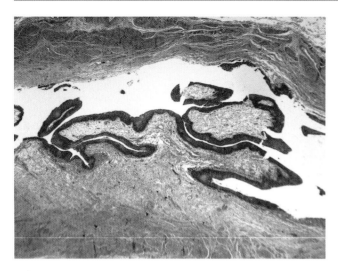

Fig. 3.12 Papillary-polypoid pyelitis. This form of mucosal inflammation is characterized by thin fingerlike and/or edematous broad-based papillary projections, and is associated with indwelling catheters or renal calculi. The pathologic changes are mostly stromal, and may include edema, chronic inflammation, and increased vascularity in the form of abundant small blood vessels or healing granulation tissue. The overlying urothelium may be normal, reactive, or denuded. This example is a section from the ureteropelvic junction in a case of congenital ureteropelvic junction obstruction, treated by nephrectomy

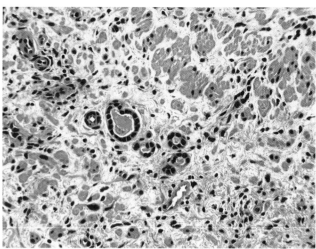

Fig. 3.14 Nephrogenic metaplasia. Closer examination of the luminal structures (*see* Fig. 3.13) shows an aggregate of small benign-appearing tubules lined by cuboidal epithelium, most consistent with nephrogenic metaplasia

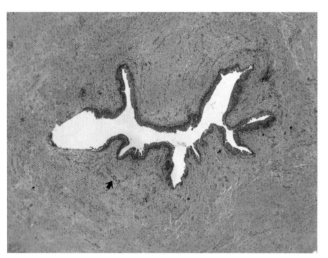

Fig. 3.13 Nephrogenic metaplasia. This is a rare finding in the ureter, most likely a reactive process. It may be subtle; *arrow* indicates small nondescript luminal structures in the ureteral wall

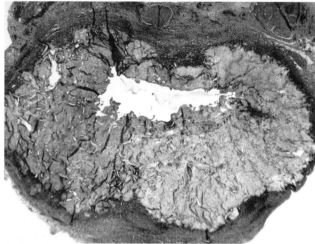

Fig. 3.15 Periureteral bulking agents. There are several clinical scenarios in which endoscopic injection of polytetrafluoroethylene or other bulking agents around the intramural portion of the distal ureter is performed to ameliorate vesicoureteral reflux. If this proves ineffective, and operative repair of reflux is done, the distal ureter and surrounding agent may be submitted for examination. This image shows a cross-section of such a ureter, with bulking agent surrounding the ureteral lumen

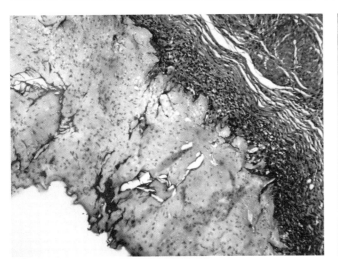

Fig. 3.16 Periureteral bulking agents. This particular amorphous agent is dextranomer/hyaluronic acid copolymer (Dx/HA). There is a mild chronic inflammatory response to the presence of the bulking agent.

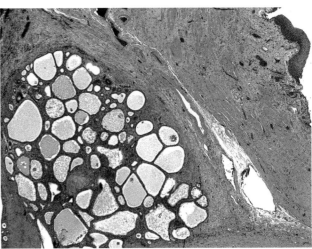

Fig. 3.18 Ureteral endometriosis. Rarely, hyperplasia and malignant transformation may occur in ureteral endometriosis. In this case, there is simple endometrial hyperplasia, characterized by crowded cystically dilated glands

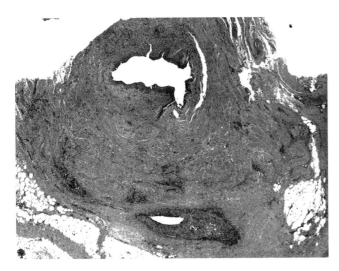

Fig. 3.17 Ureteral endometriosis. Ureteral endometriosis most commonly affects the lower third of the left ureter. Involvement of the mucosal surface, lamina propria or muscularis propria of the ureter constitutes intrinsic ureteral endometriosis, whereas involvement of the soft tissues immediately adjacent to the ureter constitutes extrinsic ureteral endometriosis. In this image, endometriosis is present in the ureter at multiple levels, and is also in adjacent soft tissues

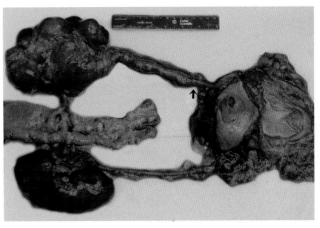

Fig. 3.19 Ureteral stricture. There are myriad causes of ureteral stricture, including congenital ureteropelvic junction obstruction, spontaneous stone passage, iatrogenic injuries, intrinsic neoplasia, and extrinsic compression by benign or malignant lesions. In this autopsy case, marked hydroureteronephrosis was found unexpectedly, proximal to a stricture in the ureter at the level of the arrow. The condition had caused no clinical symptoms, and did not contribute to the patient's demise (*Image courtesy of* Mark Costaldi, MD)

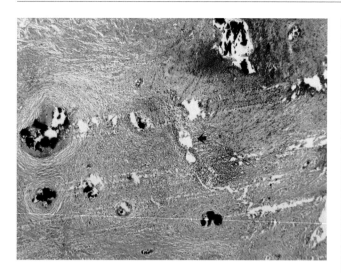

Fig. 3.20 Ureteral stricture. The ureteral lumen (*arrow*) is almost obliterated by fibrosis; chronic inflammation and multiple calcifications are present in the scar tissue

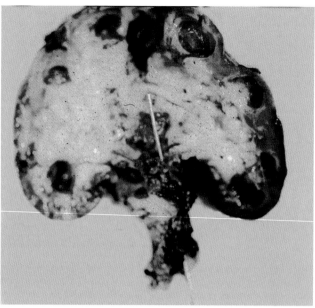

Fig. 3.22 Inflammatory myofibroblastic tumor. Patient presented with clinical signs and symptoms of ureteral obstruction, radiologically attributable to an obstructive mass lesion of indeterminate nature involving the region of the ureteropelvic junction. The metal probe is within the ureteral lumen, which was encased by a firm nondescript fibrous mass

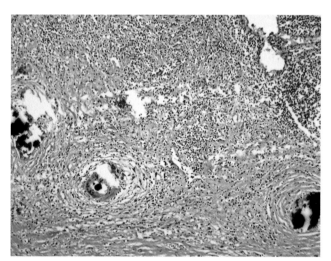

Fig. 3.21 Ureteral stricture. The inflammatory infiltrate also includes multinucleated giant cells. Special stains for fungal organisms and acid-fast bacilli were negative. The cause of the ureteral stricture was not apparent. The presence of abundant calcifications suggested that the process was a complication of prior renal calculus

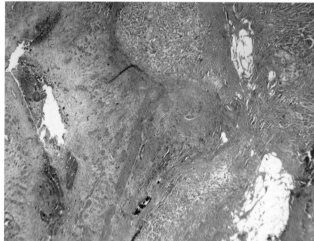

Fig. 3.23 Inflammatory myofibroblastic tumor. Section from the lesion shown in Fig. 3.22. The ureter (*left*) is encroached upon by paucicellular fibrous tissue with dense keloid-like fibrosis

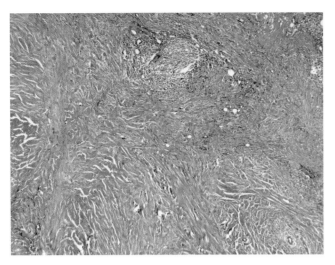

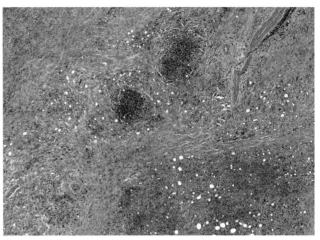

Fig. 3.24 Inflammatory myofibroblastic tumor. This lesion exhibits a spectrum of histologic changes, varying in the degree of spindle cell proliferation, inflammatory infiltration, and collagen deposition. Another section from the lesion in Fig. 3.22 shows hypocellular keloid-like fibrous tissue with patchy aggregates of chronic inflammatory cells

Fig. 3.26 Retroperitoneal fibrosis. This is an enigmatic idiopathic sclerosing process comprising inflammation and fibrosis of retroperitoneal soft tissues. Its origins are probably multifactorial; autoimmune disorders and viral infections are postulated underlying causes. Encasement and obstruction of both ureters occurs in some cases; intravenous pyelography shows medial deviation of both ureters, and varying degrees of bilateral hydronephrosis. Grossly, retroperitoneal fibrosis is a pale gray irregular plaque that encases the ureters and blood vessels. Biopsied or excised retroperitoneal tissue shows fibrosis and varying degrees of inflammation

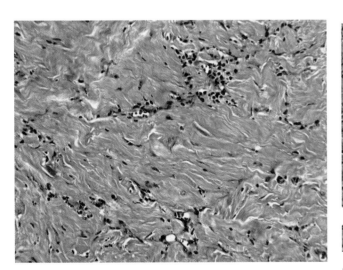

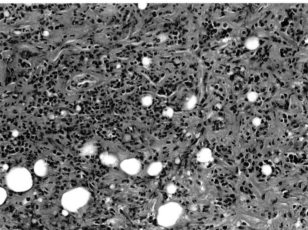

Fig. 3.25 Inflammatory myofibroblastic tumor. Despite the worrisome clinical, radiological, and gross pathologic findings related to the lesion in Fig. 3.22, only fibrosis and chronic inflammation were found, and features of malignancy were not identified

Fig. 3.27 Retroperitoneal fibrosis. The inflammatory cells infiltrating the fibrous tissue are of mixed type: neutrophils, eosinophils, lymphocytes, plasma cells, and macrophages. An important aspect of histologic evaluation is the exclusion of processes that warrant specific therapy, such as sclerosing lymphoma or metastatic carcinoma.

3.3   Renal Pelvic and Ureteral Neoplasms

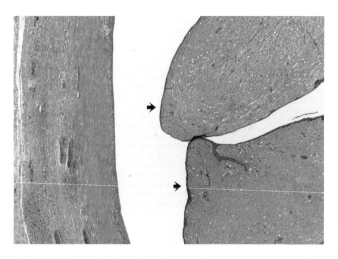

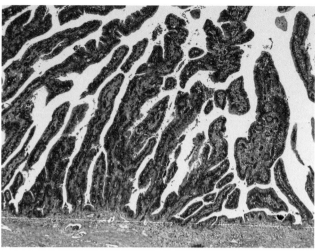

Fig. 3.30 Villous adenoma of renal pelvis. Section from the lesion shown in Fig. 3.29 shows fingerlike papillary projections lined by columnar epithelium (*Image courtesy of* Rodolfo Montironi, MD)

Fig. 3.28 Fibroepithelial polyp of ureter. This lesion occurs more often in the upper tracts than in the bladder, presenting with renal colic or hematuria in patients of all ages, most often middle-aged males. It is the commonest benign ureteral polyp in children. The lesion consists of one or more polypoid projections, lined by smooth shiny urothelium, and localized to a single site. Histologically, the polyps (*arrows*) consist of edematous, noninflamed fibrovascular cores covered by normal or ulcerated urothelium. Ureteral wall is at left (*see* MacLennan GT, Resnick MI, Bostwick DG, 2003. With permission)

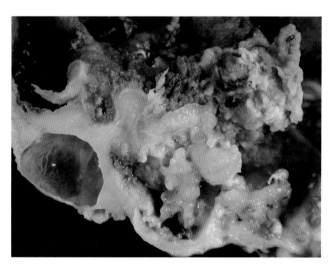

Fig. 3.29 Villous adenoma of renal pelvis. Villous adenoma can arise at various sites within the urinary system. Rarely, it may involve the renal pelvis, as in this case (*Image courtesy of* Rodolfo Montironi, MD)

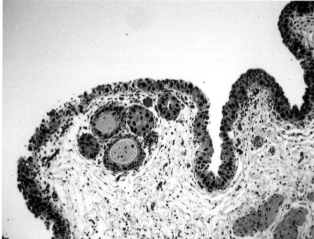

Fig. 3.31 Urothelial carcinoma in situ, at ureteropelvic junction. Section from region of ureteropelvic junction in a nephrectomy specimen, showing urothelial carcinoma in situ on the surface and extending into underlying von Brunn's nests. Patient had several selective urine cytology specimens from this renal unit showing carcinoma cells over several years, despite repeatedly negative imaging studies and ureteral endoscopies. Nephrectomy was performed on the basis of cytologic findings

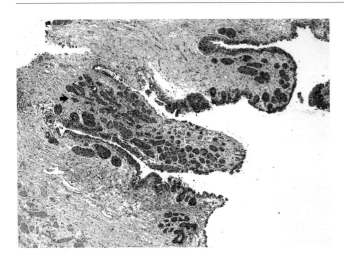

Fig. 3.32 Urothelial carcinoma, in situ and focally invasive, at uretero-pelvic junction. Section from a different area of the nephrectomy specimen described in Fig. 3.31. Surface urothelium is widely denuded, but residual surface epithelium consists almost entirely of carcinoma in situ. Focal stromal invasion is also present (*arrow*)

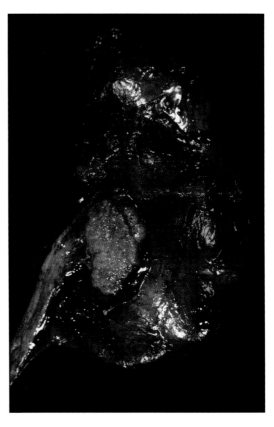

Fig. 3.34 Low-grade urothelial carcinoma of renal pelvis. Nephrectomy specimen from the patient whose renal pelvis contained the irregular filling defect shown in Fig. 3.33. The tumor is soft, shiny, and exophytic (*see* MacLennan GT, Resnick MI, Bostwick DG, 2003. With permission)

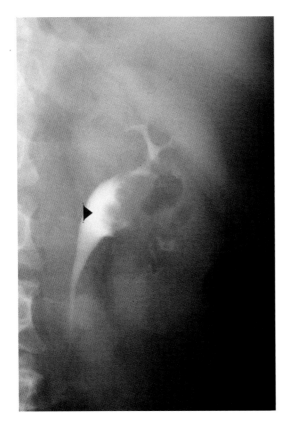

Fig. 3.33 Low-grade urothelial carcinoma of renal pelvis. An irregular filling defect is readily visible in the renal pelvis (*arrow*), suspicious for malignancy

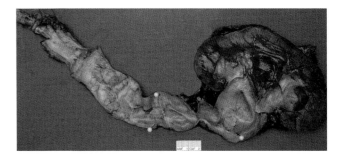

Fig. 3.35 Low-grade urothelial carcinoma of renal pelvis. This image illustrates multifocality of urothelial carcinoma, which is quite common. The tumor in the distal ureter has caused hydroureteronephrosis (*Image courtesy of* M. Carmen Frias-Kletecka, MD)

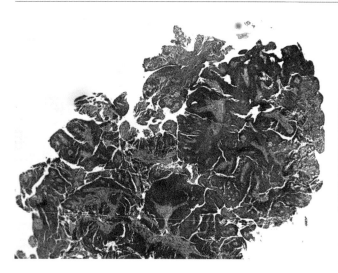

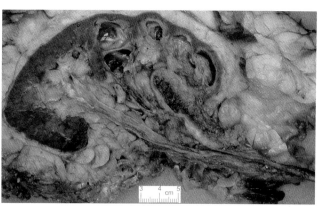

Fig. 3.36 Low-grade urothelial carcinoma of renal pelvis. The tumor is composed of complex and extensively fused papillary structures lined by multiple layers of urothelial cells, morphologically similar to lesions more commonly encountered in the bladder

Fig. 3.38 Low-grade urothelial carcinoma of renal pelvis. A somewhat unusual circumstance in which urothelial carcinoma involved only the lower pole of a partially duplicated collecting system. The ureters joined about halfway down (*Image courtesy of* Michelle Stehura, MD)

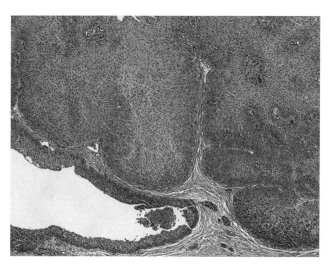

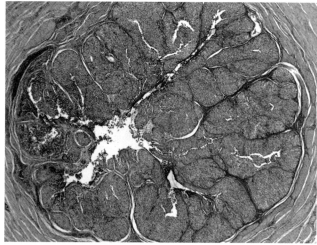

Fig. 3.37 Low-grade urothelial carcinoma of renal pelvis, with inverted growth pattern. This urothelial carcinoma had some architectural features resembling those of inverted papilloma, but the tumor cells formed broad trabeculae and expansile nodules, and there was brisk mitotic activity throughout the tumor, favoring a diagnosis of inverted urothelial carcinoma

Fig. 3.39. Low-grade urothelial carcinoma of ureter, noninvasive. This image illustrates why ureteral tumors frequently are associated with hydronephrosis: the ureter offers little room for expansion of the tumor, and becomes obstructed by the sheer bulk of the tumor, even though the tumor is noninvasive

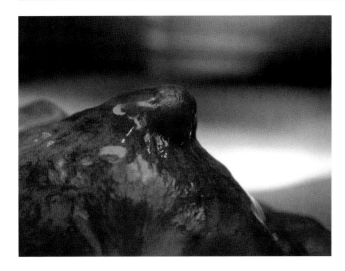

Fig. 3.40 Low-grade urothelial carcinoma of distal ureter. Patient underwent cystoprostatectomy for recurrent invasive urothelial carcinoma of the bladder, and was known to have an obstructive lesion in the distal right ureter, which accounts for the submucosal nodule at the site of the right ureteral orifice (*Image courtesy of* Alan Siroy, MD)

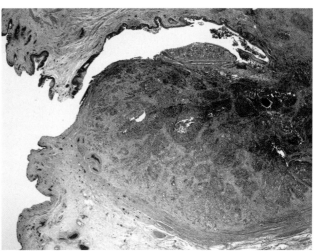

Fig. 3.42 Low-grade urothelial carcinoma of distal ureter. Microscopic section of the distal ureteral nodule shown in Fig. 3.43 shows urothelial carcinoma, invasive into the lamina propria (American Joint Committee on Cancer TNM stage T1)

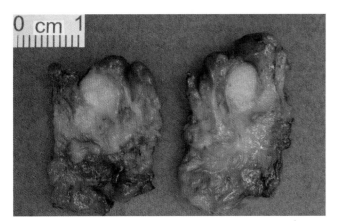

Fig. 3.41 Low-grade urothelial carcinoma of distal ureter. Section through the submucosal nodule shown in Fig. 3.42 shows urothelial carcinoma in distal ureter (*Image courtesy of* Alan Siroy, MD)

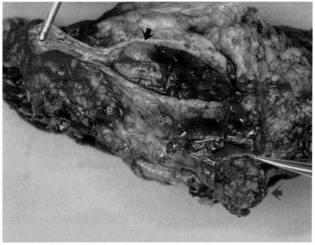

Fig. 3.43 High-grade urothelial carcinoma of renal pelvis, involving renal vein. Tumor fills the renal pelvis (*black arrow*) and also fills and expands the renal vein (*blue arrow*) (*Image courtesy of* Anaibelith Del Rio Perez, MD)

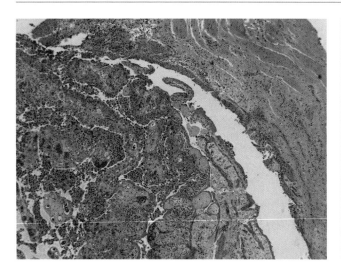

Fig. 3.44 High-grade papillary urothelial carcinoma of renal pelvis. Tumor is exophytic and has papillary architecture. Marked cellular atypia and complete loss of cellular orientation is evident even at relatively low power

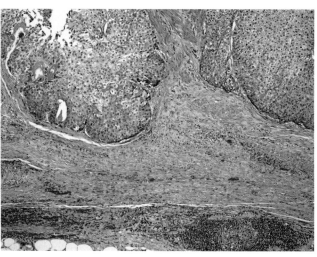

Fig. 3.46 High-grade invasive urothelial carcinoma of renal pelvis. Tumor has infiltrated lamina propria and full thickness of pelvic muscularis propria (American Joint Committee on Cancer TNM stage T2)

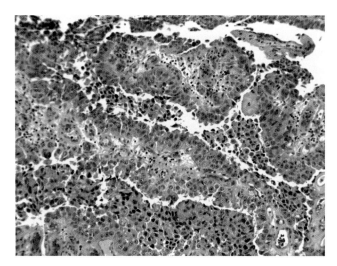

Fig. 3.45 High-grade papillary urothelial carcinoma of renal pelvis. Tumor cells are dyscohesive and lack polarity. They have large hyperchromatic nuclei with high nuclear/cytoplasmic ratios

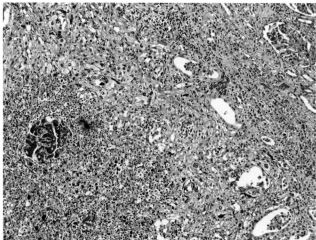

Fig. 3.47 High-grade urothelial carcinoma of renal pelvis. Poorly differentiated carcinoma cells infiltrate between renal tubules and glomeruli (American Joint Committee on Cancer TNM stage T3)

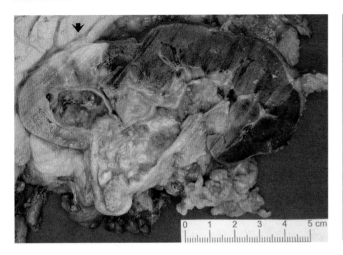

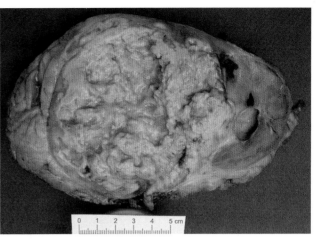

Fig. 3.48 High-grade urothelial carcinoma of renal pelvis. Almost the entire collecting system is involved by urothelial carcinoma. Much of the tumor is yellow-gray, reflecting the fact that the tumor had extensive squamous differentiation. In the region indicated by the arrow, tumor has infiltrated the full thickness of the renal parenchyma and into perirenal fat, invoking a scirrhous tissue reaction (*Image courtesy of* Zhanna Georgievskaya, MD)

Fig. 3.50 Sarcomatoid urothelial carcinoma of renal pelvis. The high-grade urothelial carcinoma had extensive necrosis and areas of sarcomatoid change. Most sarcomatoid carcinomas are at high stage when first diagnosed: this tumor obliterated much of the native renal parenchyma and extended into perirenal fat. Despite this, the patient was alive with no evidence of cancer 1 year later (*Image courtesy of* Pedro Ciarlini, MD)

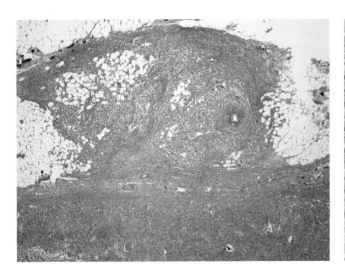

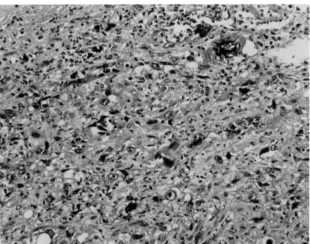

Fig. 3.49 High-grade urothelial carcinoma of renal pelvis. Histologic section from the region of grossly apparent perirenal fat invasion, confirming the presence of carcinoma in the perirenal fat (American Joint Committee on Cancer TNM stage T4)

Fig. 3.51 Sarcomatoid urothelial carcinoma of renal pelvis. Tumor is composed of cells with pleomorphic and spindled nuclei. A bizarre mitotic figure is present at upper right. Although no epithelial differentiation is apparent in this image, usually these tumors are composed of a mixture of malignant epithelial and spindle cells. The carcinoma component is most often urothelial, and less often squamous cell carcinoma, adenocarcinoma, small cell carcinoma, or mixtures of these histologic subtypes. Rarely, the carcinoma component may be represented only by carcinoma in situ

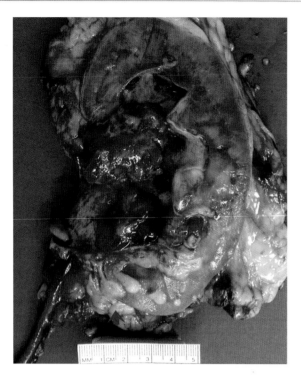

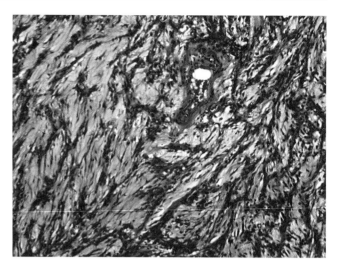

Fig. 3.54 Sarcomatoid urothelial carcinoma of renal pelvis. The tumor shown in Fig. 3.52 is composed of poorly formed fascicles of undifferentiated spindle cells set in a myxoid background. Since this component was accompanied by at least a small focus of urothelial carcinoma, the entire lesion was regarded as sarcomatoid carcinoma. Patient rapidly developed local recurrence and distant metastases and died less than 6 months after the nephroureterectomy

Fig. 3.52 Sarcomatoid urothelial carcinoma of renal pelvis. The tumor had a gelatinous appearance and although invasive into renal parenchyma and perirenal fat (*blue arrow*), it was only loosely adherent to the native renal pelvic tissue (*Image courtesy of* Amber Petrolla, MD)

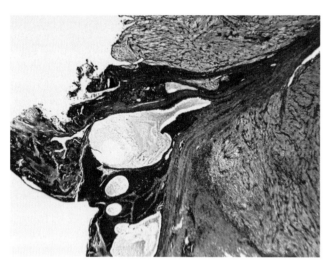

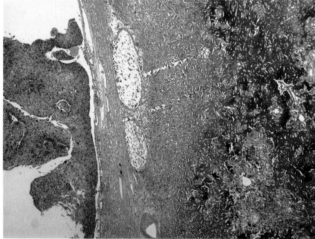

Fig. 3.53 Sarcomatoid urothelial carcinoma of renal pelvis. Section of the tumor shown in Fig. 3.52. The tumor showed only scattered foci of exophytic high-grade urothelial carcinoma; almost all of the tumor had the appearance of a myxoid sarcoma

Fig. 3.55 Sarcomatoid urothelial carcinoma of renal pelvis. In some instances, the sarcomatous component shows heterologous features, with elements recognizable as chondrosarcoma, osteosarcoma, or rhabdomyosarcoma. This patient had urothelial carcinoma with extensive squamous differentiation (*left*), as well as areas indistinguishable from osteosarcoma (*right*)

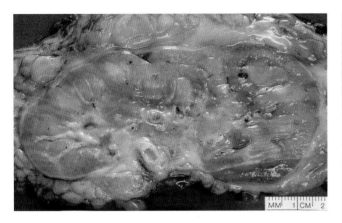

Fig. 3.56 Urothelial carcinoma of renal pelvis, post-neoadjuvant chemotherapy. This patient had high-grade urothelial carcinoma of renal pelvis, metastatic to regional lymph nodes, locally invasive into soft tissues, and clinically unresectable. Remarkably, after neoadjuvant chemotherapy, nephroureterectomy was possible, and despite extensive sampling, no tumor was found in the resected kidney, shown here. Unfortunately, the patient later showed evidence of distant metastases, and eventually died of cancer less than 2 years after surgery (*Image courtesy of* Amber Petrolla, MD)

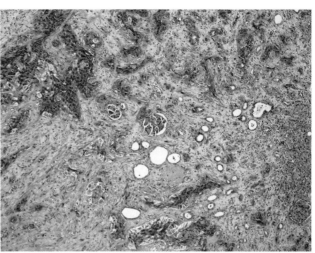

Fig. 3.58 Squamous cell carcinoma of renal pelvis. Tumor infiltrates native renal parenchyma. Whenever squamous cell carcinoma is found infiltrating renal parenchyma, the possibility of metastasis from another site, such as a lung primary, must be considered and correlated with clinical information

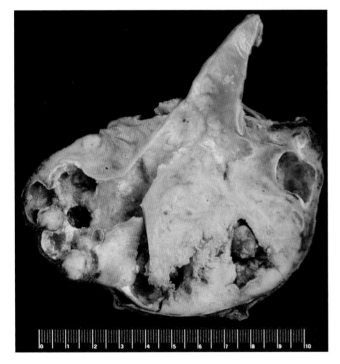

Fig. 3.57 Squamous cell carcinoma of renal pelvis. Squamous cell carcinoma accounts for 6% to 15% of cancers arising in the renal pelvis. The tumor shown here is gray-white, in keeping with abundant keratin production. High stage at the time of diagnosis is common. This tumor has obliterated almost all of the native renal parenchyma (*Image courtesy of* Rodolfo Montironi, MD)

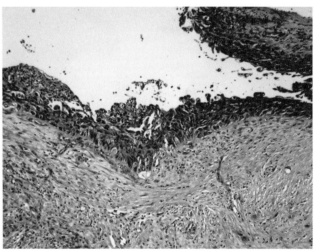

Fig. 3.59 Squamous cell carcinoma in situ of renal pelvis. This section is from a nephroureterectomy done for squamous cell carcinoma of renal pelvis. Because squamous cell carcinoma of renal pelvis is often found in a setting of urolithiasis or hydronephrosis, it is hypothesized that chronic inflammation of pelvic mucosa results in squamous metaplasia and eventually squamous malignancy; this sequence of events is difficult to validate

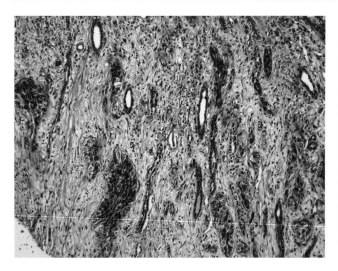

Fig. 3.60 Squamous cell carcinoma in situ of renal pelvis. In situ squamous cell carcinoma was also found in collecting ducts in the case shown in Fig. 3.59, consistent with Pagetoid spread of tumor

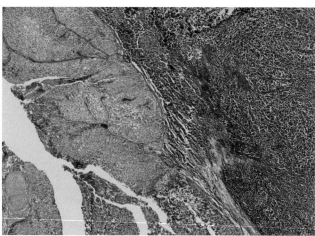

Fig. 3.62 Small cell carcinoma of ureter. There are fewer than two dozen reported cases of primary small cell carcinoma of the ureter. Some are pure small cell carcinoma; others are admixed with components of urothelial carcinoma (*left*), squamous cell carcinoma, adenocarcinoma, or sarcomatoid carcinoma.

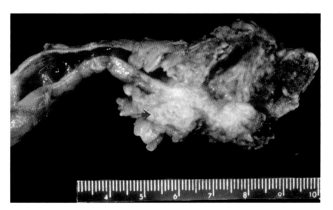

Fig. 3.61 Squamous cell carcinoma of ureter. This tumor was located in the distal ureter, at the ureterovesical junction. Extension of tumor into periureteral soft tissues is grossly evident (*arrow*)

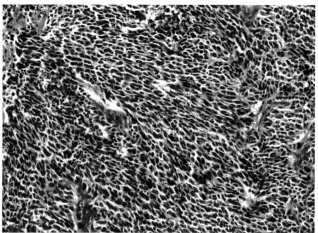

Fig. 3.63 Small cell carcinoma of ureter. As in other sites, the tumor is composed of small cells with a round to fusiform shape, nuclear molding, smoothly dispersed nuclear chromatin, inconspicuous nucleoli, scant cytoplasm, abundant mitotic activity, and abundant apoptotic cells

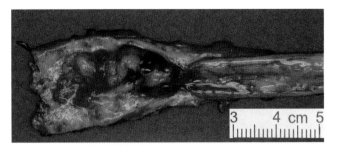

Fig. 3.64 Metastasis to ureter. Patient had previously undergone radical nephrectomy for high-grade clear cell renal cell carcinoma in the ipsilateral kidney that involved renal veins. Nine months later, gross hematuria prompted the discovery of this distal ureteral mass, which was histologically consistent with metastatic clear cell carcinoma (*Image courtesy of* Christina Bagby, MD)

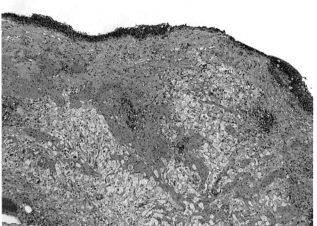

Fig. 3.66 Metastasis to ureter. Patient was a middle-aged man with a history of testicular teratoma, which was found to be recurrent 10 years later, but with an additional secondary malignancy composed of mucin-producing adenocarcinoma with a significant signet-ring cell component, which involved one ureter, as shown in this image

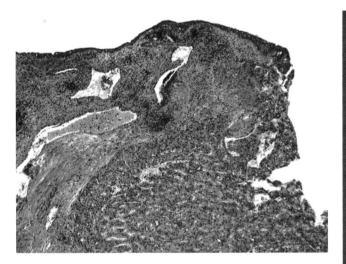

Fig. 3.65 Metastasis to renal pelvis. This patient had a renal mass lesion that impinged upon the renal pelvis. Renal pelvis was opened intraoperatively to assess for the possibility of urothelial carcinoma, which would necessitate distal ureterectomy. A spatially separate renal pelvic nodule sent for intraoperative frozen section proved to be metastatic clear cell carcinoma, occupying the lamina propria of the renal pelvis

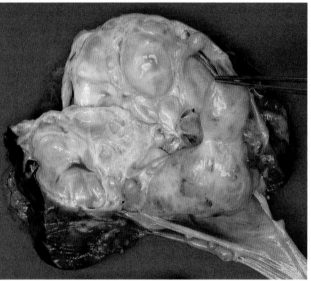

Fig. 3.67 Cystic nephroma. Not all space-occupying lesions in the renal pelvis are urothelial carcinomas. This renal mass was a cystic nephroma that had protruded into the renal pelvis (*Image courtesy of* Carmen Frias-Kletecka, MD)

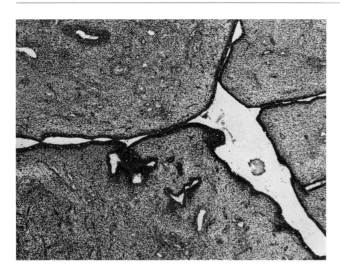

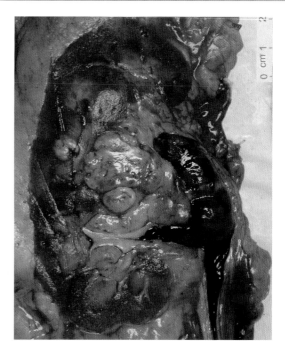

Fig. 3.68 Mixed epithelial and stromal tumor of kidney. Another example of a primary renal lesion that masqueraded as a renal pelvic mass. This was a multinodular mass protruding into the renal pelvis. It is covered by urothelium (*left*). Tumor is biphasic, consisting of variably sized glands lined by bland cuboidal epithelium, admixed with small nondescript spindled and stellate cells. Features of malignancy are absent

Fig. 3.69 Renal cell carcinoma. This is an example of a primary renal cell carcinoma, clear cell type, that protrudes extensively into the renal pelvis, similar to the lesions previously described in Figs. 3.65 and 3.67. Surgeons prefer to be assured that such lesions are not urothelial in nature; if the lesion is nonurothelial, there is no need to perform distal ureterectomy (*Image courtesy of* Khaled Sarah, MD)

The urinary bladder is a hollow muscular organ with an inner lining of lamina propria covered on its surface by urothelium three to six cell layers thick. The urinary bladder performs the physiologic functions of storage and expulsion of urine via the urethra. The bladder and urethra are the sites of an astonishing array of pathologic conditions – congenital anomalies, a host of different inflammatory conditions, a number of acquired nonneoplastic lesions, and a broad spectrum of benign and malignant neoplasms. The urachus, if it remains partially or completely patent after birth, can be the site of various pathologic conditions, as well.

4.1 Malformations, Congenital and Acquired

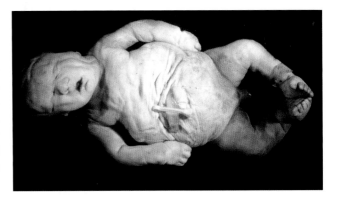

Fig. 4.2 Prune belly syndrome. Abdominal distension and prominent wrinkling of the abdominal skin are characteristic of this complex disorder, characterized by congenitally deficient abdominal musculature and urinary tract anomalies. The underlying pathophysiology is a spectrum of abnormalities, all of which have in common distension of the abdomen associated with distension of the urinary bladder

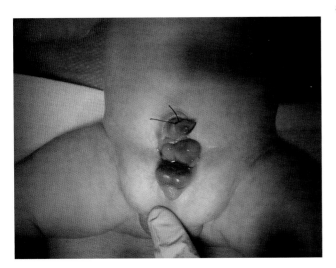

Fig. 4.1 Exstrophy of the bladder. Exstrophy is a defect in the infraumbilical portion of the anterior abdominal wall and ventral bladder wall. Posterior wall of the bladder is exposed. At the pubic level, the pubic symphysis is absent and rectus abdominis muscles are divergent. Penile deformities include epispadias and bifid glans penis (*Image courtesy of* Jonathan Ross, MD, and Katherine Hubert, MD.)

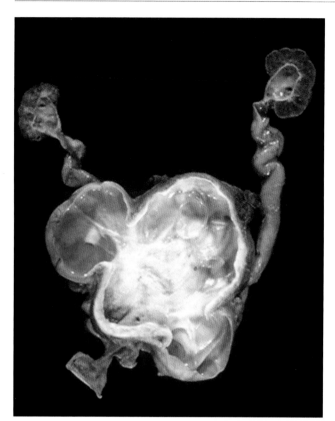

Fig. 4.3 Prune belly syndrome. In its classic form, the bladder appears distended, and there is bilateral hydroureteronephrosis. Etiology of the urinary tract distension may be multifactorial; it is unclear whether failure of bladder emptying is a mechanical or a physiologic problem. Possible mechanical obstructions include posterior urethral valves, urethral diaphragm, urethral stenosis, atresia or multiple lumina; or the bladder neck may be incompetent, forming a flaplike valve

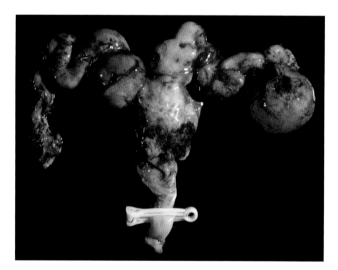

Fig. 4.4 Prune belly syndrome. The bladder is not always massively distended and thin-walled; following decompression, it may be small or normal-sized but markedly thick-walled, as in this case. Bilateral upper tract distension and renal abnormalities are readily apparent

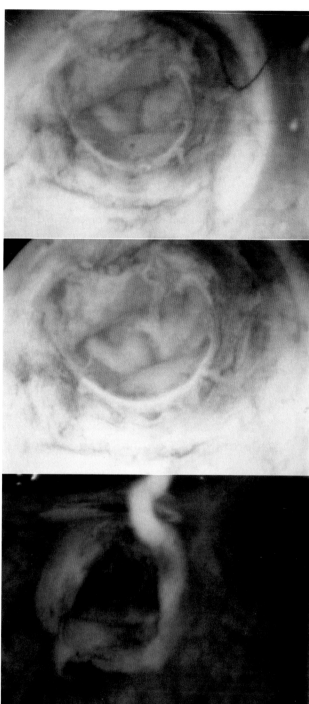

Fig. 4.5 Urachal cyst. Cysts can be found at any level of the urachus. Some are small and incidentally discovered. The largest on record contained 50 L of fluid. This urachal cyst in the bladder dome was unroofed during cystoscopy to assess microhematuria in a 45-year-old man (*Image courtesy of* Tom Leininger, MD)

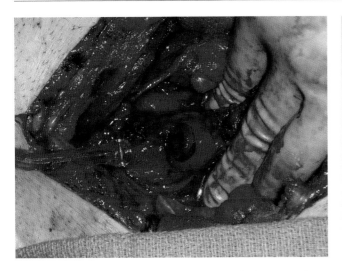

Fig. 4.6 Urachal cyst. Intraoperative photo of bladder dome cyst shown in Fig. 4.5 (*Image courtesy of* Tom Leininger, MD)

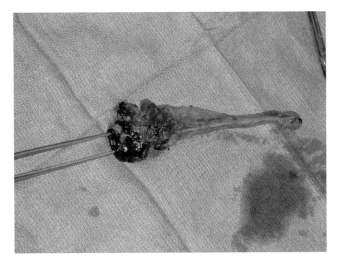

Fig. 4.7 Urachal cyst. Urachal cyst and urachal tract to the level of the umbilicus were resected (*Image courtesy of* Tom Leininger, MD)

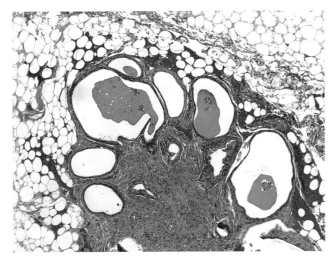

Fig. 4.8 Urachal cyst. Lesion is multilocular. Cysts are lined by flat cuboidal or columnar epithelium. No malignancy was identified

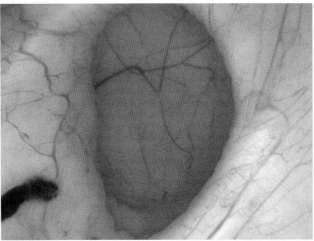

Fig. 4.9 Bladder diverticulum. This is an outpouching of bladder mucosa between the fibers of the detrusor muscle, forming a cavity outside the confines of the bladder, not lined by muscle. It is commonest in older men, and usually attributed to high voiding pressure induced by bladder outlet obstruction. Those occurring in children are attributed to localized failure of detrusor muscle development (*Image courtesy of* Allen Seftel, MD)

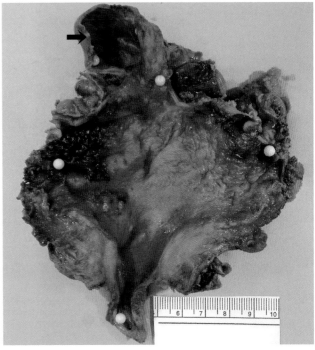

Fig. 4.10 Bladder diverticulum. *Arrow* indicates a diverticulum in this cystoprostatectomy for invasive urothelial carcinoma. The diverticulum is uninvolved by tumor

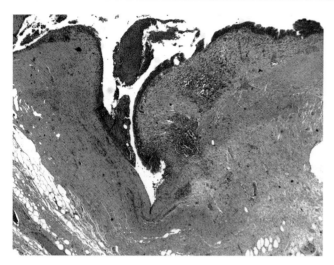

Fig. 4.11 Bladder diverticulum. At right, the intact bladder wall has a layer of muscularis propria. The lumen of the diverticulum (*left*) is separated from perivesical soft tissues only by a layer of dense fibro-connective tissue

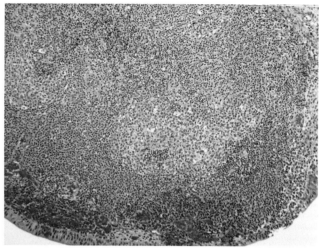

Fig. 4.13 Follicular cystitis. This lesion is seen in more than a third of patients with recurrent urinary tract infection. Endoscopically, it has the appearance of myriad small pink, white, or gray mucosal nodules. The mucosal nodules consist of lymphoid follicles, usually with germinal centers, in the lamina propria

4.2 Inflammatory Conditions

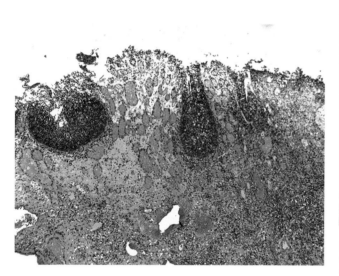

Fig. 4.12 Acute cystitis. The mucosa is thickened by edema, vascular dilatation and congestion, and infiltration of abundant acute and chronic inflammatory cells. The urothelium is partially denuded

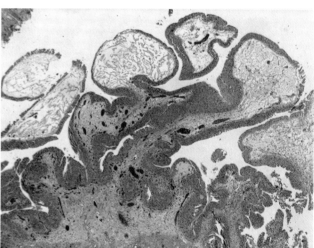

Fig. 4.14 Papillary-polypoid cystitis. This form of mucosal inflammation is characterized by thin fingerlike and/or edematous broad-based papillary projections, and is associated with indwelling catheters and vesical fistulae. The stroma in either case usually shows prominent chronic inflammation, abundant small blood vessels or healing granulation tissue, and sometimes edema fluid. The overlying urothelium may be denuded, but if present it is reactive and lacks malignant characteristics. Nonetheless, distinction of this lesion from papillary urothelial neoplasms is sometimes challenging

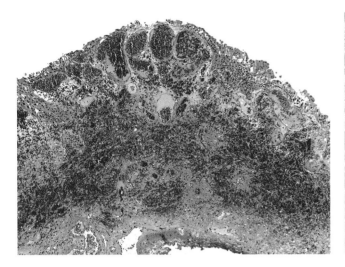

Fig. 4.15 Hemorrhagic cystitis. This condition is best known as a complication of cyclophosphamide therapy, associated with massive and sometimes intractable hematuria. Histologic findings include mucosal edema, vascular dilatation and congestion, hemorrhage in the lamina propria, and mucosal ulceration

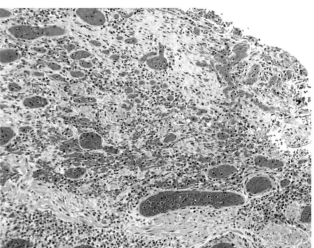

Fig. 4.17 Interstitial cystitis. Bladder biopsy shows urothelial denudation, vascular dilatation and congestion, stroma edema and hemorrhage, granulation tissue formation, and aggregates of mononuclear inflammatory cells. The findings are nonspecific. It is important to note and record that there is no evidence of transitional cell carcinoma in situ, since this is part of the clinical differential diagnosis

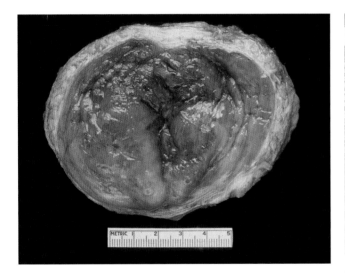

Fig. 4.16 Interstitial cystitis. The etiology and pathogenesis of this chronic idiopathic inflammatory bladder disease are unknown. The diagnosis is clinical; the pathologic findings are not pathognomonic, but help to support the clinical diagnosis and to exclude other pathologic conditions. The endpoint of this disease is a contracted, fibrotic, ulcerated bladder, as shown here, that no longer serves its intended function as a site for storage and expulsion of urine (*see* "Non-neoplastic Disorders of the Urinary Bladder" [page 229] in Bostwick and Cheng 2008. With permission)

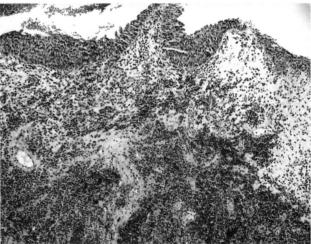

Fig. 4.18 Eosinophilic cystitis. The radiologic and endoscopic findings are often much more alarming than the pathologic findings: striking nodular and polypoid mucosal irregularities may invoke clinical concern for such entities as carcinoma or rhabdomyosarcoma. The mucosa is edematous and infiltrated by abundant eosinophils; the inflammatory infiltrate can be transmural

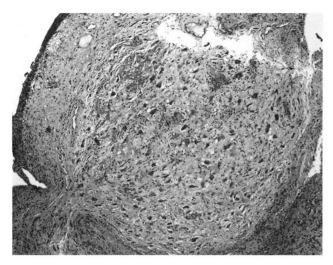

Fig. 4.19 Giant cell cystitis. The term implies the presence of numerous atypical stromal mesenchymal cells with enlarged, hyperchromatic and sometimes multiple nuclei in the lamina propria, as in this biopsy of a patient under endoscopic surveillance after previous bladder tumor resection

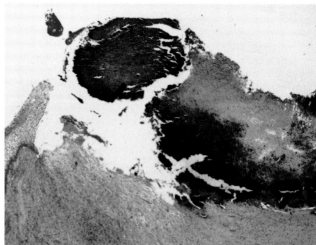

Fig. 4.21 Encrusted cystitis. This lesion occurs in a setting of infection with urea-splitting organisms that alkalinize the urea and induce deposition of inorganic salts on the mucosal surface. Calcific deposits on the surface are admixed with necrotic debris and fibrin. It is important to exclude underlying urothelial cancer, which can also undergo encrustation

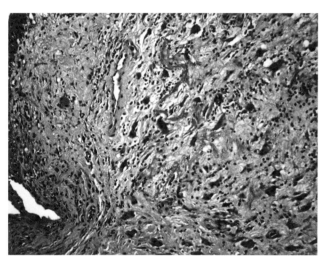

Fig. 4.20 Giant cell cystitis. The nuclei of the atypical mesenchymal cells are hyperchromatic but fairly uniform, and lack mitotic activity. The cells have bipolar or multipolar tapering eosinophilic cytoplasmic processes

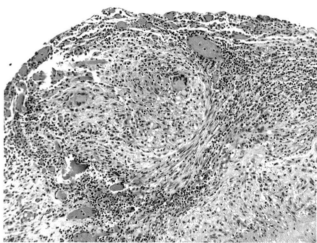

Fig. 4.22 Granulomatous cystitis related to Bacillus Calmette-Guerin (BCG) therapy. The granulomas that follow intravesical administration of BCG for treatment of carcinoma in situ are typically in the superficial lamina propria, often in a background of dense chronic inflammation. They are round or ovoid and composed of multinucleated giant cells and epithelioid histiocytes. Acid-fast stains are usually negative for organisms

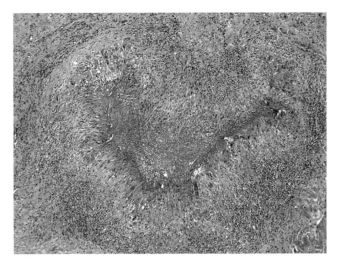

Fig. 4.23 Postsurgical necrobiotic granuloma. The use of diathermic cutting/cautery instruments during transurethral resection of bladder lesions leaves devitalized tissue that may incite formation of a necrotizing palisading granuloma as shown here. The granulomas have undulating outlines. Central amorphous necrotic material is surrounded by radially arranged (palisading) histiocytes, often accompanied by their epithelioid and multinucleated counterparts

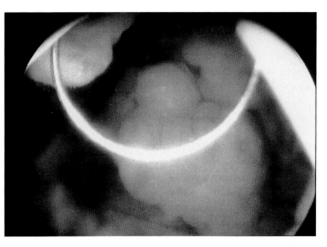

Fig. 4.25 Malakoplakia. This granulomatous condition forms soft raised nodules or plaques in the bladder mucosa that may simulate neoplasia, as shown in this endoscopic image from the bladder of a woman with a long history of recurrent urinary infection, and recent hematuria (*see* MacLennan GT, Resnick MI, Bostwick DG, 2003. With permission)

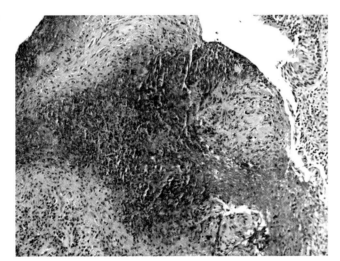

Fig. 4.24 Wegener's granulomatosis involving bladder. Bladder biopsy shows necrotizing granulomas, and in itself is nondiagnostic. Patient had similar lesions in the vagina. The diagnosis ultimately was based upon a constellation of other pathological and clinical findings

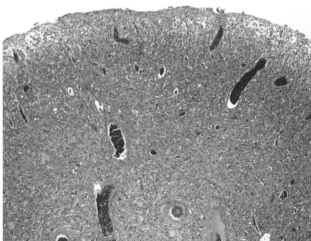

Fig. 4.26 Malakoplakia. Lamina propria is diffusely infiltrated by von Hansemann histiocytes – macrophages with abundant granular cytoplasm. Urothelium is extensively denuded

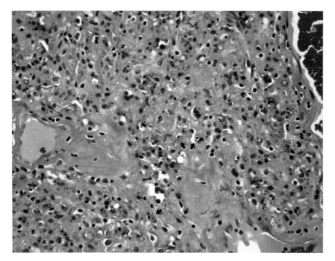

Fig. 4.27 Malakoplakia. The plaques represent mucosa that is expanded by the presence of histiocytes with a lysosomal dysfunction: ingested bacteria do not undergo the usual sequence of breakdown and lysosomal expulsion. The intracellular and extracellular target-like structures (Michaelis-Gutman bodies; *arrows*) are formed by deposition of calcium and iron phosphate on undigested bacterial components

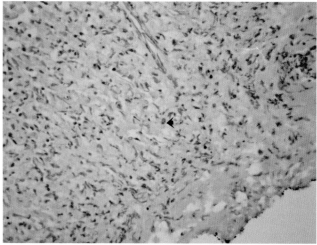

Fig. 4.29 Malakoplakia. Michaelis-Gutman bodies (*arrow*) are highlighted by Prussian blue stain for iron

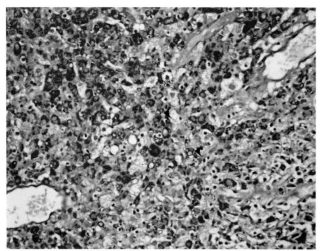

Fig. 4.28 Malakoplakia. Michaelis-Gutman bodies (*arrow*) and von Hansemann histiocytes are highlighted by periodic acid-Schiff stain

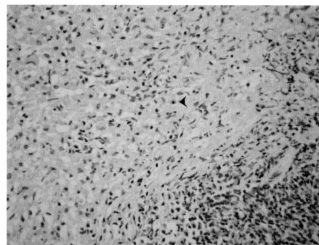

Fig. 4.30 Malakoplakia. Michaelis-Gutman bodies (*arrow*) are highlighted by von Kossa stain for calcium

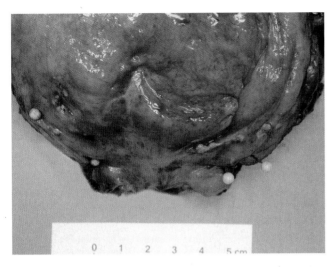

Fig. 4.31 Xanthoma. Patient had undergone transurethral resection of high-grade bladder cancers and had neo adjuvant chemotherapy prior to cystectomy. Fresh cystectomy specimen shows multiple golden-yellow submucosal nodules that appear to be in an area of prior transurethral surgery (*Image courtesy of* Zhanna Georgievskaya)

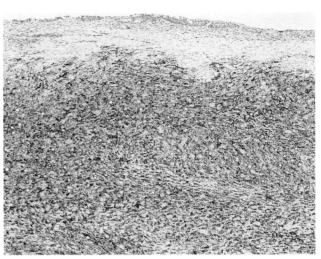

Fig. 4.33 Xanthoma. Immunostain of the section shown in Fig. 4.32. The pale cells in the lamina propria show strong diffuse immunoreactivity to antibodies against CD68, confirming that they are macrophages

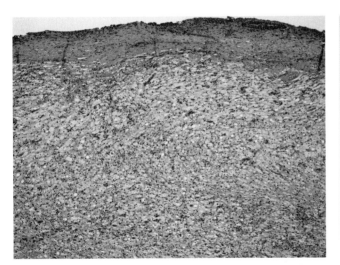

Fig. 4.32 Xanthoma. Sections from the golden-yellow nodules shown in Fig. 4.31 show sheets of foamy macrophages in the lamina propria. Despite extensive sampling, no residual in situ or invasive carcinoma was found in the specimen

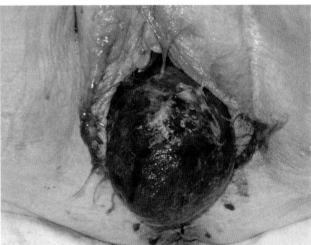

Fig. 4.34 Gangrene of bladder. Bladder gangrene may complicate debilitating illnesses such as diabetes or carcinomatosis, or compromised circulation, as in this patient who presented with bladder eversion; the bladder appears ischemic. The bladder was resituated and recovered its vascularity without additional untoward effects (*Image courtesy of* Carmin Kalorin, MD, and Elise J.B. De, MD)

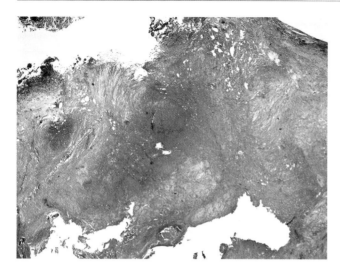

Fig. 4.35 Gangrene of bladder. This is an image from the cystectomy specimen of a man who was treated for prostate cancer with radiation therapy and developed bladder complications. The bladder wall shows evidence of extensive ischemic necrosis, presumably related to vascular injury induced by ionizing radiation

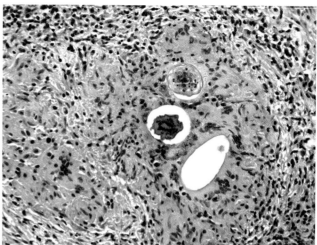

Fig. 4.37 Schistosomiasis. Adult worms of *Schistosoma haematobium* lay clusters of eggs in the venules of the lamina propria. The ova incite granuloma formation; abundant eosinophils are also present. Fibrotic reactions in the bladder and ureters can result in disabling obstructive processes, and patients are predisposed to squamous and urothelial carcinoma and adenocarcinoma

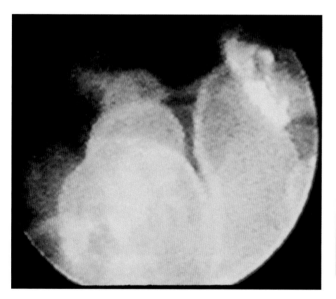

Fig. 4.36 Schistosomiasis. Various cystoscopic appearances are described: small grayish nodules, patches of granular rough mucosa ("sandy patches"), mucosal ulcers, or polyps, ranging from 2 to 20 mm in size, as shown here. The polyps consist of eggs and the surrounding tissue reaction (*see* MacLennan GT, Resnick MI, Bostwick DG, 2003. With permission)

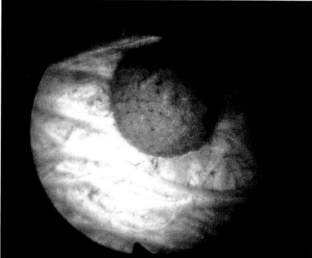

Fig. 4.38 Bladder calculus. Bladder calculi most commonly afflict men with chronic bladder outlet obstruction, and malnourished children in Asia and the Middle East. Most bladder calculi are free-floating, as shown in this cystoscopic image

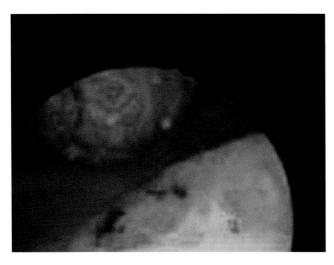

Fig. 4.39 Foreign body in bladder. This is a cystoscopic view of a surgical sponge inadvertently left in the bladder at the time of a mesh-enhanced cystocele repair (*Image courtesy of* Howard Goldman, MD)

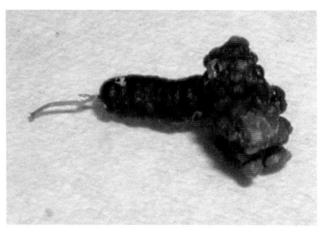

Fig. 4.41 Foreign body. The lesion shown in Fig. 4.40 was a nonabsorbable suture, errantly placed during a previous surgical procedure; calculus material had built up on the suture (*Image courtesy of* Howard Goldman, MD)

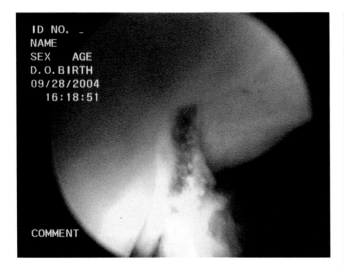

Fig. 4.40 Foreign body with calculus. Infrequently, calculi develop on foreign bodies, such as indwelling ureteral pig-tail stents, or on nonabsorbable sutures placed inadvertently through the bladder wall during pelvic surgery. This cystoscopic image shows a blue lesion dangling from the bladder dome (*Image courtesy of* Howard Goldman, MD)

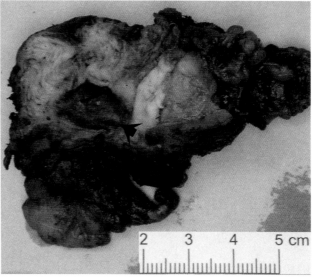

Fig. 4.42 Perivesical abscess. Common sources of perivesical abscess include urachal malformation with abscess formation and colonic diverticulitis. In the case shown here, the patient had diverticulosis and diverticulitis of the sigmoid colon, with colonic stricturing. At surgery to excise the colon segment, a mass was noted that was densely adherent to the bladder wall. Partial cystectomy was performed, with removal of the mass, which proved to be a perivesical abscess cavity, indicated by the *arrow*

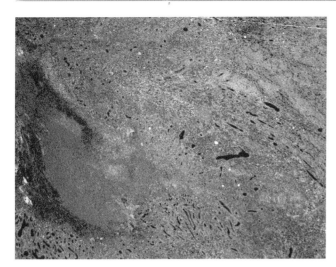

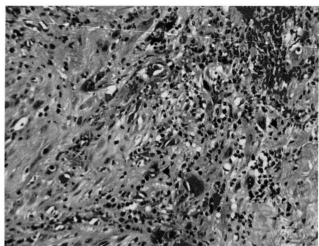

Fig. 4.43 Perivesical abscess. Section from the case shown in Fig. 4.42. An abscess is at lower left, surrounded by granulation tissue. A portion of bladder wall is at upper right

Fig. 4.45 Radiation cystitis. In the chronic phase, bladder exhibits urothelial denudation, ulceration, stromal hemorrhage and edema, fibrin deposition in stroma and blood vessels, acute and chronic inflammation, sometimes with prominent eosinophilia, and fibrosis. It is common to see atypical stromal cells with bizarre-appearing hyperchromatic smudged nuclei (*arrows*)

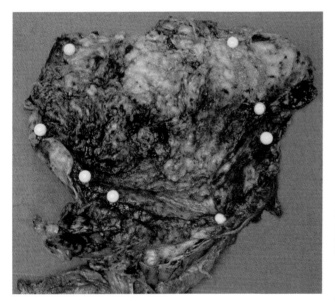

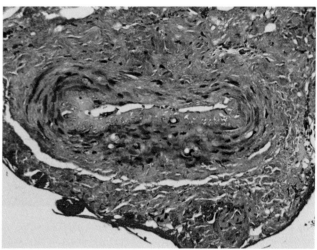

Fig. 4.46 Radiation cystitis. In the chronic phase, blood vessels may show accelerated atherosclerotic changes, characterized by myointimal thickening as well as vacuolated smooth muscle and endothelial cells

Fig. 4.44 Radiation cystitis. Incidental exposure of the bladder to radiation during therapy directed at cancer in other pelvic organs may result in bladder complications, ultimately stemming from vascular damage related to endothelial cell injury. This bladder shows mucosal edema, hemorrhage, and extensive ulceration. It was contracted and essentially nonfunctional several years after radiation therapy for prostate cancer

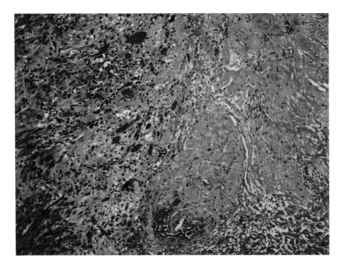

Fig. 4.47 Radiation cystitis. In the chronic phase, as vascular injury advances, mural necrosis may supervene, as shown here; as this heals by fibrosis, the bladder becomes contracted, and ultimately may no longer serve as a site for storage and expulsion of urine

4.3 Acquired Nonneoplastic Lesions

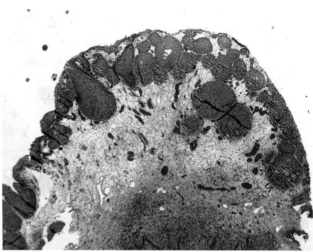

Fig. 4.49 von Brunn's nests. These are regarded as normal histologic findings in the urothelium; they consist of well-circumscribed nests of urothelial cells in the lamina propria, which represent invaginations of overlying urothelium or in some instances downward migration of urothelial cells. They may or may not be attached to overlying urothelium

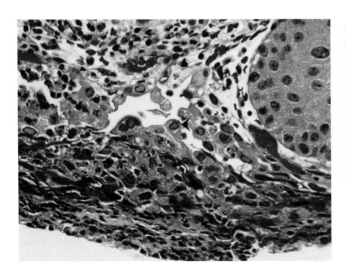

Fig. 4.48 Herpes cystitis. Biopsy from the trigone region of a 78-year-old female patient with hematuria and irritative voiding symptoms. The typical intranuclear viral inclusions are present (*arrow*). Other viruses that may infect the bladder include human papillomavirus (*see* Figs. 4.266 and 4.267), adenovirus, papovavirus, and cytomegalovirus

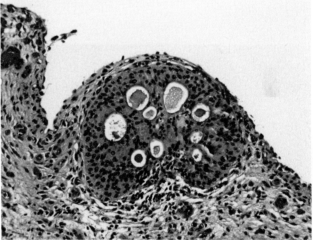

Fig. 4.50 Cystitis cystica. This is the term used to describe the presence of central cystic spaces within von Brunn's nests. The cystic spaces may be up to 5 mm; they have the appearance of submucosal cysts endoscopically, and contain clear yellow fluid. Histologically, the cystic spaces are lined by urothelium or flat cuboidal epithelium, and contain acidophilic fluid

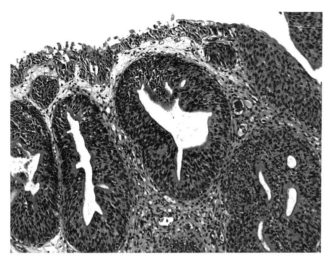

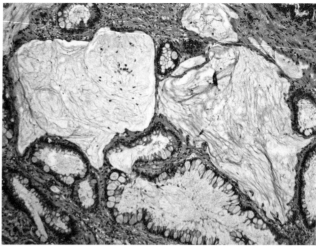

Fig. 4.51 Cystitis glandularis of the typical type. The luminal spaces within von Brunn's nests are lined centrally by columnar cells supported by one or more layers of urothelial cells. There is little or no mucin production, and goblet cells are absent. This finding is so common that it is considered normal histology

Fig. 4.53 Cystitis glandularis of the intestinal type (CGIT). In the luminal spaces of CGIT, the lining epithelium resembles intestinal epithelium, and consists of mucin-producing tall columnar epithelial cells, including occasional goblet cells, not surrounded by transitional cells as in most cases of typical cystitis glandularis. The degree of mucin production is variable, and mucin is occasionally extravasated into the stroma. CGIT differs from mucin-producing adenocarcinoma by lacking cytologic atypia of the epithelium lining luminal spaces, lacking cytologically atypical cells floating in pools of mucin, and by having a generally orderly distribution of glands that are usually, but not always, confined to the lamina propria

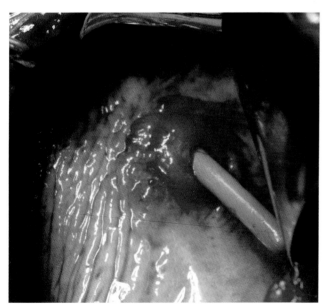

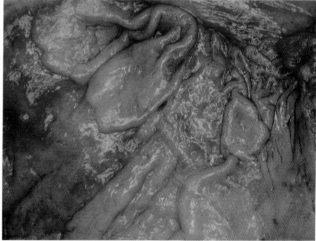

Fig. 4.54 Squamous metaplasia, nonkeratinizing. Areas of metaplasia are more pale than adjacent normal mucosa; the demarcation between normal and metaplastic epithelium may be indistinct or quite sharp, as in this case

Fig. 4.52 Cystitis glandularis of the intestinal type. This lesion most often occurs in a setting of chronic bladder inflammation: bladder exstrophy, chronically infected neurogenic bladder, and bladders chronically irritated by stones or an indwelling catheter. It takes the form of focally or diffusely inflamed edematous or polypoid bladder mucosa, as in this case. It may coexist with the typical type, or may be the dominant finding, in which case it is termed intestinal metaplasia (*see* Figler et al. 2006. With permission)

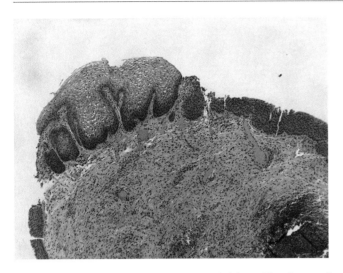

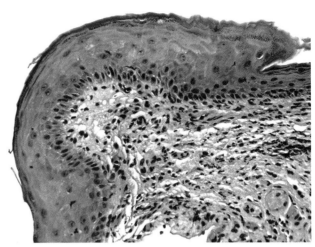

Fig. 4.55 Squamous metaplasia, nonkeratinizing. The layer of squamous epithelium at upper left is considerably thicker than the adjacent normal urothelium, accounting for its bulky gross appearance. The squamous epithelium lacks cytologic atypia

Fig. 4.57 Squamous metaplasia, keratinizing. This bladder mucosa is lined by squamous epithelium showing parakeratosis and a layer of keratin on the surface. The keratin imparts a white color to the gross appearance of the mucosa. No significant cytologic atypia is seen here, but keratinizing squamous metaplasia is regarded as a risk factor for squamous cell carcinoma of the bladder

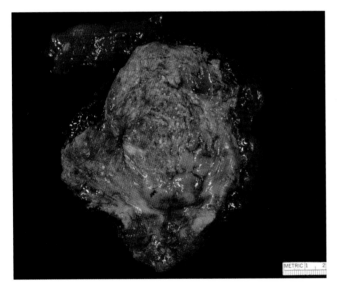

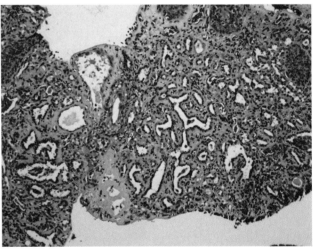

Fig. 4.56 Squamous metaplasia, keratinizing. The mucosal surface is thickened and leathery and shows extensive areas of gray or white discoloration (see MacLennan GT, Resnick MI, Bostwick DG, 2003. With permission)

Fig. 4.58 Nephrogenic metaplasia. This lesion very often arises in a setting of prior urologic surgery, calculous disease, trauma, or recent cystitis. Endoscopically, it may appear papillary, sessile, or polypoid. It is a proliferative lesion that can take a variety of architectural growth patterns: tubular, cystic, polypoid, papillary, or diffuse/solid. In this example, the outline is that of a polyp; within the polyp are numerous tubular structures of variable shape and size

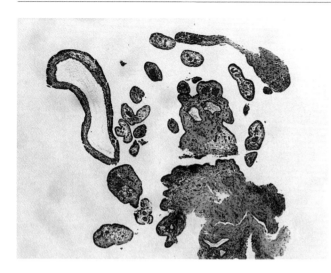

Fig. 4.59 Nephrogenic metaplasia. In this case, the metaplastic process forms predominantly papillary structures that may raise concern for papillary urothelial neoplasms. The papillary structures of nephrogenic adenoma are lined by a single layer of cuboidal or low columnar cells, in contrast to the multiple cell layers that line the papillary fronds of papillary urothelial neoplasms

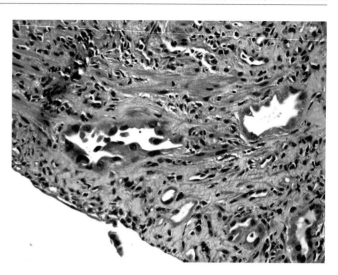

Fig. 4.61 Nephrogenic metaplasia. Cells lining the luminal structure can show mild cytologic atypia, consistent with a reactive/reparative process. The epithelium may focally have a hobnail appearance, which may raise concern for clear cell adenocarcinoma. Mitotic figures are absent or rare

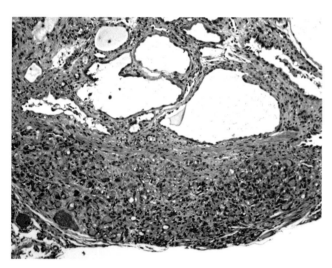

Fig. 4.60 Nephrogenic metaplasia. The architecture is a mixture of microcysts, very small tubules, and solid clusters of cells. The irregularly distributed very small tubules containing mucin can raise concern for adenocarcinoma

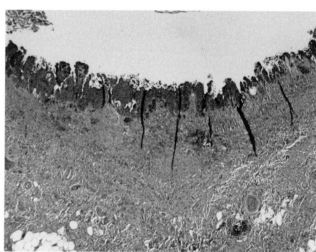

Fig. 4.62 Papillary urothelial hyperplasia. This is considered a nonspecific reactive urothelial response to an inflammatory or neoplastic process. Typically, it is not appreciable as a papillary lesion by endoscopic or gross inspection. The urothelium in this image was in a bladder diverticulum, in a male with longstanding bladder outlet obstruction. At low power, it appears as a diffuse nonspecific thickening of the urothelium

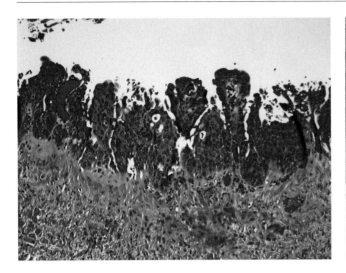

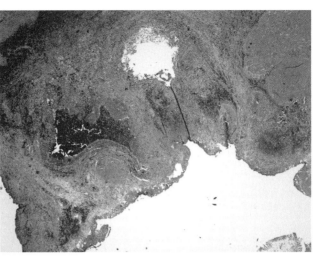

Fig. 4.63 Papillary urothelial hyperplasia. Higher power view of the urothelium in Fig. 4.62. The urothelium is thickened and shows cytologic atypia consistent with a reactive/reparative process. Focally, small fibrovascular cores are present, lined by the same thickened reactive epithelium

Fig. 4.65 Endometriosis of bladder. At low power, blood-filled endometrial glands with collars of stroma are randomly distributed between bundles of detrusor muscle. Lesions of endometriosis may involve any level of the bladder wall – serosa, muscle, or mucosa

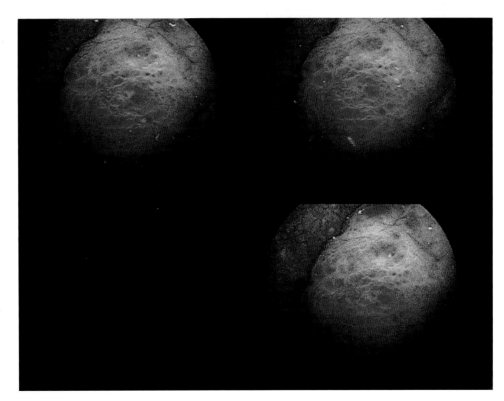

Fig. 4.64 Endometriosis of bladder. About 1% of women with endometriosis have involvement of the urinary bladder. This patient complained of voiding pain of long duration; cystoscopy showed this congested vascular mucosal nodule, which was resected endoscopically (*Image courtesy of* Donald Bodner, MD)

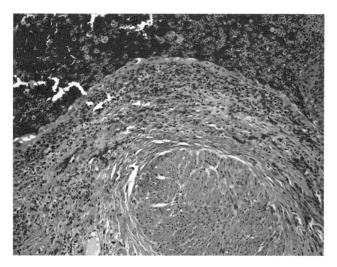

Fig. 4.66 Endometriosis of bladder. Blood-filled spaces, lined by endometrial glandular epithelium overlying endometrial stroma, adjacent to a detrusor muscle bundle

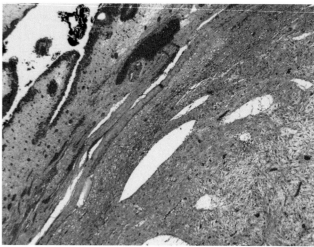

Fig. 4.68 Endometriosis of bladder, decidualized. The lesion was a circumscribed nodule in the lamina propria with features suggestive of decidual changes associated with pregnancy

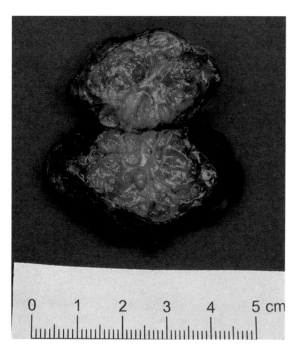

Fig. 4.67 Endometriosis of bladder, decidualized. Patient was noted to have a nodule on the dome of the bladder at the time of Caesarian section. Bladder was opened and a mucosal nodule, shown here, was shelled out, leaving the bladder essentially intact

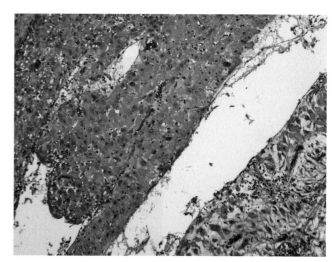

Fig. 4.69 Endometriosis of bladder, decidualized. Lesion consisted of prominently decidualized cells; findings were felt to fit best with vesical endometriosis, decidualized during pregnancy

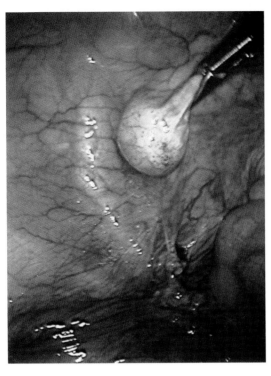

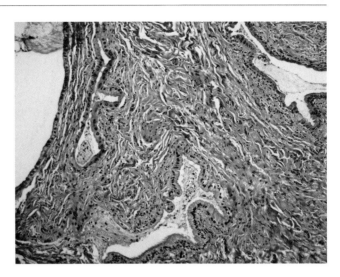

Fig. 4.72 Endocervicosis of bladder. On closer inspection, the glands are lined by a single layer of columnar cells with abundant pale cytoplasm. The glandular epithelium lacks cytologic atypia and mitotic activity. Most glands contain a modest amount of pale blue wispy mucin. The histologic features of the glands are entirely comparable to those seen in normal endocervix

Fig. 4.70 Endocervicosis of bladder. During laparoscopy to assess pelvic pain, this nodular lesion in the bladder dome was identified and resected (*Image courtesy of* Raymond Onders, MD)

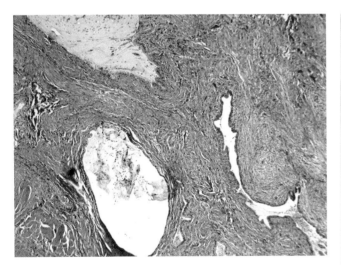

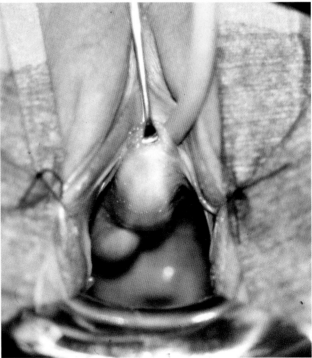

Fig. 4.71 Endocervicosis of bladder. At low power, irregular glands, some containing abundant mucin, are randomly intermingled with detrusor muscle fibers

Fig. 4.73 Suburethral Müllerian lesion. This lesion beneath the urethra, in the anterior vaginal wall, was initially thought to be a suburethral diverticulum. At surgery, it separated readily from the vaginal mucosa and the urethral wall (*Image courtesy of* Howard Goldman, MD)

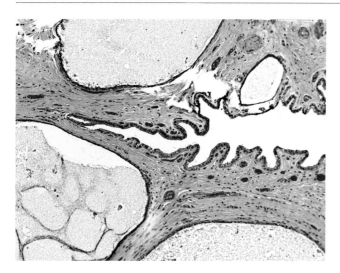

Fig. 4.74 Suburethral müllerian lesion. The lesion was composed of cystic spaces, some lined by endocervical-type epithelium and resembling endocervicosis, and some lined by tubal-type epithelium and resembling endosalpingiosis. Lesions composed of mixtures of more than one type of müllerian epithelium are appropriately designated as examples of Müllerianosis

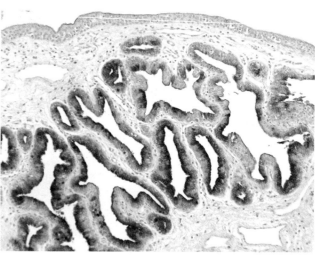

Fig. 4.76 Ectopic prostate tissue in the bladder. Confirmation that the lesion is prostatic tissue can be accomplished using appropriate immunostains; the epithelium of the glands shown here exhibits positive immunostaining for prostate-specific antigen

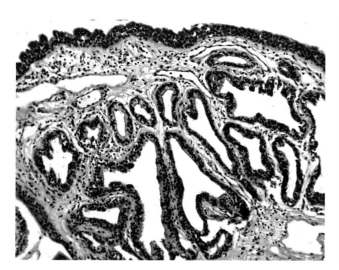

Fig. 4.75 Ectopic prostate tissue in the bladder. Prostatic-type polyps are routinely encountered in the prostatic urethra during endoscopic procedures. Infrequently, prostate tissue is found in ectopic sites, most often the bladder trigone, and less often in the lateral wall of the bladder, forming nodular, sessile, papillary or polypoid masses composed of normal prostatic glands lying beneath normal urothelium or prostatic-type epithelium

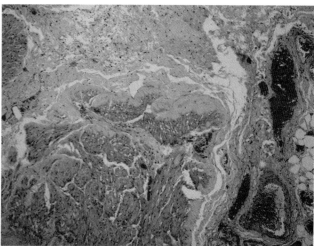

Fig. 4.77 Amyloidosis of bladder. Amyloidosis sometimes forms a tumor in the bladder, without evidence of amyloidosis elsewhere, and without evidence of a systemic disease associated with amyloidosis. At cystoscopy, sessile, polypoid, or nodular lesions, often ulcerated, are found. Histologically, amyloid deposition is present in the lamina propria and the muscularis propria. The blood vessels (*right*) appear normal

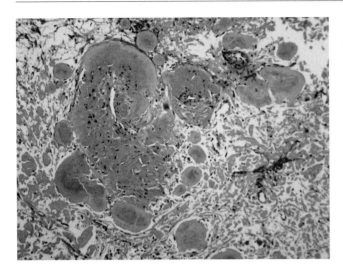

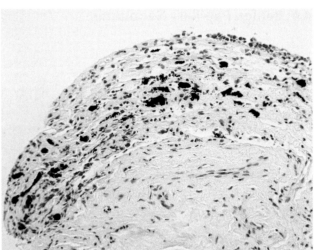

Fig. 4.78 Amyloidosis of bladder. Bladder amyloidosis in a setting of systemic diseases is less common than the occurrence of sporadic bladder amyloidosis (*see* Fig. 4.77), but may cause more pronounced hematuria. This type of amyloidosis is less likely to form a tumoral mass; it manifests as erythema or ulcerated petechiae. The amyloid deposition, shown here, mainly involves the blood vessels with less pronounced deposition in the lamina propria (*see* MacLennan GT, Resnick MI, Bostwick DG, 2003. With permission)

Fig. 4.80 Melanosis of bladder. Fontana-Masson stain highlights the presence of abundant dark granules in the lamina propria

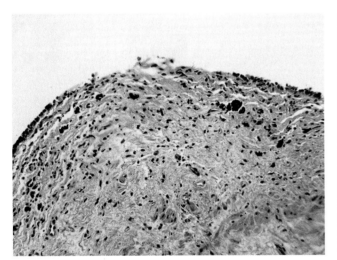

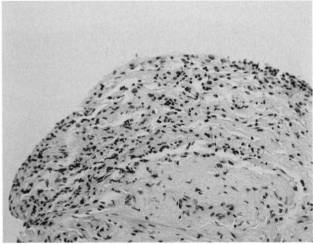

Fig. 4.79 Melanosis of bladder. Melanosis is a descriptive term for dark brown or brown-black tissue pigmentation due to melanin deposition. Fewer than a dozen cases are reported to involve the bladder. Cystoscopy may show multiple widespread areas of black or dark brown mucosal discoloration, without any particular site predilection. Microscopically, aggregates of black or dark brown granules are present in the lamina propria and sometimes also in urothelial cells

Fig. 4.81 Melanosis of bladder. After exposure to bleach, the black-staining melanin granules highlighted by Fontana-Mason stain in Fig. 4.80 have been eradicated, supporting the premise that the granules were melanin, and consistent with the diagnosis of melanosis. This case was quite unusual in that the patient subsequently developed relentlessly recurrent urothelial carcinoma and eventually required cystectomy

4.4 Benign Papillary Neoplasms

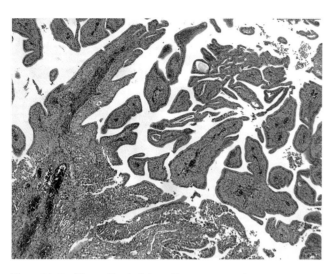

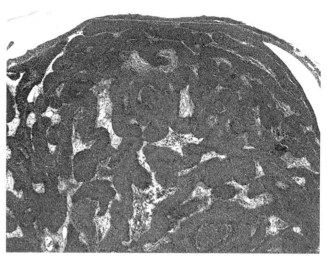

Fig. 4.82 Papilloma. Urothelial papilloma accounts for less than 1% of papillary urothelial neoplasms. It is composed of delicate fibrovascular cores lined by cytologically and architecturally normal urothelium with no more than seven layers of cells. Secondary budding of small fronds from larger simple primary papillary fronds is often noted

Fig. 4.84 Inverted papilloma. The growth pattern of inverted papilloma, rather than exophytic, is inverted, and composed of anastomosing islands and trabeculae of histologically and cytologically normal urothelial cells invaginating from the surface urothelium into the underlying lamina propria but not into the muscularis propria. An intact surface layer of normal urothelium covers most of the lesion

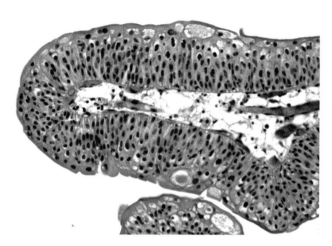

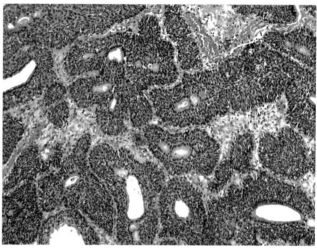

Fig. 4.83 Papilloma. The superficial cells are often prominent and may exhibit cytoplasmic vacuolization, mucinous metaplasia, eosinophilic syncytial morphology, or apocrine-like morphology. Mitotic figures are absent or rare, and restricted to the basal layer if present. The stroma may be edematous, and in some cases inflammatory cells, including foamy macrophages, may be present. Rarely, dilated lymphatics are present in the fibrovascular cores

Fig. 4.85 Inverted papilloma. The invaginating cords and trabeculae of urothelial cells demonstrate mature urothelium centrally, with darker and palisading basal cells peripherally, usually surrounded by fibrotic stroma without marked inflammation

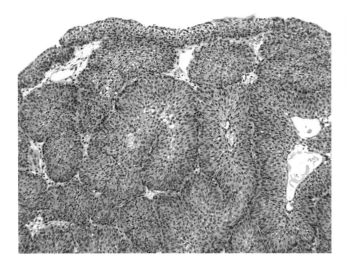

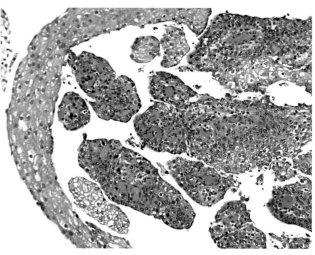

Fig. 4.86 Inverted papilloma. Inverted papilloma usually exhibits orderly central maturation of the cells comprising the invaginated trabeculae and cords. Mitotic figures, if found, are rare. Permissible findings include vacuolization and foamy xanthomatous cytoplasmic changes, focal nonkeratinizing squamous metaplasia and neuroendocrine differentiation, and focal minor cytologic atypia that is likely degenerative in nature and has no clinical significance. Findings incompatible with a diagnosis of inverted papilloma, and more in keeping with a diagnosis of inverted urothelial carcinoma include the presence of an exophytic papillary component, unequivocal tumor invasion in the lamina propria or muscularis propria, and markedly atypical cytologic findings such as nuclear pleomorphism, nucleolar prominence, and abundant mitotic activity

Fig. 4.88 Squamous papilloma. The lining squamous cells are cytologically bland, with normal maturation patterns; they lack mitotic activity or koilocytic features

4.5 Flat Intraepithelial Lesions

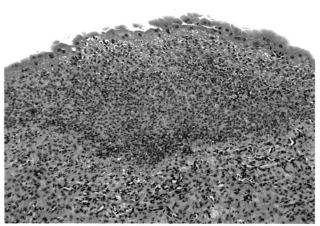

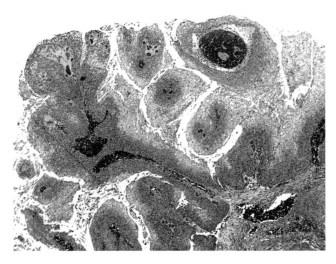

Fig. 4.87 Squamous papilloma. Squamous papilloma is a rare benign neoplasm, most often identified in elderly women and unrelated to human papillomavirus infection, possibly representing the squamous counterpart of urothelial papilloma. It is a papillary proliferation, composed of fibrovascular cores lined by multiple layers of squamous cells that show maturation from base to surface

Fig. 4.89 Flat urothelial hyperplasia (simple hyperplasia). Normal urothelium is multilayered and composed of usually less than seven cell layers, including basal, intermediate, and superficial cells. Urothelial hyperplasia is characterized by mucosal thickening and an increased number of cell layers, usually ten or more. The urothelial cells exhibit maturation from base to surface, and apart from focal slight nuclear enlargement, they show no significant cytologic abnormalities

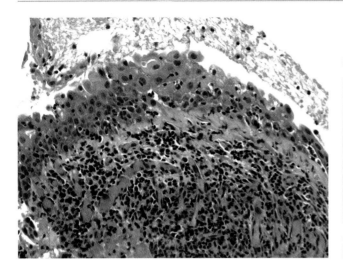

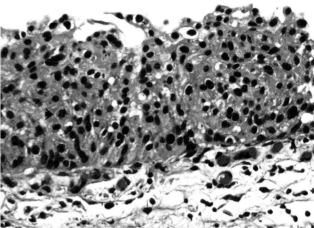

Fig. 4.90 Reactive urothelial atypia. The term *atypia* is used to denote architectural and cytologic changes in urothelium that are of lesser degree than those of dysplasia. It is a nonspecific term, and there is considerable intra- and interobserver variation in its diagnostic application. In reactive atypia, there are mild nuclear abnormalities occurring in acutely or chronically inflamed urothelium, often in a clinical setting of prior cystitis, instrumentation, infection, stones, or therapy. In all cases, inflammatory cells occupy the lamina propria and infiltrate into the urothelium, which may or may not be thickened. The urothelial cells are often larger and have more cytoplasm than normal urothelial cells, and may assume a squamoid appearance

Fig. 4.92 Urothelial dysplasia. This diagnosis is applicable when the urothelium shows significant cytological and architectural changes that cannot be attributed to inflammation or a reparative process, and yet lacks the full complement of cytologic abnormalities that characterize carcinoma in situ. Dysplasia, an example of which is shown here, is characterized by cellular crowding, loss of orderly maturation, and loss of cellular polarity, usually most conspicuous in the basal and intermediate cell layers. Mitotic figures (*arrow*) are usually but not always restricted to the lower to middle thirds. In some cases, there may be an increased number of cell layers; superficial umbrella cells can usually be found

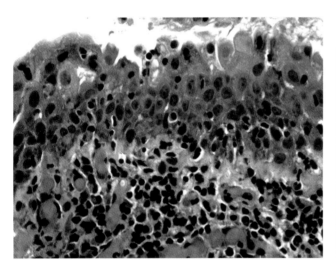

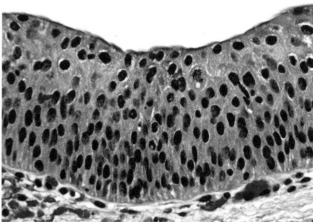

Fig. 4.91 Reactive urothelial atypia. Nuclei are vesicular, enlarged but fairly uniform in size, and often possess prominent, usually centrally located nucleoli. Mitotic figures, although often present, are confined to the basal epithelial layers

Fig. 4.93 Urothelial dysplasia. In this image, a mitotic figure is high in the urothelium; however, there is relatively good preservation of cellular polarity, and relatively good uniformity in nuclear shape and size. There are no features to suggest a reactive/reparative process. Because the urothelium lacks the full complement of features of carcinoma in situ, a diagnosis of dysplasia is reasonable

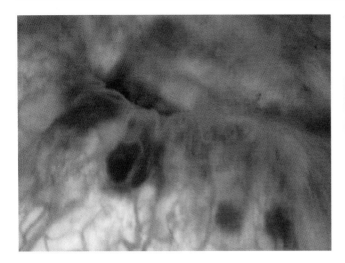

Fig. 4.94 Carcinoma in situ. Urothelial carcinoma in situ is a flat noninvasive urothelial neoplasm characterized by severe cytologic atypia. Endoscopically, as shown here, it may appear velvety, granular, or erythematous, or it may be visually undetectable (*Image courtesy of* Allen Seftel, MD)

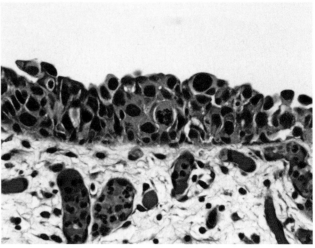

Fig. 4.96 Carcinoma in situ. There is disordered proliferation of malignant urothelial cells that demonstrate a high nuclear to cytoplasmic ratio, nuclear pleomorphism, irregular nuclear contours, and hyperchromatic or coarsely granular chromatin. Cellular polarity is lost. Vascular proliferation is often evident in the underlying stroma. Nucleoli may large, prominent, and multiple in at least some cells. Mitotic figures, which are often atypical, may be seen at any level. The diagnosis of urothelial carcinoma in situ does not require full-thickness involvement; the superficial umbrella cell layer may be intact

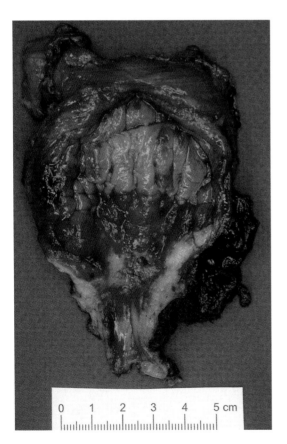

Fig. 4.95 Carcinoma in situ. Grossly, no exophytic lesion is seen. The areas of mucosal erythema is this cystectomy specimen showed extensive carcinoma in situ histologically. No invasive carcinoma was found in this specimen

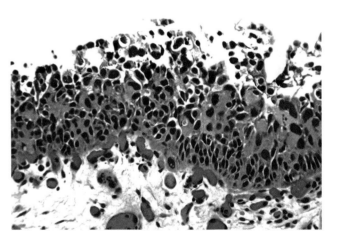

Fig. 4.97 Carcinoma in situ, large cell type. This is the commonest morphologic form of this entity. Cell nuclei are large, with nuclear pleomorphism, variably abundant cytoplasm, and anaplastic nuclear features. Note the complete loss of polarity and the stromal vascularity

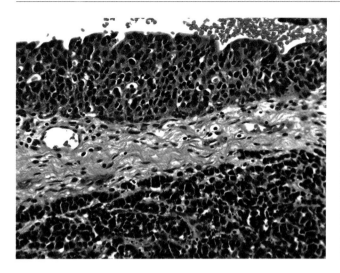

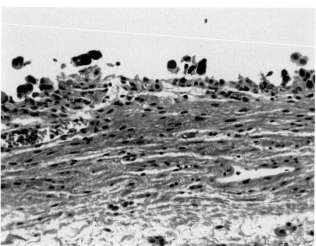

Fig. 4.98 Carcinoma in situ, small cell type. The term *small cell* in this instance refers to the size of the malignant cells, and does not imply neuroendocrine differentiation. The carcinoma cells show only modest pleomorphism; they have relatively little cytoplasm. Their nuclei are hyperchromatic, with coarse unevenly distributed chromatin; a few have prominent nucleoli. Although small cell carcinoma is present in the lamina propria in this example, associated invasive carcinomas may or may not exhibit neuroendocrine differentiation

Fig. 4.100 Carcinoma in situ, denuding type. The degree of dyscohesion and exfoliation may be of such an extent that biopsies show only a few residual carcinoma cells on the surface, or sometimes none. In some cases, the surface epithelium is entirely denuded and the only clue to the condition is the presence of carcinoma in situ in von Brunn's nests (*see* Fig. 4.94)

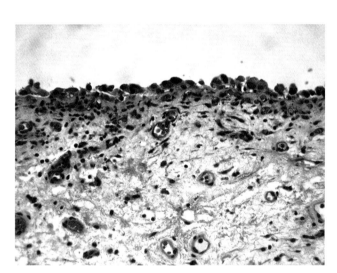

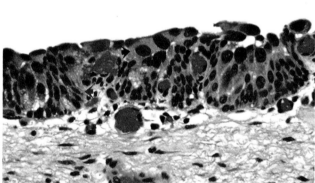

Fig. 4.99 Carcinoma in situ, clinging type. Cells comprising carcinoma in situ commonly exhibit striking loss of cohesiveness, and exfoliate readily, with the result that biopsies may show only a few residual carcinoma cells forming a patchy single cell layer on the surface, as shown here

Fig. 4.101 Carcinoma in situ with pagetoid spread. This condition, also denoted cancerization of the urothelium, can be found in up to 15% of cases of urothelial carcinoma in situ. It is characterized by the presence of carcinoma cells (*black arrow*), singly or in small clusters, subtly infiltrating otherwise normal urothelium (*blue arrow*)

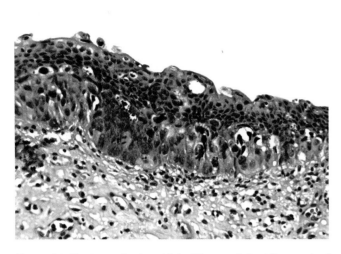

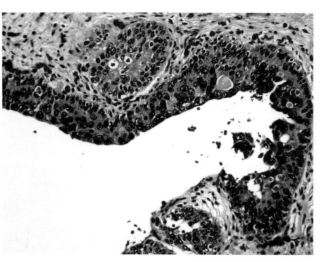

Fig. 4.102 Carcinoma in situ with lepidic spread. Lepidic growth of carcinoma in situ implies that it is overriding or undermining normal urothelium as a continuous sheet of malignant cells. In this image, a sheet of large cytologically malignant cells is separating the overlying urothelium from the underlying stroma

Fig. 4.104 Carcinoma in situ with gland-like lumina. Occasionally, otherwise typical carcinoma in situ exhibits areas of gland-like lumina, as shown in this image. Small cystic spaces containing mucin are present within what appears to be conventional urothelial carcinoma in situ. The cells lining the cystic spaces do not have a tall columnar appearance

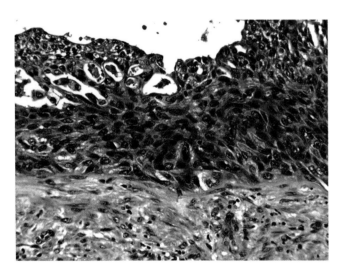

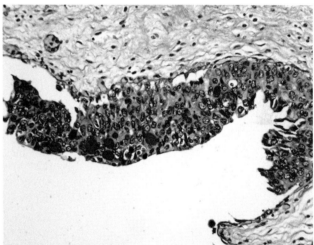

Fig. 4.103 Carcinoma in situ with squamous differentiation. Rarely, carcinoma in situ may exhibit squamous differentiation characterized by intercellular bridges and a squamoid appearance, as exemplified in this image. Carcinoma in situ with squamous features is most often associated with invasive urothelial carcinoma showing extensive squamous differentiation

Fig. 4.105 Carcinoma in situ with gland-like lumina. Section from a different area of the case shown in Fig. 4.104, stained with periodic acid-Schiff with diastase, highlighting the gland-like lumina and confirming the presence of mucin within them

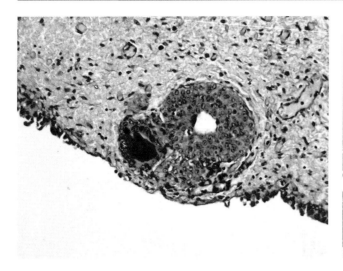

Fig. 4.106 Carcinoma in situ with gland-like lumina. This section, also stained with periodic acid-Schiff with diastase to highlight intraluminal mucin, shows carcinoma in situ with gland-like lumina involving a von Brunn's nest. The overlying urothelium is extensively denuded

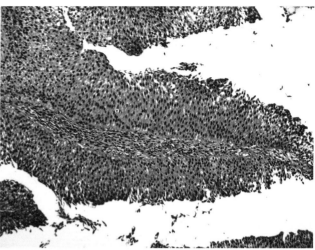

Fig. 4.108 Papillary urothelial neoplasm of low malignant potential. Low-power view of one of the papillary fronds. The fibrovascular core is lined by more than seven layers of cells, which even at this power show normal maturation and polarity. Umbrella cells are absent

4.6 Urothelial Carcinoma and Its Variants

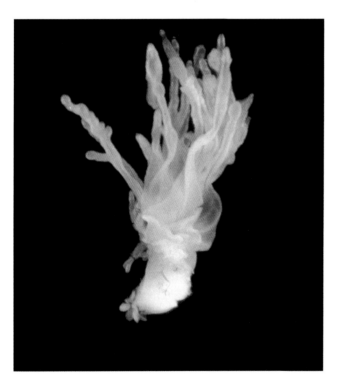

Fig. 4.107 Papillary urothelial neoplasm of low malignant potential. The lesion grows as a cluster of delicate fronds, each consisting of a fibrovascular core lined by urothelium; its endoscopic appearance has been compared with that of seaweed growing on the ocean floor (*see* MacLennan GT, Resnick MI, Bostwick DG, 2003. With permission)

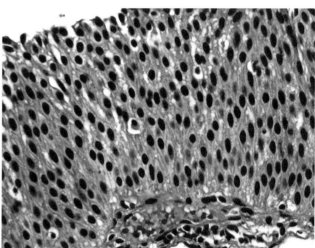

Fig. 4.109 Papillary urothelial neoplasm of low malignant potential. High-power view confirms that the lesion is composed of cells of uniform nuclear size and shape, whose polarity is well preserved. Mitotic figures are not readily found

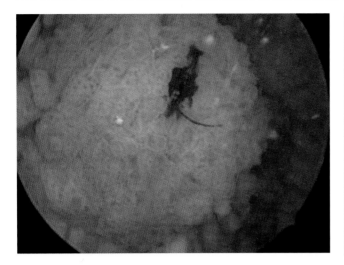

Fig. 4.110 Low-grade papillary urothelial carcinoma. At cystoscopy, the lesion is clearly papillary, but the fronds are somewhat fused and the lesion is assuming a more sessile appearance, compared with the delicate fronds seen in papillary urothelial neoplasm of low malignant potential (*Image courtesy of* Lee Ponsky, MD)

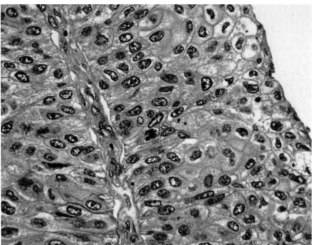

Fig. 4.112 Low-grade papillary urothelial carcinoma. At higher power, loss of cellular orientation is evident. Nuclei vary considerably in shape and size and are enlarged and irregular, with clumped chromatin; many have one or more nucleoli. Mitotic figures are readily seen, and may be found at any level

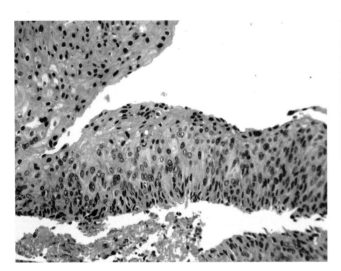

Fig. 4.111 Low-grade papillary urothelial carcinoma. At low power, there is partial loss of cell polarity. Nuclear shape and size are less uniform than in papillary urothelial neoplasm of low malignant potential

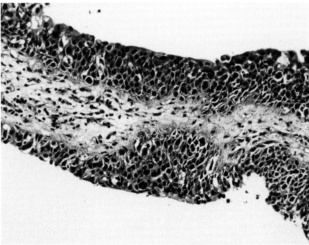

Fig. 4.113 High-grade papillary urothelial carcinoma. Marked cellular atypia is obvious even at relatively low power. There is complete loss of cellular orientation

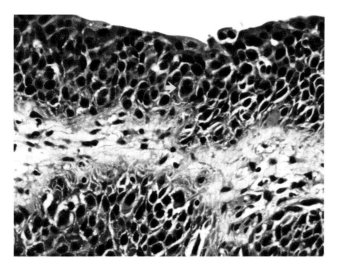

Fig. 4.114 High-grade papillary urothelial carcinoma. Nuclei are large and hyperchromatic, with high nuclear to cytoplasmic ratios, and vary considerably in shape and size. Mitotic figures are frequent, and are present at any level; *arrow* indicates a tripolar mitosis

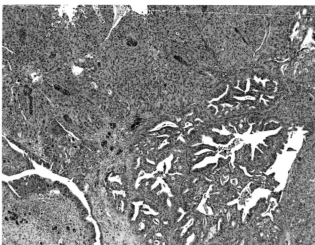

Fig. 4.116 Urothelial carcinoma with mixed differentiation. In this high-grade urothelial carcinoma, areas of true gland formation are readily apparent, a finding in about 6% of bladder urothelial carcinomas. The glands may or may not produce mucin; infrequently a colloid-mucinous pattern is found, characterized by nests of cells dispersed in extracellular mucin, occasionally with signet ring cells. Tumors composed entirely of glandular structures, without a urothelial component, are designated adenocarcinomas. Tumors composed of both urothelial and glandular element are classified as urothelial carcinoma with glandular differentiation

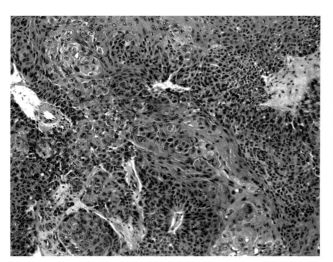

Fig. 4.115 Urothelial carcinoma with mixed differentiation. Variability in differentiation is often seen in urothelial carcinomas. This high-grade urothelial carcinoma contained areas of squamous differentiation, characterized by intercellular bridging and keratin formation, a finding that occurs in about 20% of urothelial carcinomas. In some cases of extensive squamous differentiation, the only apparent urothelial component may be carcinoma in situ

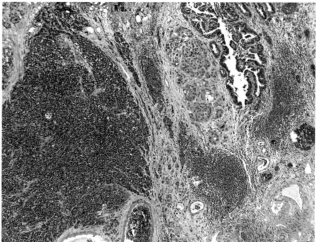

Fig. 4.117 Urothelial carcinoma with mixed differentiation. This tumor includes a small cell carcinoma component (*left*) and urothelial carcinoma (*center*). Glandular differentiation is apparent (*upper right*). Urothelial carcinomas with mixed differentiation have been shown to respond less favorably to treatment than conventional pure urothelial carcinomas of similar stage

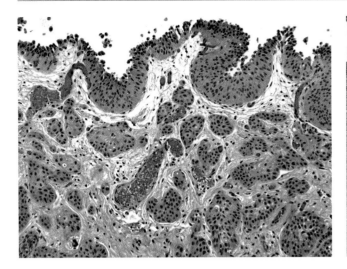

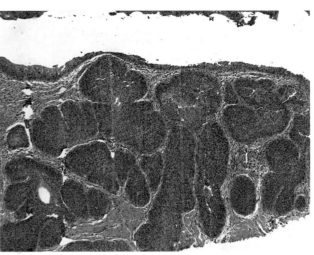

Fig. 4.118 Nested urothelial carcinoma. This uncommon cancer is subtly invasive and in limited biopsies its detection may be challenging. The tumor cells invade as small clusters and can appear "deceptively benign," because they bear some similarity to von Brunn's nests in the lamina propria. Tumor cells have abundant cytoplasm, and nuclear size and shape are fairly uniform. Nonetheless, the tumor always contains foci of unequivocal cancer in which tumor cells exhibit enlarged nucleoli and coarse nuclear chromatin

Fig. 4.120 Inverted urothelial carcinoma. This lesion bears some morphologic similarities to inverted papilloma. A partially intact layer of surface urothelium may be present, but usually an exophytic papillary component is noted. The tumor cells grow downward as thick trabeculae and cell cords of irregular width, usually without evidence of circumscription of the tumor. Obvious stromal invasion with desmoplastic reaction, if present, facilitates the diagnosis

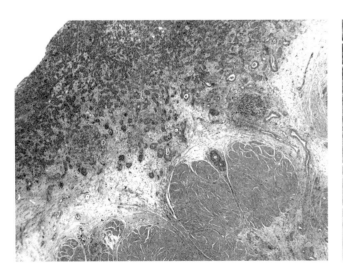

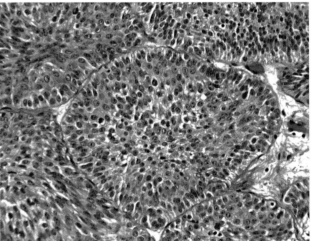

Fig. 4.119 Nested urothelial carcinoma. This low-power view of a section from a cystectomy specimen highlights the diffusely infiltrative nature of this aggressive cancer, which involves both lamina propria and deep detrusor muscle. Lumen formation is evident in deeper portions of the tumor

Fig. 4.121 Inverted urothelial carcinoma. Tumor cells show cytologic atypia. Mitotic figures are readily seen, and the trabeculae show less evident peripheral palisading and central maturation than is seen in inverted papilloma. Carcinomas with inverted growth pattern usually show positive immunostaining for Ki-67, p53, or cytokeratin 20, and also show molecular features of urothelial carcinoma on UroVysion® (Genezyme; Cambridge, MA) FISH (fluorescence in situ hybridization); inverted papillomas rarely exhibit these findings

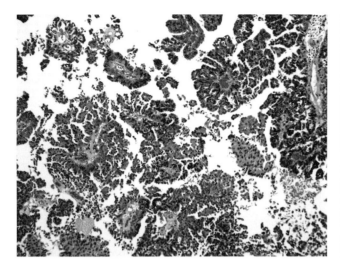

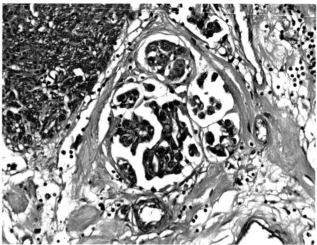

Fig. 4.122 Micropapillary urothelial carcinoma. This distinctive variant of urothelial carcinoma is uncommon; in 80% of cases, it is accompanied by conventional invasive or noninvasive urothelial cancer. At low power, as shown here, its exophytic component consists of delicate papillary structures lined by tumor cells, clusters of which appear to float freely. It bears a striking resemblance to papillary serous carcinoma of the ovary

Fig. 4.124 Micropapillary urothelial carcinoma. The lacunae in which the tumor cell clusters lie can be shown to lack lining endothelial cells. This cancer is aggressive, commonly exhibiting high pathologic and clinical stage when initially diagnosed

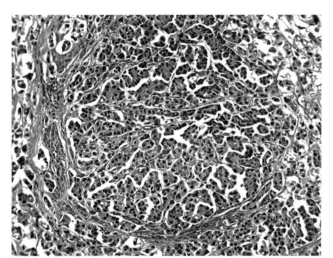

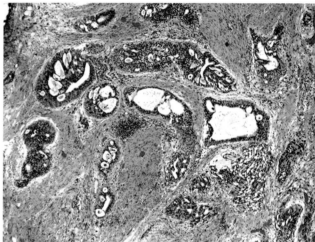

Fig. 4.123 Micropapillary urothelial carcinoma. The invasive component consists of infiltrating delicate filiform processes or small tight papillary tumor cell clusters lying within lacunae that resemble lymphovascular spaces

Fig. 4.125 Microcystic urothelial carcinoma. This invasive variant is characterized by microcysts and macrocysts that may reach up to 2 cm in diameter. The cysts and tubules display irregular outlines and incite a stromal reaction; they may contain mucin or necrotic debris, or may be empty

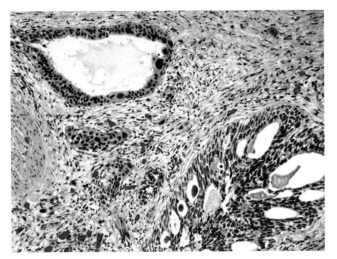

Fig. 4.126 Microcystic urothelial carcinoma. The cells lining the tubules and infiltrating the stroma are cytologically malignant. The microcystic variant of urothelial carcinoma may resemble other entities, including florid polypoid cystitis cystica and glandularis, nephrogenic metaplasia, and nested variant of urothelial carcinoma with tubular differentiation

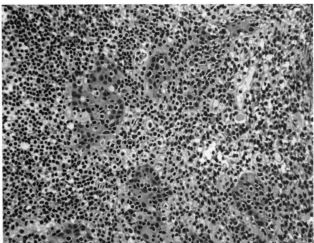

Fig. 4.128 Lymphoepithelioma-like urothelial carcinoma. The undifferentiated carcinoma cells are arranged in sheets, nests, and cords

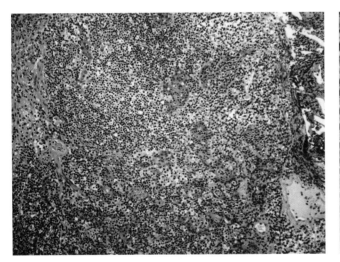

Fig. 4.127 Lymphoepithelioma-like urothelial carcinoma. This variant histologically resembles lymphoepithelioma of the nasopharynx. At low power, the most prominent feature is the presence of abundant lymphocytes (both B- and T- cell types), admixed with plasma cells, histiocytes, and occasional neutrophils and eosinophils. Almost inconspicuous in this background are epithelial cells

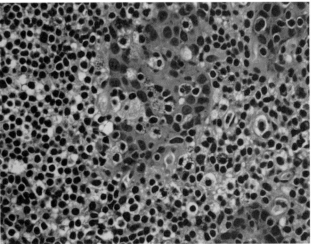

Fig. 4.129 Lymphoepithelioma-like urothelial carcinoma. The carcinoma cells have large nuclei and prominent nucleoli. They have relatively abundant pink cytoplasm, and indistinct cell borders, imparting a syncytial appearance

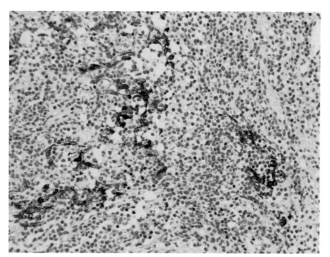

Fig. 4.130 Lymphoepithelioma-like urothelial carcinoma. Immunostain for keratin AE1/AE3 highlights the presence of epithelial cells in the background of inflammatory cells. In these tumors, components of readily apparent conventional urothelial carcinoma may also be present

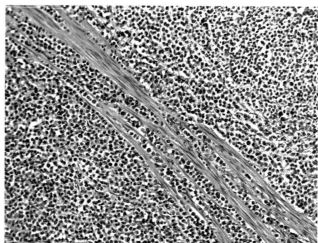

Fig. 4.132 Lymphoma-like/plasmacytoma-like urothelial carcinoma. Tumor cells freely infiltrate between and around fibers of detrusor muscle

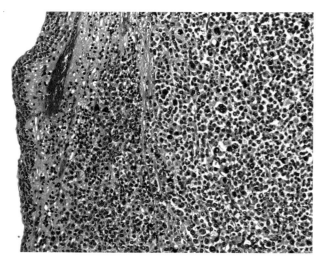

Fig. 4.131 Lymphoma-like/plasmacytoma-like urothelial carcinoma. The lamina propria is diffusely infiltrated by a sheet of rather monotonous undifferentiated cytologically malignant cells. The overlying urothelium is unremarkable. The findings at low power are suggestive of lymphoma

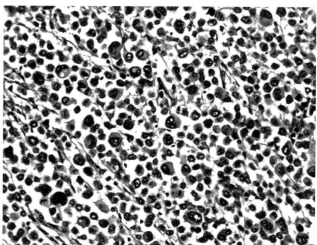

Fig. 4.133 Lymphoma-like/plasmacytoma-like urothelial carcinoma. Tumor cells are medium-sized, with limited amounts of eosinophilic cytoplasm. Nuclei are somewhat pleomorphic and irregular, with clumped chromatin, and mitotic activity is brisk. Nuclei of many tumor cells are eccentrically placed, imparting a plasmacytoid appearance

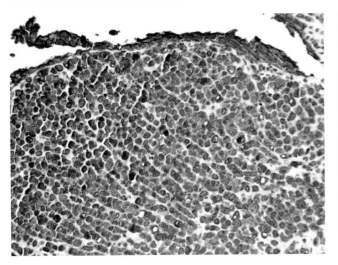

Fig. 4.134 Lymphoma-like/plasmacytoma-like urothelial carcinoma. Immunostain for keratin AE1/AE3 confirms the epithelial nature of the malignancy

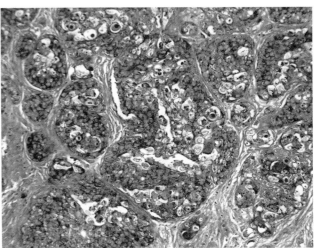

Fig. 4.136 Clear cell (glycogen-rich) urothelial carcinoma. Staining for glycogen using a periodic acid-Schiff stain highlights the presence of abundant cytoplasmic glycogen. After diastase digestion, glycogen staining was lost

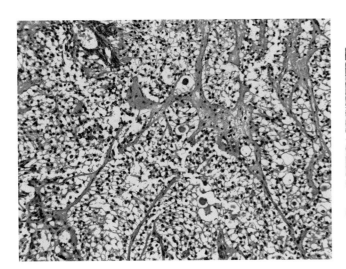

Fig. 4.135 Clear cell (glycogen-rich) urothelial carcinoma. About two-thirds of urothelial carcinomas have focal areas of cytoplasmic clearing due to glycogen accumulation. In some tumors, the extent of this finding is such that other entities, such as metastatic renal cell carcinoma, or clear cell adenocarcinoma of bladder, must be considered. The tumor shown here had extensive areas of clear cell change. Tumor cells have abundant optically clear cytoplasm and fairly well-defined cell membranes

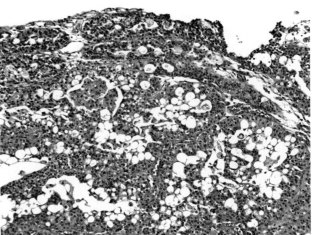

Fig. 4.137 Lipoid cell urothelial carcinoma. In this variant, in a background of an otherwise conventional urothelial carcinoma, 10–30% of the tumor cells have morphologic features comparable to those of signet-ring lipoblasts, as shown here

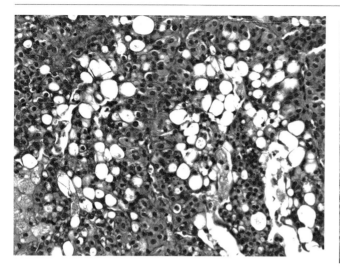

Fig. 4.138 Lipoid cell urothelial carcinoma. Due to the paucity of reported cases, it is unclear whether this neoplasm represents a distinct entity worthy of separate classification. The lipoid cells show positive immunostaining for keratin markers; hence, it is unlikely that this lesion qualifies as a sarcomatoid carcinoma/carcinosarcoma

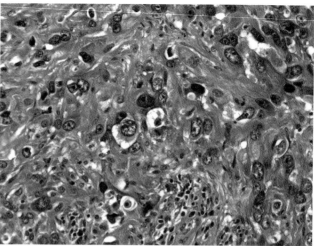

Fig. 4.140 Large cell undifferentiated urothelial carcinoma. Tumor cells have large pleomorphic nuclei, prominent nucleoli, and abundant amphophilic cytoplasm. They dwarf the red cells and lymphoid cells scattered through the tumor

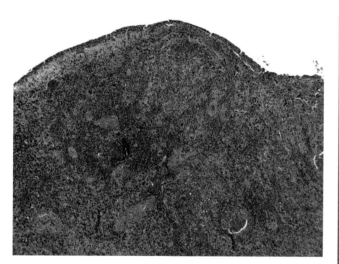

Fig. 4.139 Large cell undifferentiated urothelial carcinoma. The defining characteristic of these cancers is that they are entirely composed of very large undifferentiated tumor cells, and do not resemble other well-defined variants of urothelial carcinoma. In this low-power view, the lamina propria is diffusely infiltrated by an undifferentiated tumor; the large size of the tumor cells is obvious even at this low power

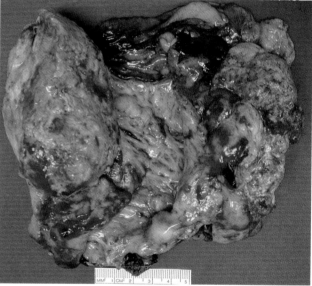

Fig. 4.141 Sarcomatoid urothelial carcinoma. These are malignant neoplasms that exhibit morphologic or immunohistochemical evidence of both epithelial and mesenchymal differentiation. Bladder carcinomas with sarcomatoid change tend to be bulky (*Image courtesy of* Paul Grabenstetter, MD)

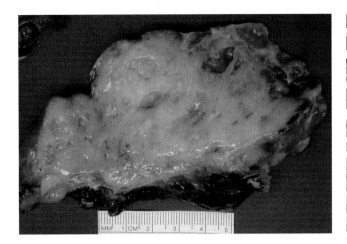

Fig. 4.142 Sarcomatoid urothelial carcinoma. The cut surface is fleshy. The tumor has infiltrated full thickness of bladder wall and occupies all of the perivesical space to the level of the inked surgical margin (*Image courtesy of* Paul Grabenstetter, MD)

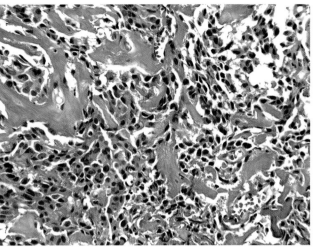

Fig. 4.144 Sarcomatoid urothelial carcinoma. Heterologous elements are often seen in sarcomatoid urothelial carcinoma. The commonest is osteosarcoma, shown here

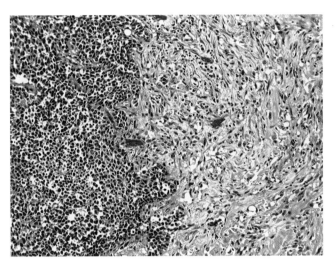

Fig. 4.143 Sarcomatoid urothelial carcinoma. Conventional urothelial carcinoma is present on the left. On the right is the sarcomatoid component, in the form of a high grade undifferentiated spindle cell neoplasm

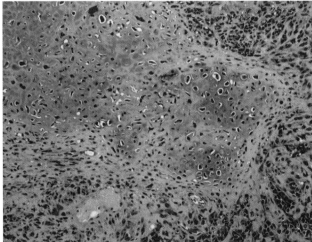

Fig. 4.145 Sarcomatoid urothelial carcinoma. The second most common heterologous element in these tumors is chondrosarcoma

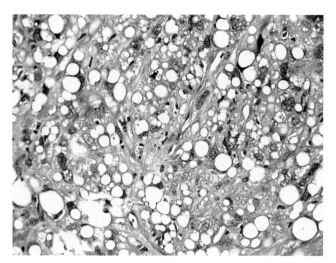

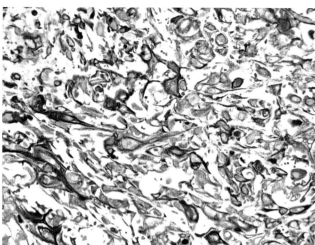

Fig. 4.146 Sarcomatoid urothelial carcinoma. Liposarcoma, shown here, is an infrequent heterologous component of these tumors. Other uncommon heterologous elements are rhabdomyosarcoma, leiomyosarcoma, angiosarcoma, and mixed mesenchymal neoplasms

Fig. 4.148 Sarcomatoid urothelial carcinoma. Immunostaining of a section from the tumor shown in Fig. 4.147 with antibodies against keratin AE1/AE3 highlights the spindled and pleomorphic cells, supporting a diagnosis of sarcomatoid carcinoma, rather than undifferentiated sarcoma

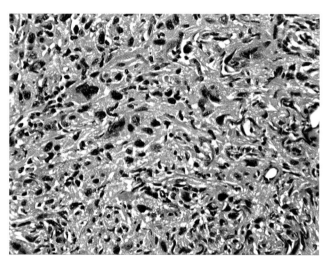

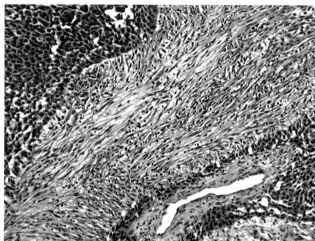

Fig. 4.147 Sarcomatoid urothelial carcinoma. Some of these tumors are entirely composed of sarcomatoid elements, raising the question of whether the neoplasm is a true bladder sarcoma. This bladder tumor was entirely composed of spindled and pleomorphic cells; no recognizable carcinomatous component was found, despite extensive sampling

Fig. 4.149 Urothelial carcinoma with pseudosarcomatous stromal reaction. Infiltrating urothelial carcinoma may incite stromal reactive processes, such as this spindle cell proliferation, which may cause concern for sarcomatoid differentiation. Features favoring a reactive process include the presence of inflammatory cells, the relative lack of cytologic atypia, and the absence of mitotic figures

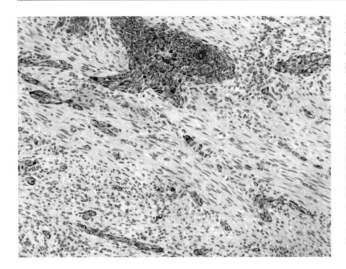

Fig. 4.150 Urothelial carcinoma with pseudosarcomatous stromal reaction. Immunostain for keratin AE1/AE3 highlights the infiltrating carcinoma cells. The reactive stromal cells show no immunoreactivity for this marker

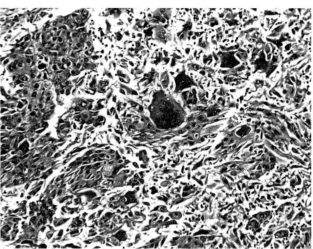

Fig. 4.152 Urothelial carcinoma with osteoclast-like giant cells. This invasive high-grade urothelial carcinoma contained many giant cells with numerous small round nuclei and abundant eosinophilic cytoplasm. There is no evidence that this finding has any prognostic significance

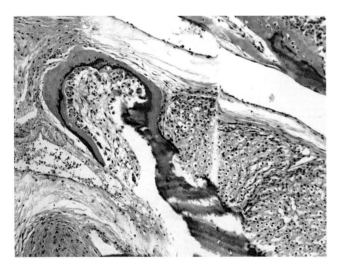

Fig. 4.151 Urothelial carcinoma with stromal osseous metaplasia. This is an unusual stromal reactive process. The metaplastic bone has a lamellar architecture. The osteocytes in the lacunae and rimming the bone have small bland nuclei and are distinctly different from the mesenchymal cells in the adjacent stroma

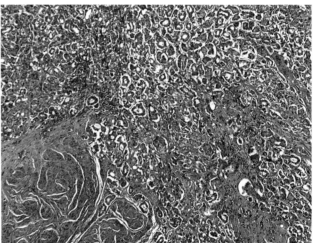

Fig. 4.153 Urothelial carcinoma with acinar/tubular differentiation. The morphology of this uncommon variant raises concern for adenocarcinoma, metastatic or infiltrating from an adjacent organ

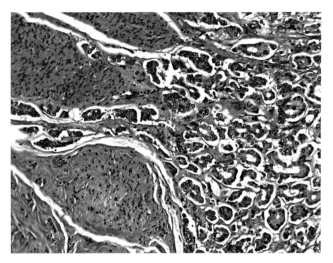

Fig. 4.154 Urothelial carcinoma with acinar/tubular differentiation. A rare finding in otherwise conventional urothelial carcinomas, in which there are areas of small crowded glands lined by a single layer of cells with prominent nucleoli. Tumor cells show negative immunostaining for prostate specific antigen and prostatic acid phosphatase, and positive immunostaining for cytokeratins 7, 20 and 34βE12

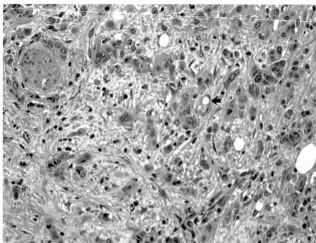

Fig. 4.156 Urothelial carcinoma with dyscohesive growth pattern. Varying numbers of tumor cells containing prominent intracytoplasmic vacuoles are usually present (*arrow*). The findings can closely mimic metastatic gastric carcinoma or lobular breast carcinoma, necessitating clinical assessment for those entities. Almost invariably, patients with breast or gastric cancer metastatic to the bladder have a history of the prior malignancy

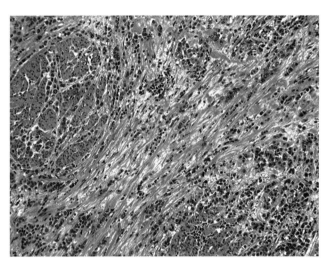

Fig. 4.155 Urothelial carcinoma with dyscohesive growth pattern. In this section from a cystectomy specimen, this portion of the tumor exhibits a diffusely infiltrative growth pattern, arranged in some areas in linear single-cell files (Indian-file pattern) and in other areas there are aggregates of loosely cohesive cells

4.7 Glandular Neoplasms

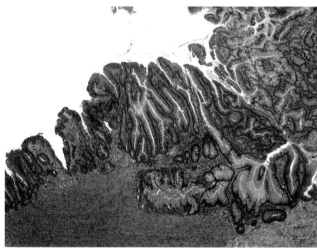

Fig. 4.157 Villous adenoma. Villous adenoma is an uncommon benign exophytic glandular epithelial neoplasm, often associated with urachal adenocarcinoma, and most commonly found in the urachus, bladder dome, or trigone. Villous adenoma of the bladder is morphologically identical to villous adenoma of the colon, with mucin-producing cells showing at least low-grade dysplasia, lining delicate fibrovascular stalks. No invasive component is present (*see* MacLennan GT, Resnick MI, Bostwick DG, 2003. With permission)

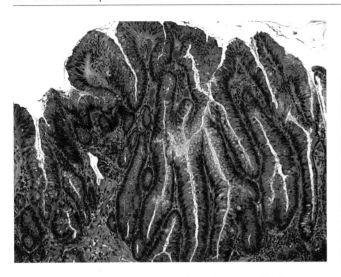

Fig. 4.158 Villous adenoma. The lining columnar cells show pseudostratification, crowding, occasional prominent nucleoli, and hyperchromasia, as in the colon

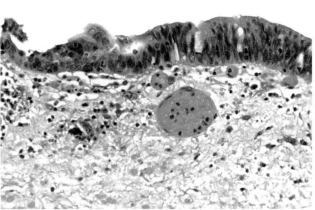

Fig. 4.160 Adenocarcinoma in situ of bladder. In the flat form of adenocarcinoma in situ, a single layer of moderately pleomorphic pseudostratified tall columnar mucin-producing cells line the surface of the bladder, as shown here

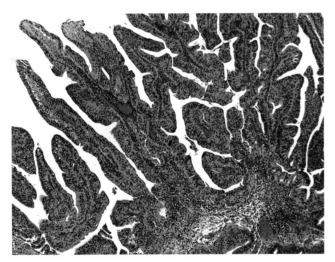

Fig. 4.159 Adenocarcinoma in situ of bladder. In situ adenocarcinoma of the bladder demonstrates three architectural patterns: papillary, flat, and cribriform. The papillary type, shown here, closely resembles papillary urothelial carcinoma, but on close inspection, the fibrovascular cores are lined by tall columnar cells characteristic of glandular differentiation, rather than multiple layers of urothelial cells

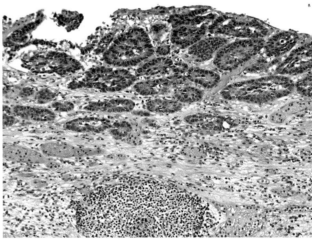

Fig. 4.161 Adenocarcinoma in situ of bladder. This is an example of the cribriform type of adenocarcinoma is situ of bladder. True glandular spaces with cribriform architecture are lined by moderately pleomorphic columnar cells with apical cytoplasm

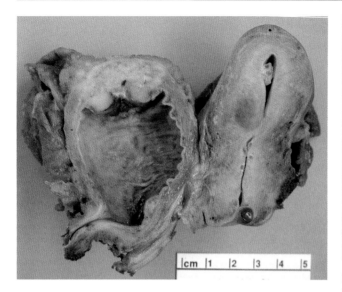

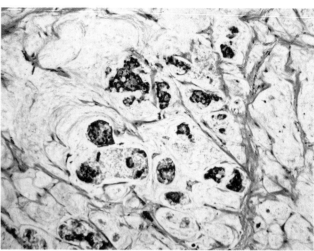

Fig. 4.164 Adenocarcinomas of urachus and bladder. Tumors that show carcinoma cell clusters apparently floating in pools of mucin are classified as mucinous (colloid) type

Fig. 4.162 Adenocarcinoma of urachus and bladder. Urachal adenocarcinoma and adenocarcinoma of the bladder differ in that there are certain criteria that must be met to diagnose urachal adenocarcinoma: (1) tumor in the bladder dome; (2) a sharp demarcation between the tumor and the surface urothelium; and (3) exclusion of primary adenocarcinoma located elsewhere that has involved the bladder secondarily. Urachal carcinoma usually involves the muscular wall of the bladder dome, with or without destruction of the overlying mucosa. Its cut surface often exhibits a glistening appearance, reflecting its mucinous contents

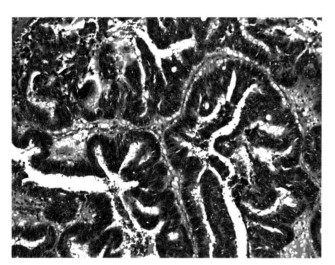

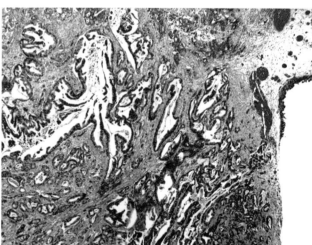

Fig. 4.163 Adenocarcinomas of urachus and bladder show a variety of histologic growth patterns: (1) enteric (colonic) type; (2) adenocarcinoma not otherwise specified (NOS); (3) mucinous (colloid) type; (4) signet ring cell type; (5) clear cell type; (6) hepatoid type; and (7) mixed forms, which are commonly encountered. The enteric type, shown here, closely resembles colonic adenocarcinoma

Fig. 4.165 Adenocarcinomas of urachus and bladder. Tumors exhibiting a nonspecific glandular growth pattern are designated adenocarcinoma not otherwise specified. This particular adenocarcinoma arose in a setting of carcinoma in situ with gland-like lumina (*see* Fig. 4.104)

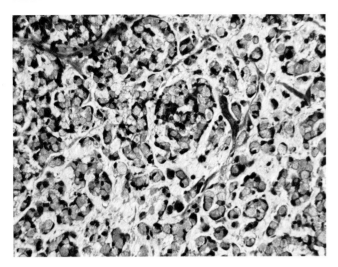

Fig. 4.166 Adenocarcinomas of urachus and bladder. Signet ring cell adenocarcinoma is morphologically similar to signet-ring adenocarcinomas occurring at other sites; it may have a monocytoid or plasmacytoid phenotype and it carries the worst prognosis among different histologic types of adenocarcinoma found in bladder or urachus

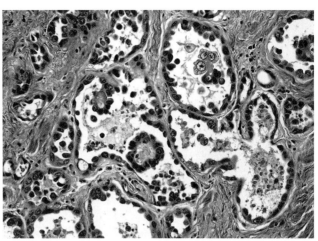

Fig. 4.168 Clear cell adenocarcinoma of bladder and urethra. Clear cell adenocarcinoma is distinctive histologically and exhibits a variety of architectural patterns. It often forms tubulocystic structures that vary in size and may contain either basophilic or eosinophilic secretions. The tumor cells may be flat, cuboidal, or columnar, and they may have either clear or eosinophilic cytoplasm. Hobnail cells are frequently seen in tubules. Tumor cells show moderate to severe atypia, and mitotic figures are frequently observed

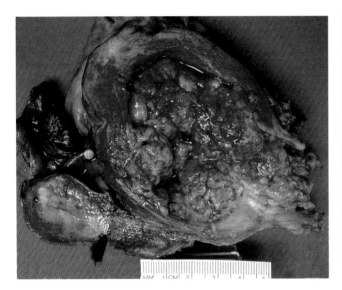

Fig. 4.167 Clear cell adenocarcinoma of bladder and urethra. Tumors may be bulky and exophytic, nodular, or sessile in appearance. This cystectomy is from a 63-year-old woman who had undergone transurethral resection of the primary lesion 18 months previously. The lesion initially was in the urethra and at the bladder neck, but the recurrent tumor involved the bladder much more extensively

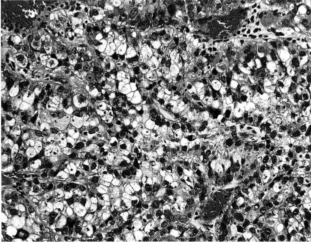

Fig. 4.169 Clear cell adenocarcinoma of bladder and urethra. Tumor cells may grow in diffuse solid sheets or may form papillary structures; the papillae are usually small and their fibrovascular cores may be extensively hyalinized. The cytoplasm often contains glycogen, imparting a clear cell appearance. In some cases, clear cell adenocarcinoma coexists with conventional urothelial carcinoma; there is now very compelling evidence that clear cell adenocarcinoma of the bladder and urethra is of urothelial origin

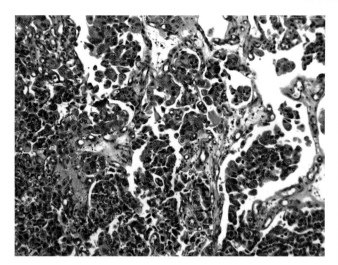

Fig. 4.170 Hepatoid adenocarcinoma. The pathological diagnosis of this rare cancer is based on a combination of histological features resembling hepatocellular carcinoma and positive immunostaining for alpha-fetoprotein. Tumor cells are polygonal, with abundant granular eosinophilic cytoplasm, vesicular nuclei and prominent nucleoli, arranged in nests and trabecular structures, imparting an appearance similar to hepatocellular carcinoma

4.8 Squamous Cell Neoplasms

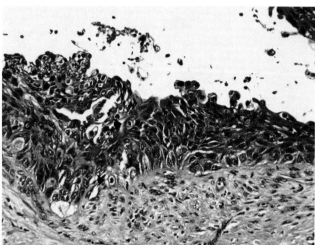

Fig. 4.172 Squamous cell carcinoma in situ. Noninvasive proliferation of dysplastic squamous cells with markedly impaired maturation and abundant mitotic figures, present basally and in the middle to upper thirds as well (*arrows*)

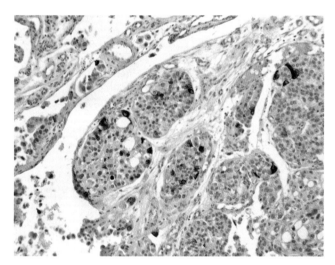

Fig. 4.171 Hepatoid adenocarcinoma. A proportion of the tumor cells show immunoreactivity for α-fetoprotein, as shown here. Tumor cells also show positive immunostaining for keratin Cam 5.2, α-1- antitrypsin, albumin, hepatocyte paraffin-1, epithelial membrane antigen, and a striking canalicular staining pattern with polyclonal anticarcinoembryonic antigen, features indicative of hepatocellular differentiation; this is further supported by the demonstration of albumin gene mRNA in tumor cells by non-isotopic in situ hybridization

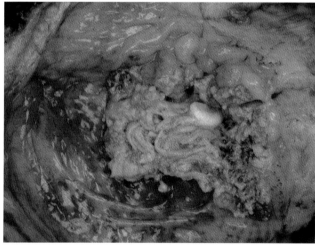

Fig. 4.173 Invasive squamous cell carcinoma. Pale white 5 cm tumor in a cystectomy specimen, fresh state. Patient had a remote history of tobacco smoking but no other known risk factors for squamous cell carcinoma (*Image courtesy of* Pedro Ciarlini, MD)

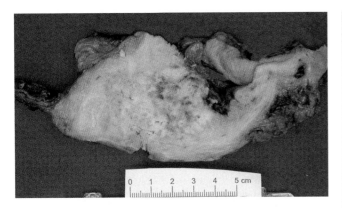

Fig. 4.174 Invasive squamous cell carcinoma. After fixation and sectioning, the tumor in Fig. 4.173 shows extensive white areas due to keratin production. The tumor infiltrates full thickness of detrusor muscle into perivesical fat, but does not reach the serosal margin grossly (*Image courtesy of* Pedro Ciarlini, MD)

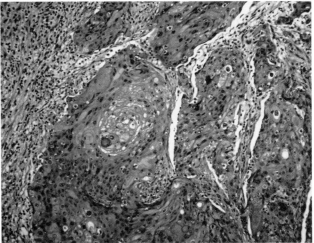

Fig. 4.176 Invasive squamous cell carcinoma, well differentiated. Tumor shows well-defined islands of squamous cells with keratinization, keratin pearls, prominent intercellular bridges, and minimal nuclear pleomorphism

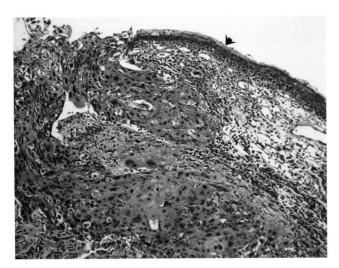

Fig. 4.175 Invasive squamous cell carcinoma. Tongues of malignant squamous cells infiltrate into lamina propria. Keratinizing squamous metaplasia (*arrow*) is evident in the epithelium adjacent to the invasive carcinoma

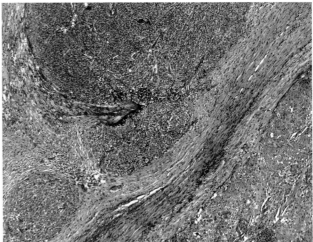

Fig. 4.177 Invasive squamous cell carcinoma, basaloid type. Readily recognizable moderately differentiated invasive squamous carcinoma is present (*lower right*). The cancer (*upper left*) appears poorly differentiated; it is composed of variably sized nests of small dark cells in a desmoplastic stroma

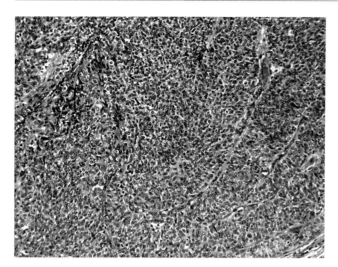

Fig. 4.178 Invasive squamous cell carcinoma, basaloid type. The tumor is composed of small basaloid cells with a high nuclear to cytoplasmic ratio and dense hyperchromatic nuclei, arranged with peripheral palisading. Numerous mitotic figures and apoptotic bodies are present

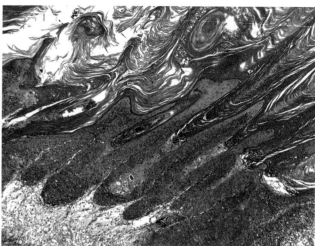

Fig. 4.180 Squamous cell carcinoma, verrucous type. This example shows more florid hyperkeratosis than the tumor shown in Fig. 4.179

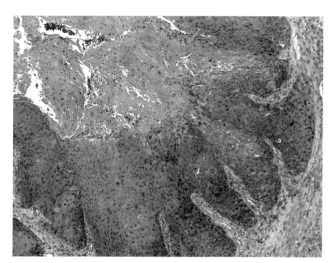

Fig. 4.179 Squamous cell carcinoma, verrucous type. These tumors are grossly described as "warty;" most, but not all, are associated with schistosomiasis. Tumors show epithelial acanthosis and papillomatosis, minimal nuclear and architectural atypia and rounded pushing deep borders. It is recommended that tumors with these features, but with an obvious invasive component, should be diagnosed as regular squamous cell carcinoma

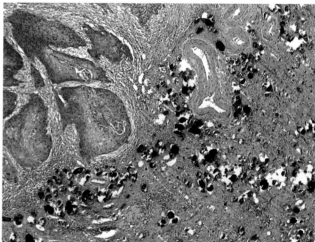

Fig. 4.181 Squamous cell carcinoma associated with schistosomiasis. As noted previously, schistosomiasis is a risk factor for the development of invasive squamous cell carcinoma. Schistosoma-associated squamous cell carcinomas are typically exophytic and large, polypoid or solid with visible necrosis and keratin debris; others are ulcerated infiltrating tumors. Very often, the adjacent flat epithelium shows keratinizing squamous metaplasia, dysplasia or carcinoma in situ. Schistosoma-associated squamous cell carcinomas vary from well to poorly differentiated; most are well-differentiated, with prominent keratinization, intercellular bridge formation, and minimal nuclear pleomorphism. In this image, numerous calcified *Schistosoma haematobium* eggs are present in the stroma at right

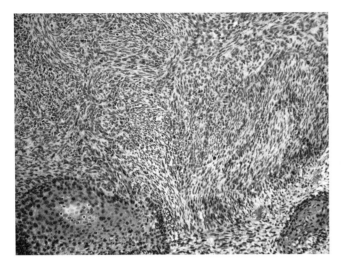

Fig. 4.182 Squamous cell carcinoma with sarcomatoid change. Sarcomatoid change can be found in pure squamous cell carcinomas, as in this case. There is molecular and morphologic evidence that sarcomatoid carcinoma is a common final pathway of all forms of epithelial bladder tumors

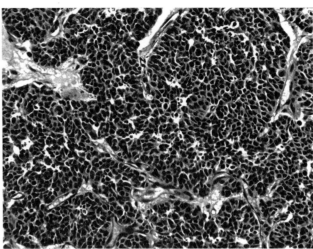

Fig. 4.184 Small cell carcinoma. Tumor is composed of sheets or nests of small or intermediate-sized cells with nuclear molding, scant cytoplasm, inconspicuous nucleoli, and evenly dispersed finely stippled chromatin. Usually mitotic figures are readily found; geographic or punctate necrosis is common. Vascular invasion is always apparent, and the great majority of tumors extensively infiltrate the detrusor muscle

4.9 Neuroendocrine and Neural Neoplasms

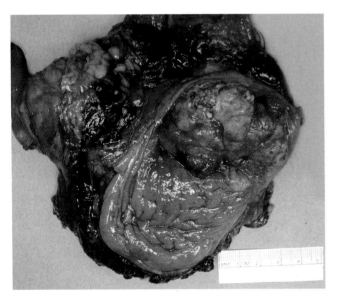

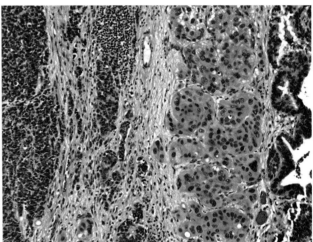

Fig. 4.185 Small cell carcinoma. About one third of cases are purely small cell carcinoma; the remainder are mixtures of small cell carcinoma with carcinoma in situ, conventional urothelial carcinoma, adenocarcinoma, squamous cell carcinoma, or sarcomatoid carcinoma. This image shows small cell carcinoma (*left*), conventional urothelial carcinoma (*center*), and adenocarcinoma (*right*)

Fig. 4.183 Small cell carcinoma. Most tumors form a single large, solid, polypoid mass. Less often, the tumor is sessile, ulcerated, and deeply infiltrative. Commonest sites are lateral walls and dome of the bladder (*Image courtesy of* Paul Grabenstetter, MD)

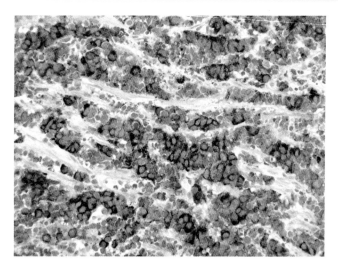

Fig. 4.186 Small cell carcinoma. Tumor cells show positive immunostaining for chromogranin

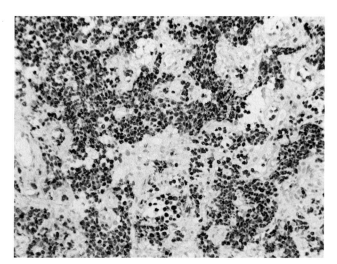

Fig. 4.187 Small cell carcinoma. Tumor cells show positive immunostaining for thyroid transcription factor-1

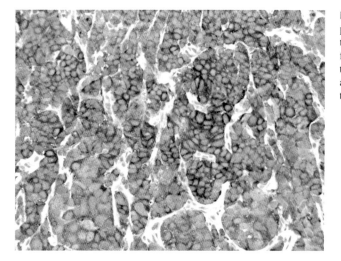

Fig. 4.188 Small cell carcinoma. Tumor cells show positive immunostaining for synaptophysin

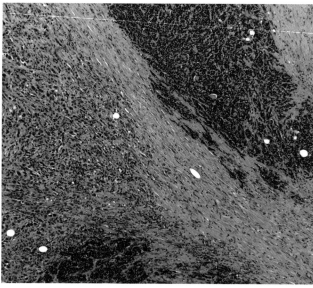

Fig. 4.189 Small cell carcinoma. This tumor had areas of sarcomatoid differentiation (*left*)

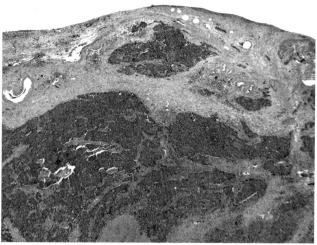

Fig. 4.190 Large cell neuroendocrine carcinoma. This is a high-grade poorly differentiated neuroendocrine neoplasm, morphologically indistinguishable from its pulmonary counterpart, occurring either in pure form, or admixed with other types of bladder carcinoma. Its architecture may be organoid, nested, palisaded, or trabecular. It is aggressive, and as shown in this low-power image, is often deeply invasive at the time of diagnosis

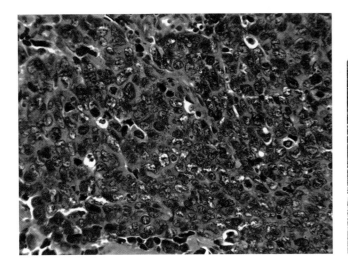

Fig. 4.191 Large cell neuroendocrine carcinoma. Tumor cells are large compared with those of small cell carcinoma, polygonal, with more cytoplasm. Cell borders are indistinct. Nuclear chromatin is more clumped and nucleoli are present in many cells. Abundant apoptotic bodies and mitotic figures are present

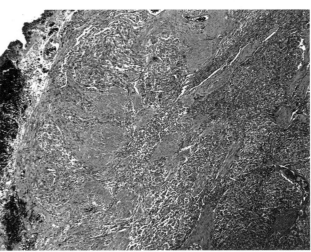

Fig. 4.193 Paraganglioma. It is hypothesized that paragangliomas of the bladder originate from paraganglionic cells that migrated into the bladder wall. Endoscopically, they are small (<3 cm) dome-shaped nodules, usually in the trigone, dome, or lateral wall, covered by normal mucosa. At least 94% of paragangliomas involve detrusor muscle, as illustrated in this image; normal mucosa is at upper left

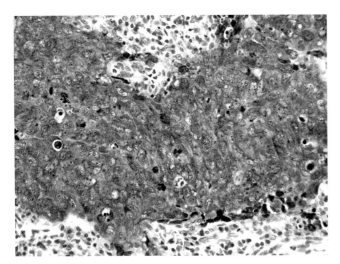

Fig. 4.192 Large cell neuroendocrine carcinoma. Tumor cells show immunoreactivity for one or more neuroendocrine markers (chromogranin A, CD56, neuron-specific enolase, or synaptophysin [shown here]), and for one or more cytokeratin markers (Cam 5.2, AE1/AE3, and/or epithelial membrane antigen)

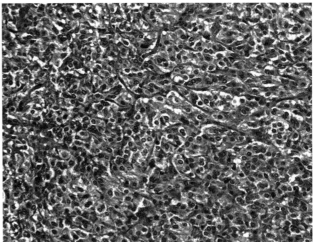

Fig. 4.194 Paraganglioma. Similar to their counterparts elsewhere, tumors consist of round or polygonal epithelioid cells with abundant eosinophilic or granular cytoplasm, typically arranged in discrete nests (zellballen), with intervening vascular septa. Tumor cell nuclei are vesicular with finely granular chromatin; mitotic figures, necrosis, and vascular invasion are usually absent. Only the occurrence of regional or distant metastases allows a diagnosis of malignancy; this occurs in about 20% of bladder paragangliomas

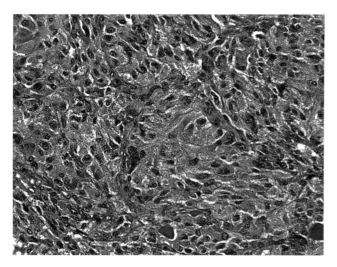

Fig. 4.195 Paraganglioma. In some cases, the tumor cells are arranged in sheets and their cytoplasm acquires a lavender tint due to the presence of numerous cytoplasmic granules

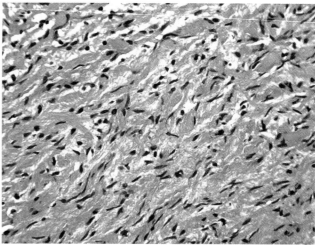

Fig. 4.197 Neurofibroma. Tumors are composed of a hypocellular proliferation of loosely arranged spindle cells with wavy bland nuclei, loosely arranged into fascicles with scattered "shredded carrot" bundles of collagen. Individual cells have wavy, bland nuclei

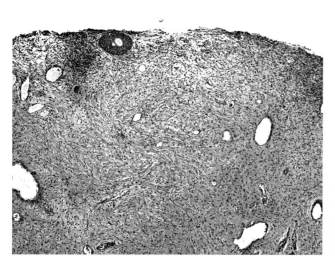

Fig. 4.196 Neurofibroma. Neurofibroma is a benign proliferation of various nerve sheath cells, including Schwann cells, perineurium-like cells, fibroblasts, and intermediate type cells. Most that involve the bladder occur in patients with neurofibromatosis type 1 rather than as isolated sporadic lesions. Bladder involvement tends to be transmural with both diffuse and plexiform growth patterns. This image shows diffuse lamina propria effacement by neurofibroma

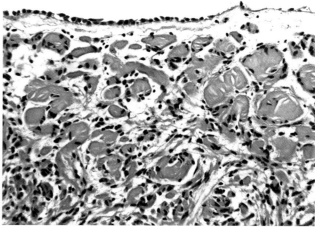

Fig. 4.198 Neurofibroma. In this example, there is a band-like subepithelial collection of pseudo-meissnerian corpuscles

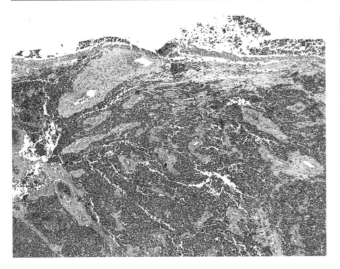

Fig. 4.199 Primitive neuroectodermal tumor. This is extremely rare in the bladder, and behaves aggressively. Lamina propria is diffusely infiltrated by a small round blue-cell tumor

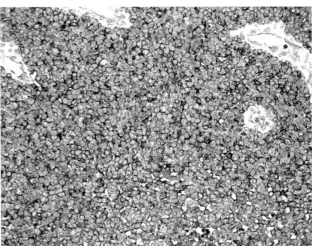

Fig. 4.201 Primitive neuroectodermal tumor. Tumor cells show strong diffusely positive immunostaining for CD99, as shown in this image. Cells of primitive neuroectodermal tumor also frequently show positive immunostaining for FLI-1, vimentin, and CD117 (c-kit), and focally positive immunostaining for cytokeratin and S-100 protein

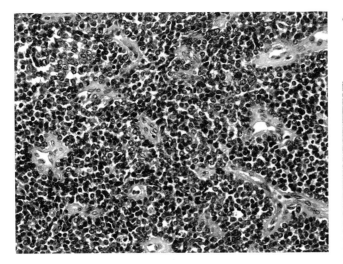

Fig. 4.200 Primitive neuroectodermal tumor. Tumor is composed of undifferentiated small round blue cells. Although rosette formation is sometimes seen in these tumors, none is apparent in this case

4.10 Soft Tissue/Myofibroblastic Proliferations

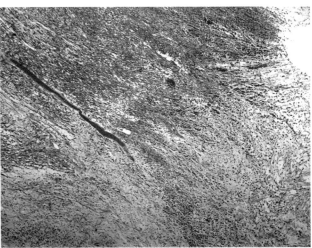

Fig. 4.202 Inflammatory myofibroblastic tumor. In the bladder, this tumor usually takes the form of a polyp or a submucosal nodule. Three histologic patterns have been recognized, the commonest being the "nodular fasciitis-like" pattern with myxoid, vascular, and inflammatory areas. This is a low power view of the "nodular fasciitis-like" pattern. The tumor shows a variable degree of cellularity. At least part of the tumor has a myxoid background; prominent blood vessels and abundant inflammatory cells are present

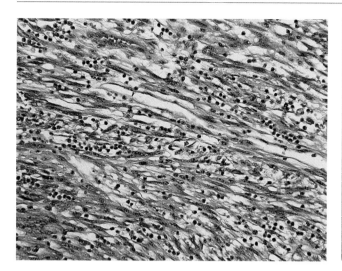

Fig. 4.203 Inflammatory myofibroblastic tumor. Higher power view of the "nodular fasciitis-like" pattern, showing a myxoid background and numerous inflammatory cells, predominantly neutrophils and eosinophils. A few extravasated red blood cells are present. Tumor is composed of spindle cells with elongated eosinophilic cytoplasmic processes; they bear some resemblance to cells in tissue cultures. Tumor cell nuclei are uniform and lack significant nuclear atypia or mitotic activity

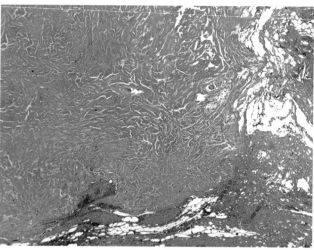

Fig. 4.205 Inflammatory myofibroblastic tumor. The third pattern, described as "scar or desmoid-like," has dense collagen with fewer spindled and inflammatory cells. At low power, this bladder lesion almost entirely consists of dense hyalinized collagen.

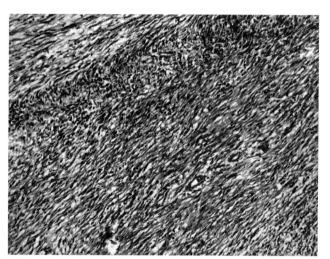

Fig. 4.204 Inflammatory myofibroblastic tumor. A second pattern, designated "fibrous histiocytoma-like," is shown here. It consists of a more compact spindle cell proliferation, with chronic inflammatory cells, mainly lymphocytes, plasma cells, or eosinophils, scattered throughout

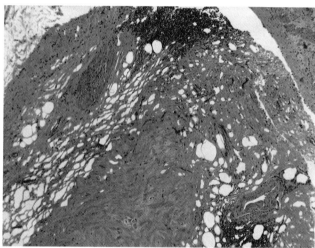

Fig. 4.206 Inflammatory myofibroblastic tumor. A higher power view of the desmoid-like form of this lesion shows the dense collagen and clusters of chronic inflammatory cells that characterize this lesion

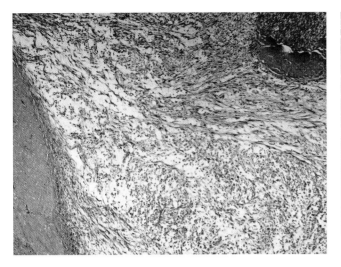

Fig. 4.207 Inflammatory myofibroblastic tumor. An element that complicates distinction of inflammatory myofibroblastic tumor from myxoid leiomyosarcoma is that both entities can show surface ulceration and necrosis, both can infiltrate into the detrusor muscle, and both can exhibit necrosis deep in the bladder wall. This is an inflammatory myofibroblastic tumor that is infiltrating between two large bundles of detrusor muscle

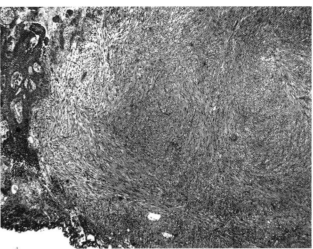

Fig. 4.209 Postoperative spindle cell nodule. Classically, this lesion arises in the lower genital tract and lower urinary tract in males and females some months after surgical instrumentation or resection. It forms nodules up to 4 cm in diameter, and clinically may raise concern for malignancy. At low power, it is a spindle cell proliferation that has indistinct and apparently infiltrative margins

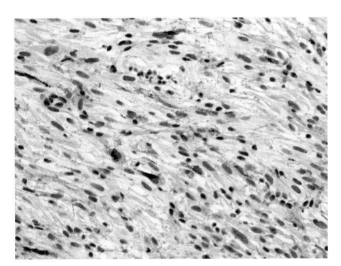

Fig. 4.208 Inflammatory myofibroblastic tumor. Positive cytoplasmic immunostaining for anaplastic lymphoma kinase (ALK-1) has been identified in 89% of inflammatory myofibroblastic tumor in the bladder, as exemplified here. ALK-1 overexpression correlates with identification by fluorescence in situ hybridization of a fusion gene resulting from translocation of the ALK gene on chromosome 2p23 to the clathrin heavy chain region on chromosome 17q23. Bladder leiomyosarcomas and rhabdomyosarcomas exhibit neither ALK-1 staining nor translocation of the ALK-1 gene

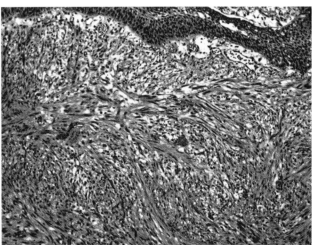

Fig. 4.210 Postoperative spindle cell nodule. Histologically, the nodules are composed of intersecting fascicles of uniform plump spindle cells with delicate vessels, focal hyalinization, and moderate collagen deposition

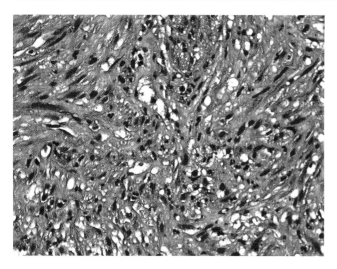

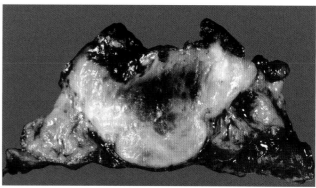

Fig. 4.213 Leiomyoma. Most are well circumscribed white nodules without necrosis, ranging from 1.6 to 5.8 cm in diameter (*see* MacLennan GT, Resnick MI, Bostwick DG, 2003. With permission)

Fig. 4.211 Postoperative spindle cell nodule. The spindle cells have variable amounts of eosinophilic cytoplasm. The nuclei vary only slightly in size and there is no significant cytologic atypia. The number of mitotic figures ranges from 1 to 25 per 10 HPF; no abnormal mitotic figures are seen. Surface ulceration is always present; acute inflammatory cells are found in the ulcer bed, as well as scattered chronic inflammatory cells in deeper areas

4.11 Benign Soft Tissue Neoplasms

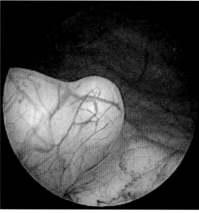

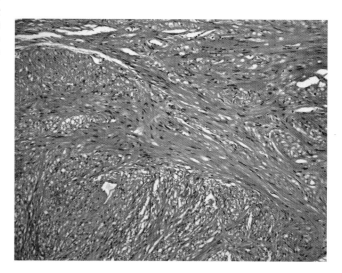

Fig. 4.214 Leiomyoma. Leiomyoma consists of intersecting bundles of smooth muscle cells with oval to cigar-shaped, centrally located and blunt-ended nuclei, and moderate to abundant eosinophilic cytoplasm. Cell nuclei lack significant nuclear atypia and mitotic activity. Typically, cellularity is limited, and myxoid change and necrosis are absent

Fig. 4.212 Leiomyoma. This is one of the commonest benign bladder neoplasms. Most protrude into the bladder lumen and are covered by normal mucosa, as does this one, viewed endoscopically. Some are predominantly in the detrusor muscle, and others extend outside the bladder (*Image courtesy of* Lee Ponsky, MD)

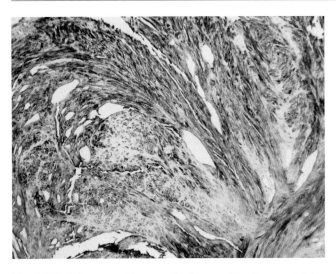

Fig. 4.215 Leiomyoma. Tumor cells show positive immunostaining for desmin, a smooth muscle marker

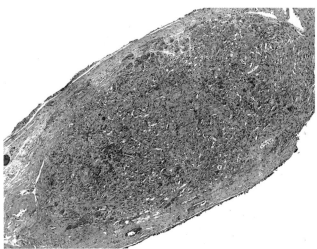

Fig. 4.217 Capillary hemangioma. Capillary hemangioma is less common than cavernous hemangioma in the bladder. The tumor shows lobular growth. It is composed of plump endothelial cells lining vascular spaces with small inconspicuous lumens

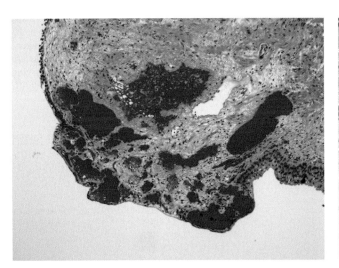

Fig. 4.216 Cavernous hemangioma. Most bladder hemangiomas present with hematuria; endoscopically, they appear as sessile, blue, elevated mucosal nodules on the posterior and lateral walls of the bladder, usually less than 7 mm in diameter. Microscopically, they resemble hemangiomas elsewhere. The commonest type is cavernous hemangioma, shown here, composed of large, dilated, blood-filled vessels lined by small, inconspicuous, endothelial cells

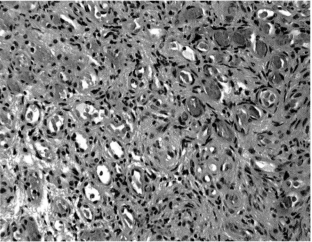

Fig. 4.218 Capillary hemangioma. Some vascular lumens are inconspicuous; others are well-canalized and lined by flattened endothelium

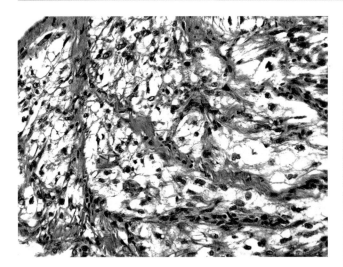

Fig. 4.219 Perivascular epithelioid cell tumor (PECOMA). The PECOMA family is a group of mesenchymal tumors composed of histologically and immunohistochemically distinctive perivascular epithelioid cells. Rare examples occur in the bladder. Tumors are composed of sheets and fascicles of epithelioid and spindled cells with clear to eosinophilic cytoplasm, separated by delicate strands of vascular stroma. Mitotic figures are inconspicuous

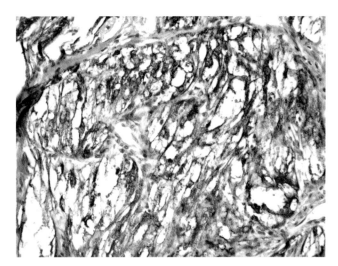

Fig. 4.220 Perivascular epithelioid cell tumor (PECOMA). Tumor cells of bladder PECOMA show positive immunostaining for HMB-45 (shown here) and smooth muscle actin, but negative immunostaining for S-100 protein, Melan-A, desmin, and pancytokeratin

4.12 Malignant Soft Tissue Neoplasms

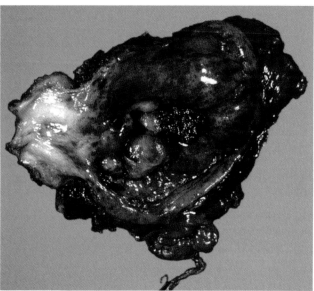

Fig. 4.221 Leiomyosarcoma of bladder. Leiomyosarcoma is the commonest malignant mesenchymal tumor of the urinary bladder in adults. It arises most often in the dome of the bladder, and less frequently in the lateral walls. It is typically large and polypoid with surface ulceration, and usually infiltrates all layers of the bladder wall. Cut surfaces are firm or fleshy, with a fibrous or myxoid appearance, and with varying amounts of hemorrhage and necrosis (*see* MacLennan GT, Resnick MI, Bostwick DG, 2003. With permission)

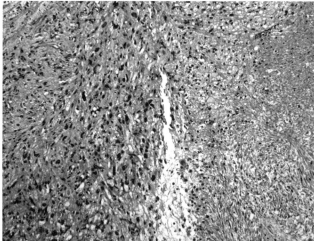

Fig. 4.222 Leiomyosarcoma of bladder. Tumors are composed of interlacing bundles and fascicles of elongated, eosinophilic cytoplasmic processes and spindled to elongate hyperchromatic nuclei. High-grade lesions have significant nuclear pleomorphism with hyperchromasia and irregular nuclear membranes, and may show abundant necrosis, as in the image shown here

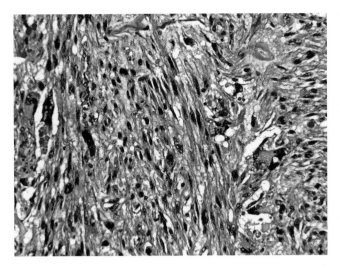

Fig. 4.223 Leiomyosarcoma of bladder. High-grade leiomyosarcomas exhibit pleomorphic nuclei, often with macronucleoli, interspersed with some multinucleate giant cells. The pleomorphism of high-grade leiomyosarcoma is usually evident even at low power, along with necrosis and infiltration of the muscularis propria

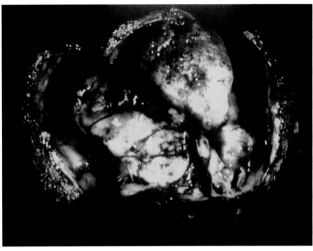

Fig. 4.225 Rhabdomyosarcoma. Rhabdomyosarcoma is the most common type of bladder sarcoma in children. Bladder rhabdomyosarcoma is classically a polypoid gelatinous and lobulated mass protruding into the bladder lumen, with variable amounts of hemorrhage and necrosis. This shiny, lobulated, grape-like appearance prompted the use of the descriptive term "sarcoma botryoides." Most tumors are covered by urothelium (*see* MacLennan GT, Resnick MI, Bostwick DG, 2003. With permission)

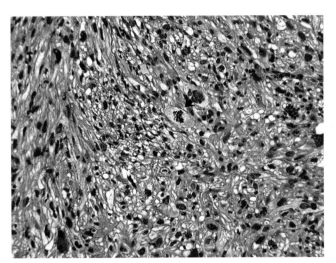

Fig. 4.224 Leiomyosarcoma of bladder. Frequent and often bizarre mitotic figures (*arrow*) are a common finding in high-grade tumors

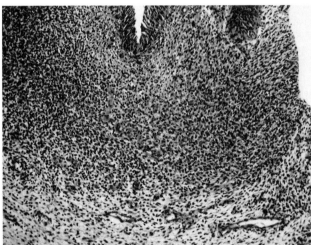

Fig. 4.226 Rhabdomyosarcoma (RMS). The majority of rhabdomyosarcomas are of embryonal type, a category that includes conventional embryonal rhabdomyosarcoma and two variants – botryoid rhabdomyosarcoma and spindle cell rhabdomyosarcoma. Alveolar rhabdomyosarcoma is rare in the bladder. The botryoid subtype of embryonal RMS is characterized by a "cambium" layer, or condensed layer of small round rhabdomyoblasts under the intact epithelium, as shown here. Much of the underlying tumor bulk may consist of mixtures of paucicellular myxoid tumor and more cellular areas

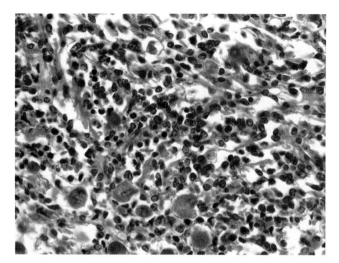

Fig. 4.227 Rhabdomyosarcoma. Embryonal rhabdomyosarcoma is usually composed of small dark round, ovoid, or spindle-shaped cells with minimal cytoplasm, admixed with a variable proportion of cells resembling rhabdomyoblasts

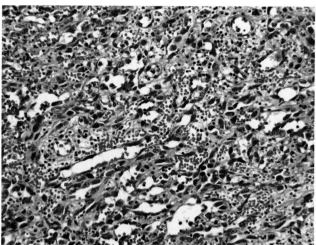

Fig. 4.229 Angiosarcoma. Angiosarcoma of the bladder is composed of anastomosing vascular channels lined by abnormal endothelial cells that are often pleomorphic with large hyperchromatic nuclei, prominent nucleoli and abundant mitotic figures. The malignant endothelial cells may protrude into the lumen, imparting a hobnail appearance. There may be little or no intervening stroma. The vascular channels vary in size, from capillaries to sinusoidal spaces

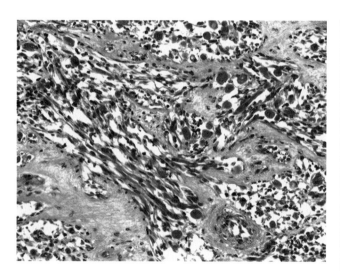

Fig. 4.228 Rhabdomyosarcoma. Well differentiated tumor cells are large round or oval cells with abundant eosinophilic cytoplasm, containing granular material or stringy or filamentous material. Elongated cytoplasmic processes may impart an appearance of striated muscle. Cross-striations can be seen in about half of cases

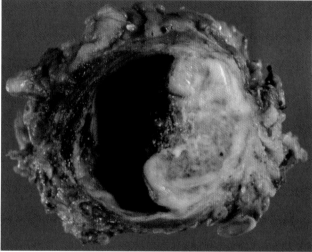

Fig. 4.230 Malignant fibrous histiocytoma. Tumors are typically bulky and nodular, and involve all layers of the bladder as well as perivesical soft tissues (*see* MacLennan GT, Resnick MI, Bostwick DG, 2003. With permission)

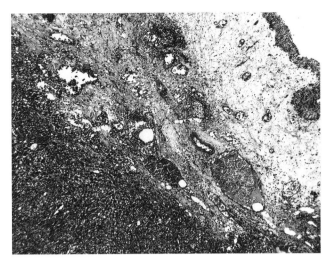

Fig. 4.231 Malignant fibrous histiocytoma. A spindle cell neoplasm obliterates tissues deep to the lamina propria

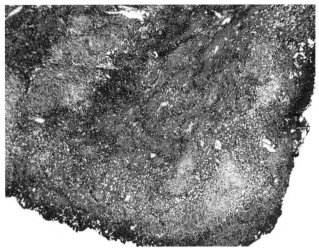

Fig. 4.233 Osteosarcoma. Osteosarcoma arising in the bladder is typically a solitary, large, polypoid, gritty, often deeply invasive, variably hemorrhagic mass, often located in the trigone. This image is from a transurethrally resected high-grade urothelial carcinoma, partially visible at upper left, that had large components of osteosarcoma and malignant spindle cells, and consequently was best diagnosed as sarcomatoid carcinoma

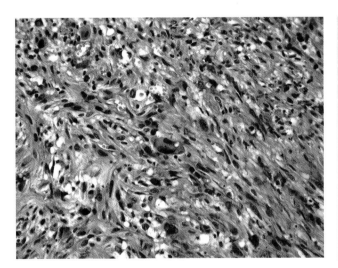

Fig. 4.232 Malignant fibrous histiocytoma. Tumor is composed of pleomorphic and spindled cells and multinucleated giant cells with abundant mitotic activity. The differential for such tumors is broad and includes sarcomatoid carcinoma of the bladder, but an epithelial component immunoreactive to cytokeratin and epithelial membrane antigen is usually identifiable in sarcomatoid carcinoma, but not in malignant fibrous histiocytoma

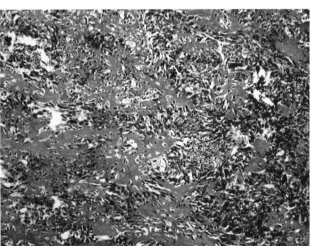

Fig. 4.234 Osteosarcoma. Higher power view of the tumor shown in Fig. 4.233. This part of the tumor consists of cytologically malignant cells surrounding variably calcified, woven bone lamellae. Cytologic atypia of the surrounding tumor cells confirms that this is osteosarcoma, rather than stromal osseous metaplasia, which occurs in some urothelial carcinomas

4.13 Malignant Melanoma

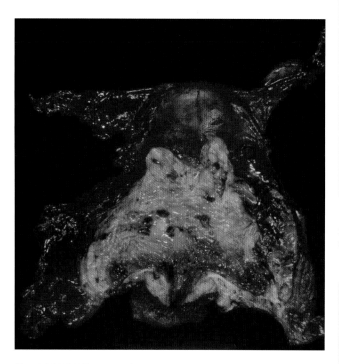

Fig. 4.235 Malignant melanoma. Malignant melanomas found in the bladder may be primary or metastatic; the latter is far more common than the former. This cystectomy specimen contained a primary melanoma, accounting for the scattered areas of dark mucosal pigmentation (*see* MacLennan GT, Resnick MI, Bostwick DG, 2003. With permission)

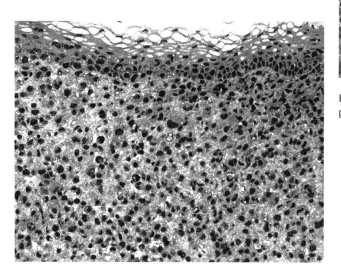

Fig. 4.236 Malignant melanoma. The entire lamina propria is occupied by poorly differentiated malignant cells. Cystectomy specimen contained a primary melanoma, accounting for the scattered areas of dark mucosal pigmentation

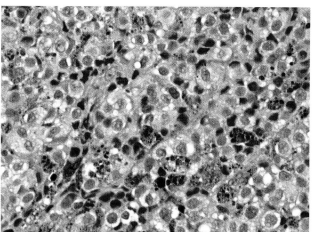

Fig. 4.237 Malignant melanoma. Tumor consists of cells with pleomorphic nuclei, spindle and polygonal cytoplasmic contours, and intracytoplasmic melanin pigment

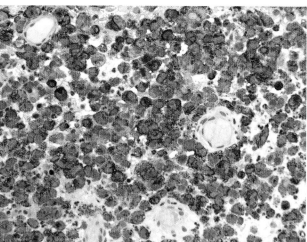

Fig. 4.238 Malignant melanoma. Tumor cells show strong diffusely positive immunostaining with HMB-45, a melanocytic marker

4.14 Germ Cell Neoplasms

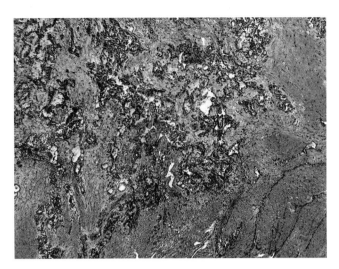

Fig. 4.239 Yolk sac tumor of urachus. Germ cell neoplasms that have been reported to arise in the bladder include dermoid cyst, teratoma, seminoma, choriocarcinoma, and yolk sac tumor. This infiltrating tumor in the dome of the bladder has a complex papillary and glandular architecture and a myxoid background

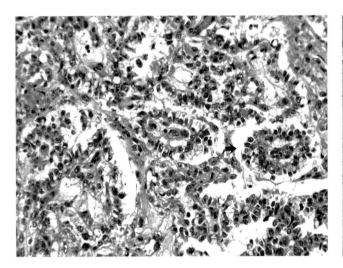

Fig. 4.240 Yolk sac tumor of urachus. Tumor shows an endodermal sinus pattern. A Schiller-Duval body is evident (*arrow*). Tumor cells showed positive immunostaining for α-fetoprotein

4.15 Hematopoietic and Lymphoid Neoplasms

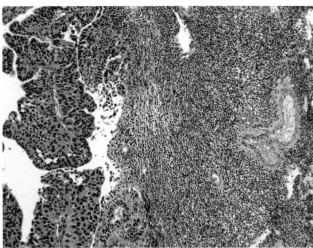

Fig. 4.241 Lymphoma. Lymphoma in the bladder may be primary or a component of systemic disease. Endoscopically, lymphoma forms solitary or multiple nodules in the mucosa, usually covered by intact urothelium. Occasionally, lymphoma coexists with papillary urothelial neoplasms, as in the case shown here: noninvasive papillary urothelial carcinoma is at left, and small lymphocytic lymphoma diffusely involves the lamina propria at right

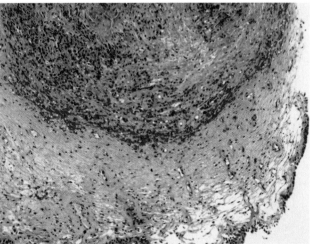

Fig. 4.242 Multiple myeloma. Patient was a 50-year-old man with AIDS, and an 8-year history of anaplastic multiple myeloma, who developed bilateral ureteral obstruction and a large pelvis mass. At cystoscopy, bladder had multiple nodular masses, which were biopsied, and showed cellular infiltrates in the lamina propria

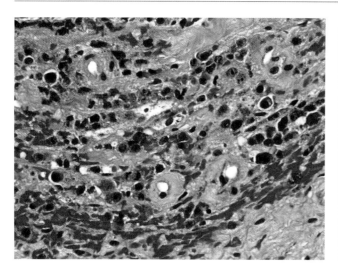

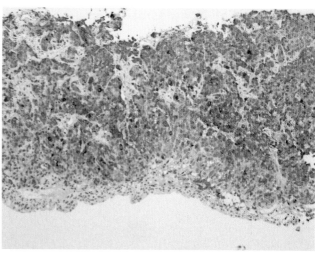

Fig. 4.243 Multiple myeloma. High-power view of infiltrate noted in Fig. 4.242. Diagnosis was lambda-restricted plasma cell infiltrate consistent with involvement by multiple myeloma. Biopsy of the retroperitoneal/pelvic mass showed similar findings

Fig. 4.245 Bladder involvement by direct extension of adjacent cancer. The cancer shown in Fig. 4.244 shows positive immunostaining for prostatic acid phosphatase, consistent with direct extension of prostatic adenocarcinoma into the bladder

4.16 Cancers Involving Bladder by Direct Extension or Metastasis

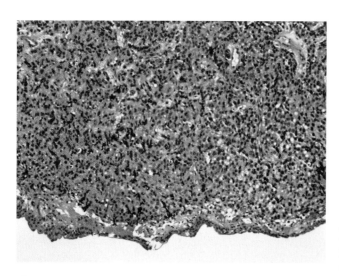

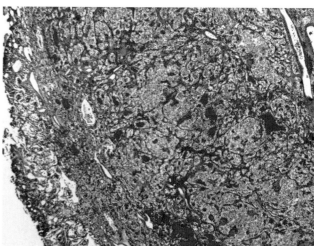

Fig. 4.246 Bladder involvement by metastatic carcinoma. Patient had a radical nephrectomy for high-grade clear cell renal cell carcinoma that had involved the renal vein. Six months later, patient developed hematuria, and was found to have a red mucosal nodule near the orifice on the side of the nephrectomy. The nodule is composed of clear cell carcinoma, consistent with vascular metastasis, possibly via ureteral veins

Fig. 4.244 Bladder involvement by direct extension of adjacent cancer. This is an example of local extension of prostatic adenocarcinoma into bladder. The lamina propria is diffusely infiltrated by a poorly differentiated neoplasm

4.17 Congenital Urethral Malformations

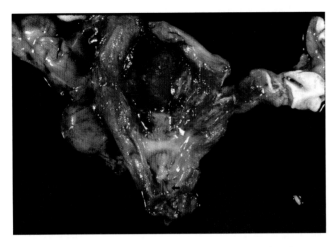

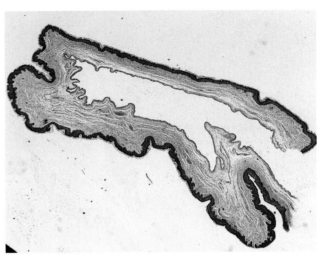

Fig. 4.249 Urethral meatal cyst. Lesion is an uninflamed epithelial-lined cyst

Fig. 4.247 Posterior urethral valves. Posterior urethral valves are mucosal folds located in the region of the verumontanum; they are the commonest cause of congenital urethral obstruction. Various forms of valves are described: a diaphragm with a central pinhole, and bivalvular forms as represented in this photograph are the commonest. Regardless of their form, they can cause marked and even life-threatening bladder outlet obstruction, with upper tract deterioration

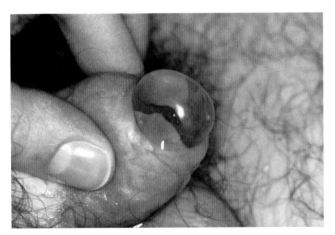

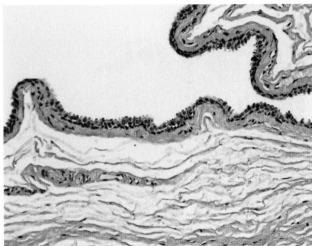

Fig. 4.248 Urethral meatal cyst. Urethral meatal cyst is a median raphe cyst arising at the urethral meatus. This cyst may be unilocular or multilocular (*see* MacLennan GT, Resnick MI, Bostwick DG, 2003. With permission)

Fig. 4.250 Urethral meatal cyst. These cysts are lined by pseudostratified columnar epithelium and contain serous or mucinous material

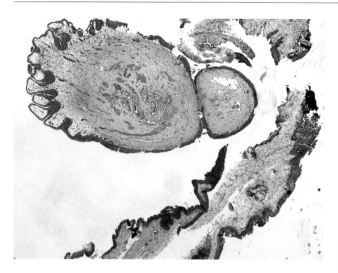

Fig. 4.251 Congenital urethral polyp. An uncommon lesion found only in males, most of whom present between the ages of 6 and 9 years with obstructive or irritative voiding symptoms, hematuria, or urethral bleeding. Some of these polyps arise in the distal urethra, but most lesions originate in the prostatic urethra near the verumontanum. If the stalk of the polyp is long enough, as in this case, the polyp prolapses down into the penile urethra

4.18 Nonneoplastic Urethral Lesions

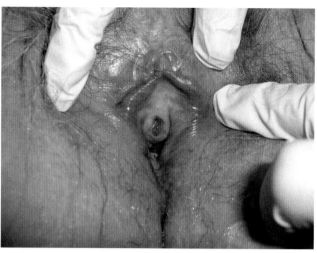

Fig. 4.253 Urethral caruncle. This lesion occurs only in females, most of whom are postmenopausal. The etiology is uncertain, but may be related to mucosal prolapse and/or obstructive/inflammatory changes in paraurethral glands and stroma. The lesion may be asymptomatic, or may cause pain or bloody spotting. Grossly, caruncle is a red or pink, polypoid or pedunculated lesion immediately adjacent to the urethral meatus (*Image courtesy* of Howard Goldman, MD)

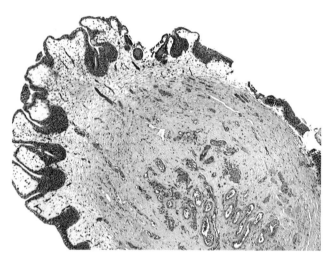

Fig. 4.252 Congenital urethral polyp. The polyp is composed of a stalk containing blood vessels, loose fibrous tissue, and sometimes smooth muscle, covered by urothelium, which may show reactive or reparative features, or ulceration

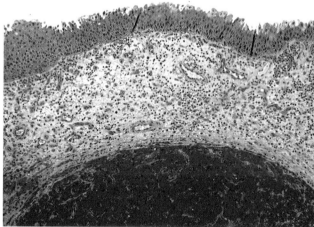

Fig. 4.254 Urethral caruncle. Lesion is composed of variable components of proliferative epithelium, neovascularity, and inflammatory infiltrate. Evidence of recent or remote stromal hemorrhage is often evident. Reactive atypical stromal cells and glandular elements derived from preexisting paraurethral glands are sometimes present. Caruncles have no association with neoplasia

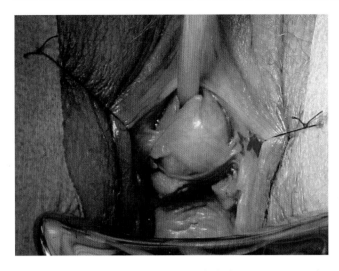

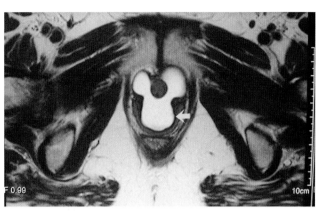

Fig. 4.255 Infected Skene's gland cyst. The lesion presents as a painful periurethral swelling. Skene's glands (periurethral glands) are tubuloalveolar mucus glands that line the urethral wall, located posterolaterally in the mid and distal third of the urethra. Most drain into the distal urethra. Blocked drainage results in swelling due to mucus accumulation and/or infection (*Image courtesy of* Howard Goldman, MD)

Fig. 4.257 Urethral diverticulum. This is a localized variably sized saccular outpouching of urethral mucosa into the anterior vaginal wall. Although it may occasionally be congenital in origin, the vast majority are probably acquired as a result of repetitive infection and inflammation superimposed on obstruction and dilatation of paraurethral glands. Urethral pain, drainage of urine or purulent material, or irritative voiding symptoms draw attention to the lesion, which may be visible and palpable. In this MRI scan, the white structure indicated by the *arrow* is a periurethral fluid collection (*Image courtesy of* Howard Goldman, MD)

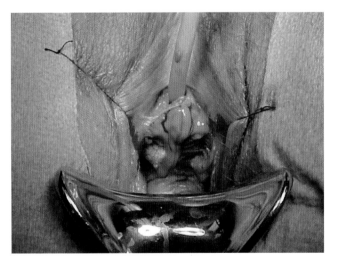

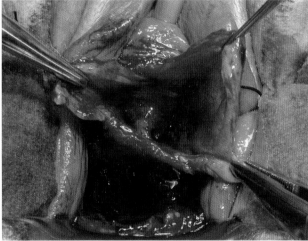

Fig. 4.256 Infected Skene's gland cyst. The lesion contains purulent material. The relationship between Skene's gland infection and urethral diverticulum is discussed in the section concerning urethral diverticulum (*Image courtesy of* Howard Goldman, MD)

Fig. 4.258 Urethral diverticulum. This is the interior of the suburethral diverticulum shown in Fig. 4.257. A Foley catheter is in the urethra, which lies at the base of the opened cystic lesion (*Image courtesy of* Howard Goldman, MD)

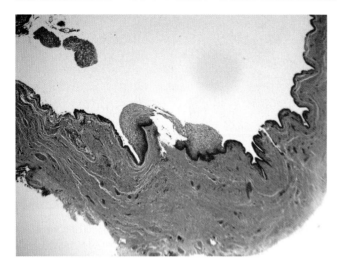

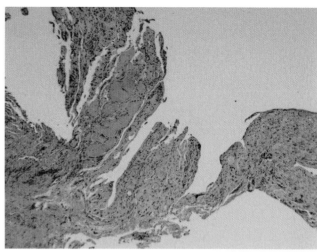

Fig. 4.259 Urethral diverticulum. The diverticulum is a fibrous-walled cyst lined by epithelium

Fig. 4.261 Urethral diverticulum, with nephrogenic metaplasia of lining epithelium. This is a reactive process, discussed in Figs. 4.58–4.61. The lesion is vaguely polypoid

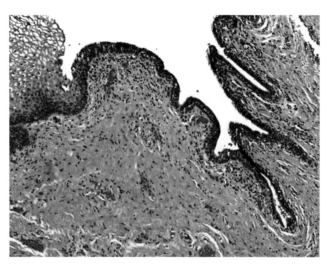

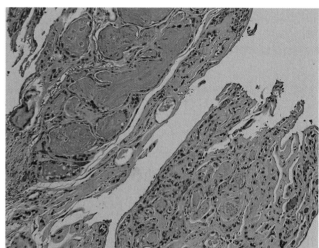

Fig. 4.260 Urethral diverticulum. Usually, there is acute and chronic inflammation in the soft tissues surrounding the diverticulum. Diverticula are lined by urothelium; however, the development of squamous, glandular, or nephrogenic metaplasia is quite common. Stones sometimes form in diverticula, and various types of carcinoma within diverticula have been reported: urothelial, squamous, conventional adenocarcinoma, or clear cell adenocarcinoma

Fig. 4.262 Urethral diverticulum, with nephrogenic metaplasia of lining epithelium. The metaplastic process forms tubules lined by flat nondescript cuboidal epithelium, and containing mucin. The absence of nuclear atypia and mitotic activity favor a reactive process, rather than adenocarcinoma

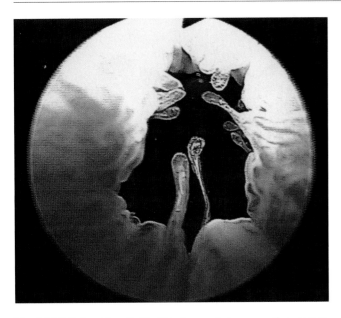

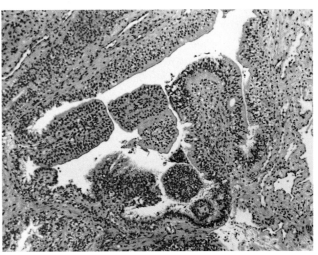

Fig. 4.265 Polypoid urethritis. At higher power, the lesion consists of papillary/polypoid structures composed of abundant edematous stroma supported by prominent blood vessels and infiltrated by acute and chronic inflammatory cells. The overlying urothelium is benign, but may show reactive or metaplastic changes

Fig. 4.263 Polypoid urethritis. This is regarded as a reactive process, often attributed to recurrent infection or the presence of a foreign body, such as an indwelling catheter. In this endoscopic image, fronds of edematous mucosa are present at the bladder neck in a female (*Image courtesy of* Howard Goldman, MD)

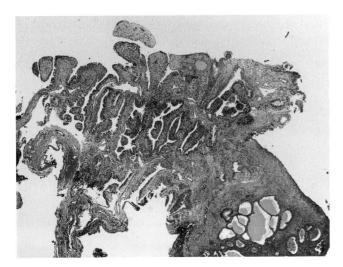

Fig. 4.264 Polypoid urethritis. The lesion has arisen in the prostatic urethra (benign prostatic tissue is present at lower right). Its papillary architecture mimics that of a papillary urothelial neoplasm endoscopically, prompting transurethral resection

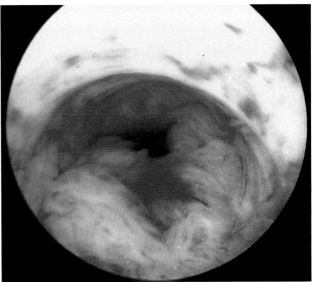

Fig. 4.266 Urethral condyloma acuminatum. These lesions are usually but not always associated with similar lesions in the mucocutaneous surfaces of anus, perineum, or external genitalia. Although easily recognized in this urethroscopic view, urethral condyloma may be hard to recognize if they are flat rather than papillary (*Image courtesy of* Martin Resnick, MD)

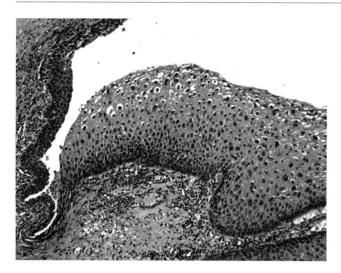

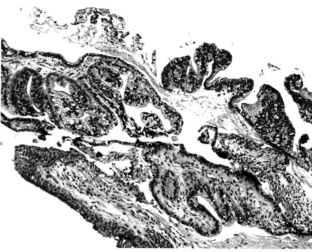

Fig. 4.267 Urethral condyloma acuminatum. The squamous epithelium is hyperplastic but shows somewhat delayed maturation. The nuclei of the squamous cells are eccentric, hyperchromatic, and moderately pleomorphic (koilocytic atypia), and many have clear perinuclear halos due to cytoplasmic retraction away from the nucleus

Fig. 4.269 Ectopic prostatic tissue in urethra. In contrast to polypoid urethritis, the papillary fronds that comprise this lesion are lined by typical prostatic acinar-type epithelium with small basally located round or oval nuclei, lacking nucleoli, and clear or eosinophilic apical cytoplasm

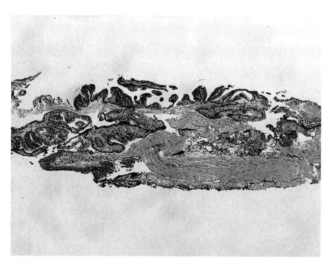

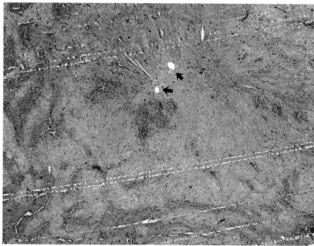

Fig. 4.268 Ectopic prostatic tissue in urethra. Ectopic prostate tissue may be found incidentally in the urethra during endoscopic procedures, usually appearing as delicate papillary structures or roughened mucosa

Fig. 4.270 Acquired urethral stricture. Urethral strictures can occur at any point in the urethra, due to a broad spectrum of etiologic entities, including infection and prior trauma; some are idiopathic in origin. The endpoint is urethral scarring and diminution of the caliber of the urethra. The stricture shown here followed an endoscopic procedure; the lumen is reduced to two tiny pinholes (*arrows*) surrounded by fibrosis and chronic inflammation

4.19 Urethral Neoplasms

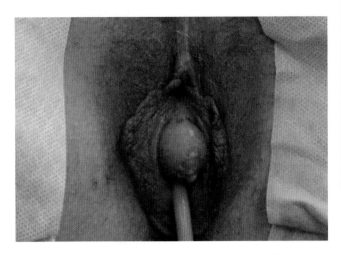

Fig. 4.271 Leiomyoma of urethra. Paraurethral or urethral leiomyomas occur almost exclusively in women. They generally present as an anterior vaginal wall mass or a mass that protrudes from the urethral meatus, as exemplified here. This lesion was resected locally and its histology was typical of leiomyoma (*Image courtesy of* Howard Goldman, MD)

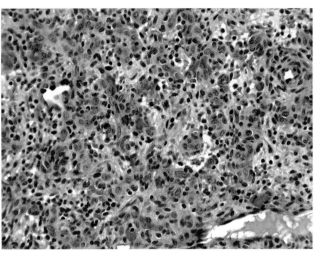

Fig. 4.273 Lobular capillary hemangioma of urethra. The vascular lumens are very small and inconspicuous; only a few are canalized. Lumens are enclosed by plump endothelial cells

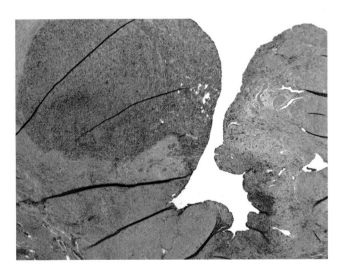

Fig. 4.272 Lobular capillary hemangioma of urethra. Lesion was present in a urethral diverticulum. It has a well circumscribed edge in keeping with a lobular growth pattern

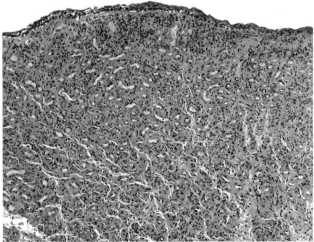

Fig. 4.274 Capillary hemangioma of urethra. Lesion is a capillary hemangioma, consisting of abundant closely spaced small blood vessels whose lumens are well-canalized and lined by flattened endothelium

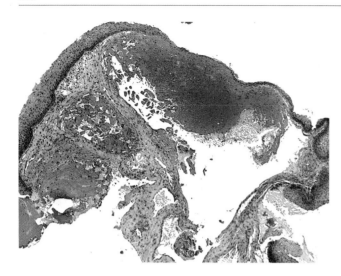

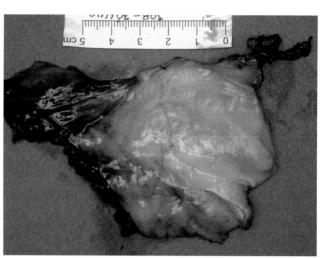

Fig. 4.275 Cavernous hemangioma of urethra, with papillary endothelial hyperplasia. Lesion is composed of large dilated blood-filled vessels lined in most areas by small inconspicuous endothelial cells. In some areas, there are coarse papillae with fibrin cores

Fig. 4.277 Periurethral aggressive angiomyxoma. This is an uncommon neoplasm of the perineum and genital area. It is usually poorly circumscribed, and can be quite large. Its cut surface is usually smooth and homogeneous, and the tumor is soft and edematous or gelatinous. The lesion shown here was adjacent to the urethra in a female. Tumors are usually locally infiltrative, and sometimes recur after excision

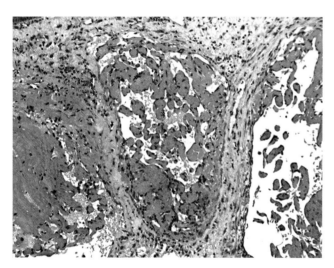

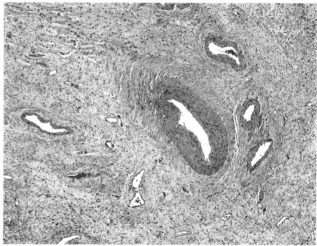

Fig. 4.276 Cavernous hemangioma of urethra, with papillary endothelial hyperplasia. Innumerable small papillae project into the lumen; they consist of collagenized fibrin cores lined by a single layer of bland endothelial cells. This is a form of organizing thrombus. The simple fact that the process appears to be confined to a vascular lumen helps to differentiate it from angiosarcoma

Fig. 4.278 Periurethral aggressive angiomyxoma. Lesion is composed of blood vessels of variable caliber, dispersed in a hypocellular myxoid stroma sparsely populated by evenly dispersed spindled and stellate cells

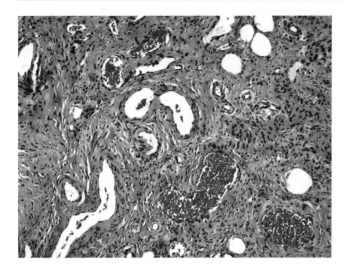

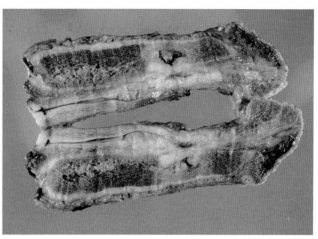

Fig. 4.279 Periurethral aggressive angiomyxoma. The spindled and stellate tumor cells have small oval uniform nuclei with dense chromatin and indistinct nucleoli. They lack pleomorphism and mitotic figures are absent or rare. In all cases, arteries, veins, venules, arterioles and capillaries are abundantly and randomly distributed throughout

Fig. 4.281 Primary urothelial carcinoma of urethra. It is rare to develop invasive urothelial carcinoma in the urethra, without a prior urothelial carcinoma elsewhere in the urinary system. Many such patients have a predisposing condition such as diverticulum, fistula, or stricture. A gray-white poorly circumscribed tumor is evident in this specimen, deeply invasive into the adjacent corpora cavernosa

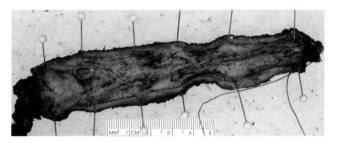

Fig. 4.280 Urothelial carcinoma in situ. This patient was at high risk of having urothelial carcinoma in the urethra, having previously undergone cystoprostatectomy and unilateral nephroureterectomy for widespread multifocal carcinoma in situ and superficially invasive high-grade urothelial carcinoma. The urethra contained many areas of carcinoma in situ, but no invasive tumor (*Image courtesy of* Francisco Paras, MD)

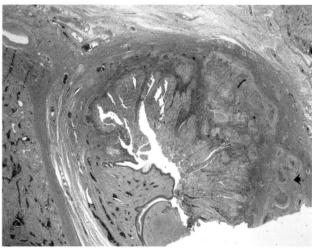

Fig. 4.282 Primary urothelial carcinoma of urethra. Section from the lesion shown in Fig. 4.281. A papillary carcinoma protrudes into the urethral lumen and infiltrates corpus spongiosum (*arrow*)

Fig. 4.283 Primary squamous cell carcinoma of urethra. Patient was a 27-year-old male, with no prior history of malignancy. The gray-white lesion (*arrow*) infiltrated periurethral soft tissues. There were no known predisposing conditions prior to discovery of this lesion (*see* MacLennan et al. 2003. With permission)

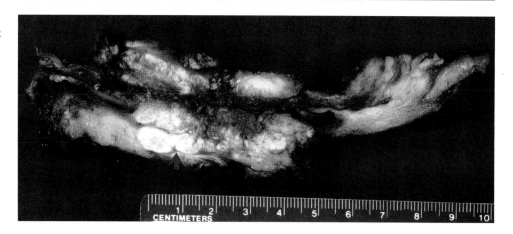

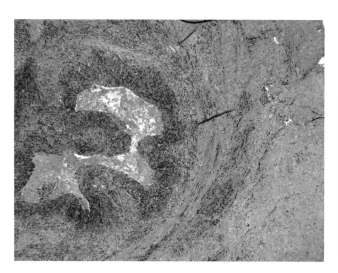

Fig. 4.284 Primary squamous cell carcinoma of urethra. Patient underwent excision of a lesion that was clinically a suburethral diverticulum. The lining of the diverticulum was thickened and irregular, an unexpected finding

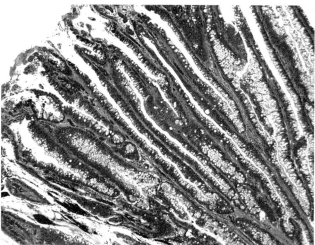

Fig. 4.286 Villous adenoma of urethra. Female patient who presented with urethral bleeding. A polypoid urethral lesion was resected. It is composed of long, delicate, fingerlike structures. No invasive component was present

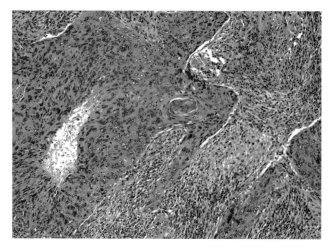

Fig. 4.285 Primary squamous cell carcinoma of urethra. Another section from the specimen shown in Fig. 4.284. Infiltrating squamous cell carcinoma was found, shown here

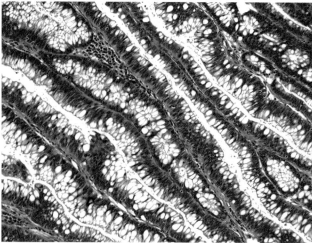

Fig. 4.287 Villous adenoma of urethra. The lesion is similar in appearance to colonic villous adenomas

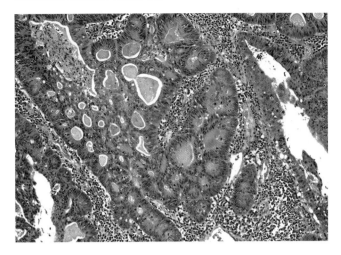

Fig. 4.288 Primary adenocarcinoma of urethra. Women are more prone to develop urethral adenocarcinoma than men. It may arise in sites of glandular metaplasia or in periurethral glands, and often there is a setting of chronic inflammation or irritation. Tumors tend to be polypoid or papillary. Urethral adenocarcinomas have predominantly glandular architecture, as in the image shown here; some are papillary, and some are mucin-producing adenocarcinomas

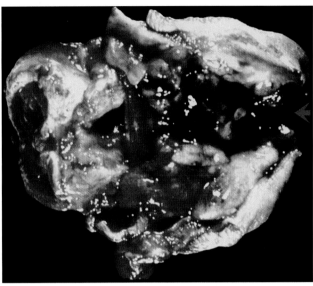

Fig. 4.290 Urethral melanoma. A darkly pigmented nodular neoplasm is present in the distal urethra (*see* "Penis and scrotum" [page 930] in Bostwick and Cheng 2008. With permission)

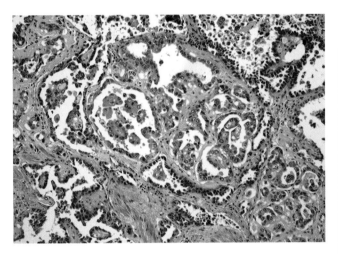

Fig. 4.289 Clear cell adenocarcinoma. This malignancy, almost certainly of urothelial origin, can arise primarily in the urethra. It forms polypoid to papillary masses ranging from 0.6 to 7 cm in diameter. The tumor cells most often have tubulocystic and papillary architecture; growth in diffuse sheets is less common (*see* Figs. 4.168 and 4.169). Tumor cells may be flat, cuboidal or hobnail type. Most tumors have at least some cells with abundant clear to faintly eosinophilic cytoplasm

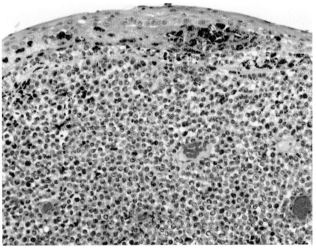

Fig. 4.291 Urethral melanoma. The lamina propria is entirely occupied by sheets of poorly differentiated cells, many of which contain dark-brown melanin granules, particularly those just below the surface urothelium

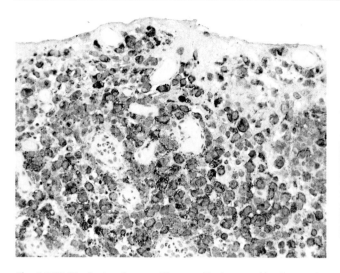

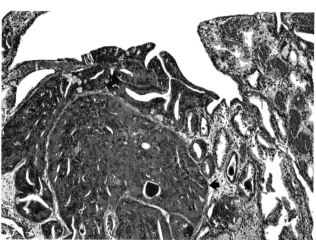

Fig. 4.292 Urethral melanoma. Tumor cells show positive immunostaining for melanin marker HMB-45

Fig. 4.293 Prostatic adenocarcinoma arising in a prostatic urethral polyp. This aggregate of small crowded and fused glands (*arrow*) lined by cells with large hyperchromatic nuclei and prominent nucleoli stands out in sharp contrast to the architecture of the prostatic urethral polyp in which it arose

Prostate

The prostate surrounds the urethra in the region between the bladder neck and the urogenital diaphragm. Its ducts and the ejaculatory ducts empty into the urethra. Maldevelopments of the prostate are rare. The prostate is a problematic organ that arguably accounts for more doctor's visits by men than any other organ. Inflammatory conditions are troublesome from late youth onward, and problems with benign prostatic hyperplasia and prostate cancer are remarkably common in older men.

5.1 Normal Findings

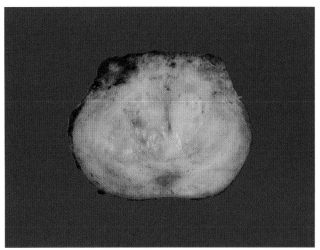

Fig. 5.2 Cross section of the prostate. Note distinct peripheral and transition zone

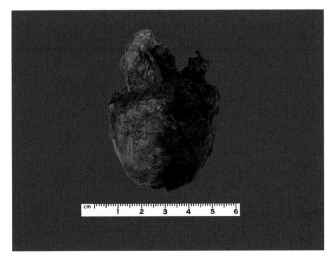

Fig. 5.1 The prostate. This is a specimen from a patient who underwent radical prostatectomy for prostate cancer. The left side is inked black; the right side is inked yellow. The prostate is a muscular, walnut-sized gland that lies just below the bladder. The seminal vesicles are paired accessory sex glands located in the posterolateral aspect of the prostate

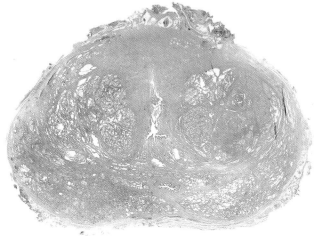

Fig. 5.3 Whole mount cross section of the prostate. The prostate is composed of tubules and acinar structures supported by fibromuscular stroma

G. MacLennan and L. Cheng, *Atlas of Genitourinary Pathology*,
DOI: 10.1007/978-1-84882-395-2_5, © Springer-Verlag London Limited 2011

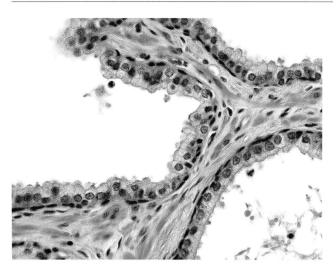

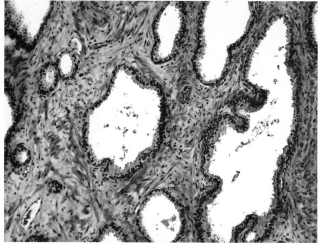

Fig. 5.4 Normal prostatic acinus. The epithelial lining is composed of secretory cells and basal cells. The secretory cells are cuboidal to columnar with pale to clear cytoplasm. Nuclei are small and round with inconspicuous nucleoli. The normal acini are surrounded by outer layer of flattened basal cells and have smooth rounded contours. The basal cells are elongated with small hyperchromatic nuclei. One of the hallmarks of prostatic adenocarcinoma is the lack of basal cells in malignant acini

Fig. 5.6 Peripheral zone. The acini are lined by columnar cells surrounded by flattened basal cell layers

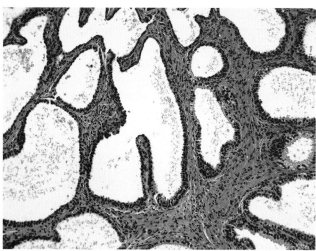

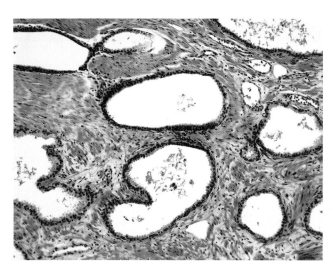

Fig. 5.7 Transition zone. It consists of simple acini in compact stroma

Fig. 5.5 Peripheral zone. It consists of simple acini in a loose stroma. The acini are dilated

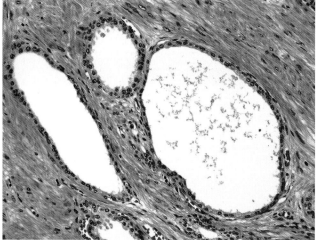

Fig. 5.8 Transition zone. The acini are lined by cuboidal cells. Proteinaceous intraluminal secretion is present

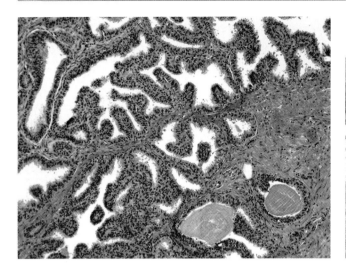

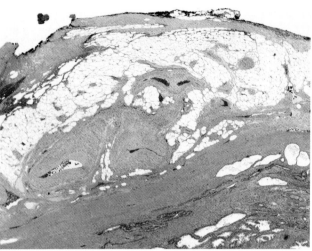

Fig. 5.9 Central zone. Central zone acini are surrounded by compact muscular stroma. The acini are large and complex with intraluminal ridges and papillary infoldings

Fig. 5.11 Neurovascular bundle. Large neurovascular bundles are present in the posterolateral aspect of the prostate, surrounded by abundant adipose tissue. Invasion into periprostatic adipose tissue or large neurovascular bundles is considered extraprostatic extension (pathologic stage pT3a). True prostatic capsule does not exist. Invasion into the peripheral dense fibromuscular stroma does not constitute extraprostatic extension

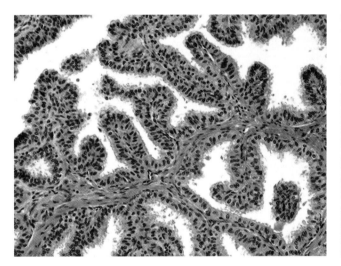

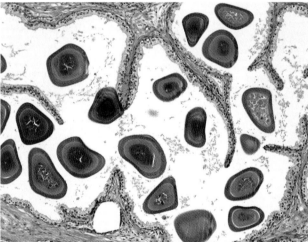

Fig. 5.10 Central zone. The epithelial lining is columnar with small uniform nuclei. Nucleoli are inconspicuous. Basal cell layers are present

Fig. 5.12 Corpora amylacea. These intraluminal eosinophilic secretions have a concentrically lamellated appearance

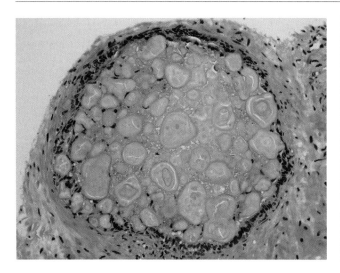

Fig. 5.13 Corpora amylacea. The duct is expanded by eosinophilic concentrical lamellae intermixed with epithelial cells, reminiscent of collagenous spherulosis of the breast

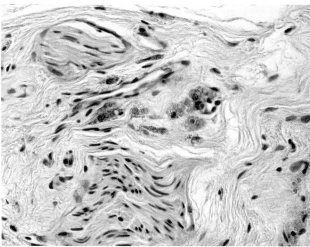

Fig. 5.16 Lipofuscin pigment depositions in the stroma

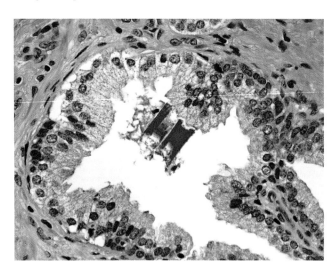

Fig. 5.14 Crystalloids in benign glands. These crystalloids are more commonly seen in malignant glands

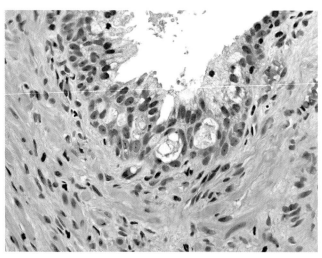

Fig. 5.17 Mucin in benign glands. Atypical basal cells are also noted

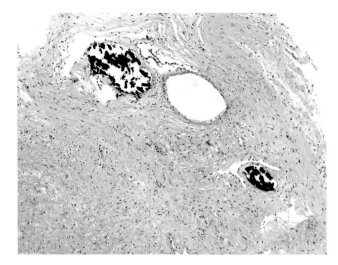

Fig. 5.15 Microcalcifications. Stromal calcification is noted. It is more commonly seen after radiation or hormonal therapy

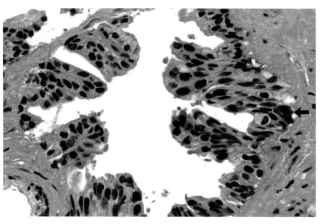

Fig. 5.18 Neuroendocrine cells in benign epithelium. These cells have large intracytoplasmic eosinophilic granules and have been designated "Paneth cell-like change" (PCLC)

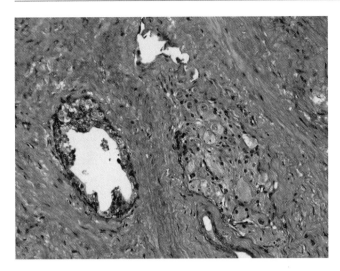

Fig. 5.19 Ganglion cells in the prostate. These cells have voluminous pale cytoplasm with low nuclear to cytoplasmic ratio. Eccentrically located nuclei are present. Prominent nucleoli may be seen

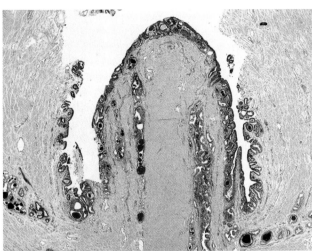

Fig. 5.22 Verumontanum. There is an elevation or protuberance in the posterior urethra where the ejaculatory ducts enter the prostatic urethra

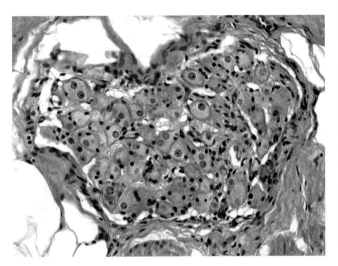

Fig. 5.20 Paraganglion in periprostatic tissue

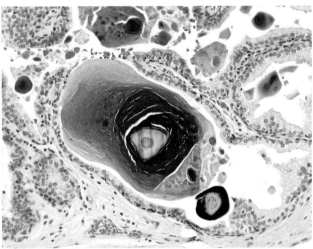

Fig. 5.23 Verumontanum. Corpora amylacea in verumontanum glands often have yellow-gold or orange coloration

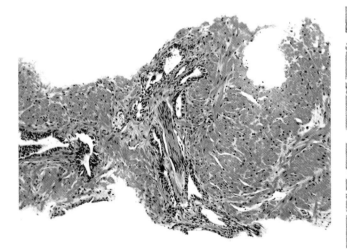

Fig. 5.21 Benign glands abutting a nerve. This is an uncommon finding and must be distinguished from perineural invasion by prostatic adenocarcinoma

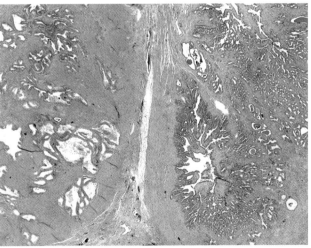

Fig. 5.24 Normal junction between seminal vesicle and prostate proper. The seminal vesicles are paired accessory sex glands located in the posterolateral aspect of the prostate. The glands are complex and convoluted

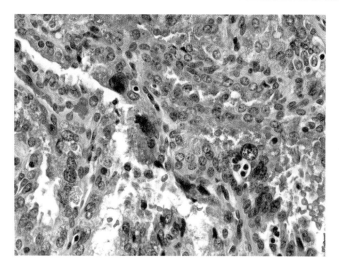

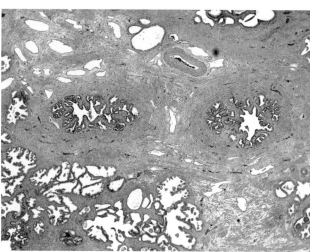

Fig. 5.25 Seminal vesicle. The secretory cells of seminal vesicles contain bright golden lipofuscin granules and have degenerative changes. Some cells may exhibit prominent cytologic atypia including nuclear hyperchromasia, nuclear pleomorphism, multinucleation, and nucleomegaly

Fig. 5.28 Ejaculatory ducts. Paired ejaculatory ducts are surrounded by attenuated thin muscular walls, embedded within the prostatic parenchyma

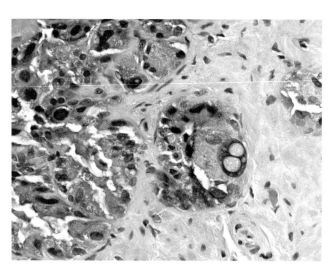

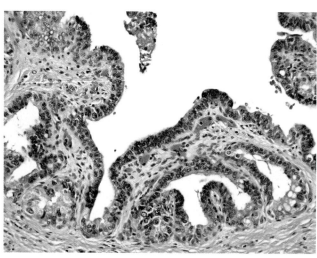

Fig. 5.26 Seminal vesicle. Intranuclear inclusions are noted

Fig. 5.29 Ejaculatory ducts. The epithelial lining is similar to that of the seminal vesicle. Note prominent lipofuscin pigments

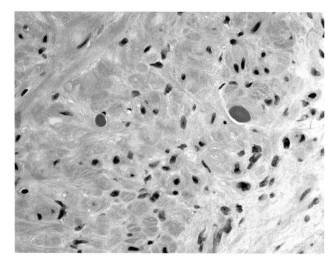

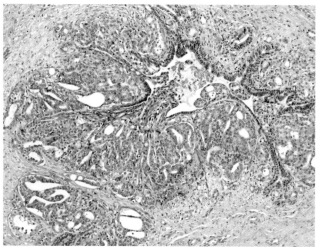

Fig. 5.27 Seminal vesicle. Eosinophilic globules are seen in the muscular wall of seminal vesicles. These hyaline globules probably are derived from degenerated smooth muscle cells

Fig. 5.30 Ejaculatory duct invasion by prostate cancer. This does not qualify for advanced prostate cancer (pT3)

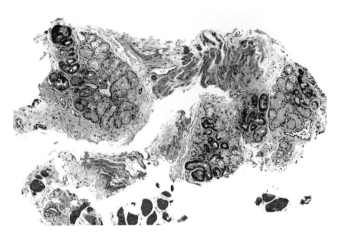

Fig. 5.31 Cowper's gland. Cowper's glands are small, paired bulbomembranous urethral glands that are occasionally sampled inadvertently at the time of needle biopsy. They are composed of well-circumscribed lobules of closely packed acini

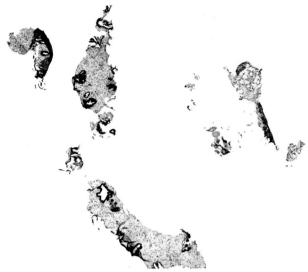

Fig. 5.34 Cowper's gland. Immunostain for prostate-specific antigen is negative in Cowper's gland epithelium. The adjacent benign prostatic epithelium shows positive immunostaining

5.2 Inflammatory Entities

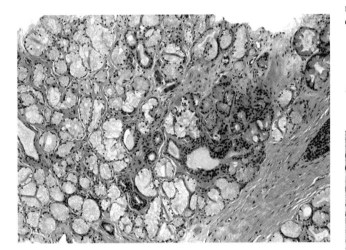

Fig. 5.32 Cowper's gland. These acini are clustered around central ducts and are lined by cytologically benign mucin-producing cells

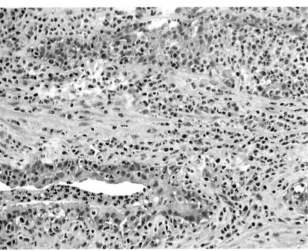

Fig. 5.35 Acute prostatitis. There are diffuse neutrophilic infiltrates in both prostatic epithelium and stroma. The acini are disrupted by the inflammatory process

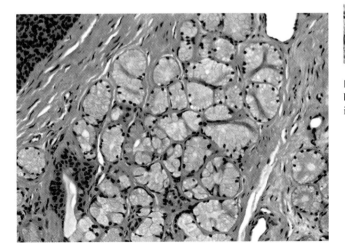

Fig. 5.33 Cowper's gland. The cells have abundant apical mucinous cytoplasm. Nuclei are small with inconspicuous nucleoli

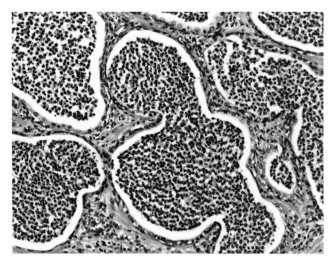

Fig. 5.36 Acute prostatitis. The luminal space is filled with neutrophils

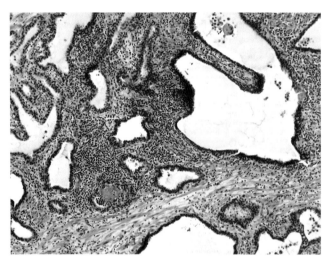

Fig. 5.37 Chronic prostatitis, nonspecific. There is prominent periductal inflammation. The inflammatory infiltrate is composed of lymphocytes and histiocytes

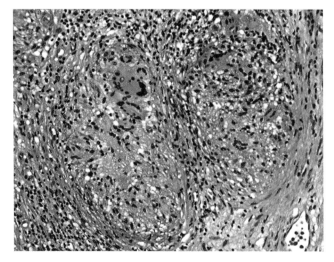

Fig. 5.38 Granulomatous prostatitis, nonspecific. There is a polymorphous infiltrate of lymphocytes, macrophages, plasma cells, neutrophils, multinucleated giant cells, and occasional eosinophils

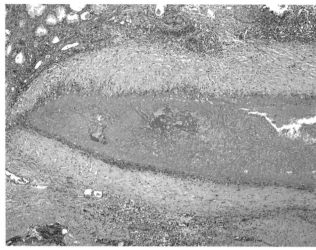

Fig. 5.39 Necrotizing palisading granuloma, status post needle biopsy. There is a central zone of fibrinoid necrosis surrounded by sheets of histiocytes

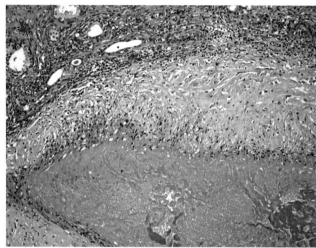

Fig. 5.40 Necrotizing palisading granuloma, status post needle biopsy. This is a higher power view of previous image (*see* Fig. 5.39)

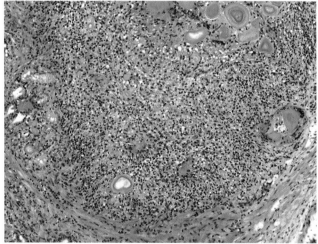

Fig. 5.41 Post-transurethral resection granuloma. The granuloma has a nodular appearance and is well-circumscribed

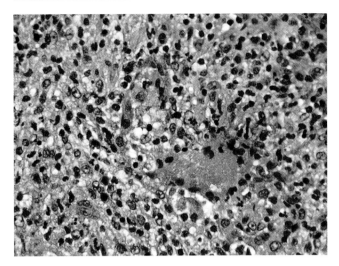

Fig. 5.42 Post-transurethral granuloma. Multinucleated giant cells and sheets of epithelioid histiocytes are present

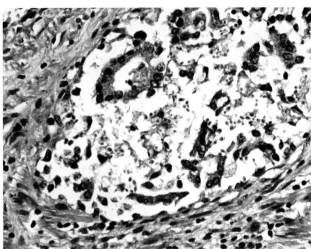

Fig. 5.45 Fungal prostatitis (*Cryptococcosis*). Numerous cryptococcal organisms are present

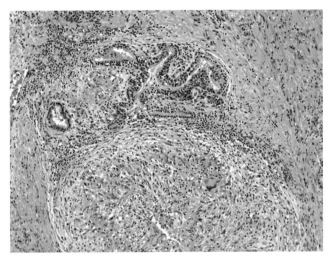

Fig. 5.43 Bacillus Calmette-Guérin (BCG)-induced granuloma. This patient was previously treated with BCG for urothelial carcinoma

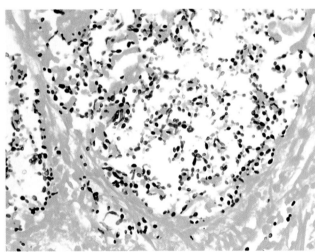

Fig. 5.46 Fungal prostatitis (*Cryptococcosis*). Gomori methenamine silver stain highlights *Cryptococcus neoformans*

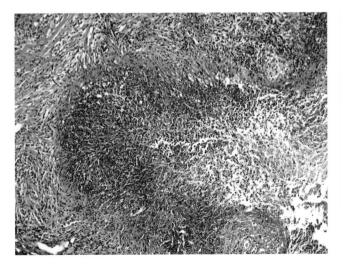

Fig. 5.44 Wegener's granulomatosis. A necrotizing granuloma is present. Histiocytes and fibroblasts are aligned at right angles to the area of central necrosis

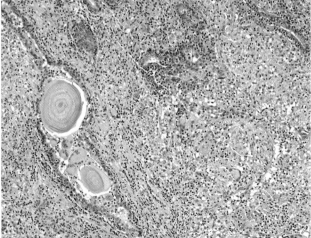

Fig. 5.47 Xanthogranulomatous prostatitis. There are sheets of histiocytes surrounding the prostatic ducts. Numerous intraepithelial lymphocytes are noted

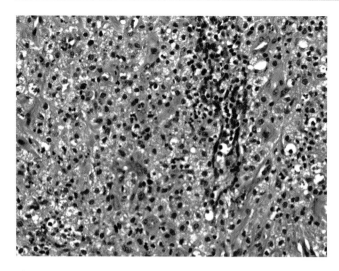

Fig. 5.48 Xanthogranulomatous prostatitis. The prostatic duct is ruptured

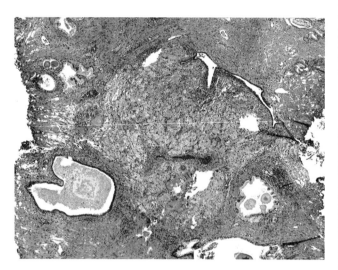

Fig. 5.49 Xanthoma. Xanthoma is a rare form of idiopathic granulomatous prostatitis that consists of a localized collection of cholesterol-laden macrophages

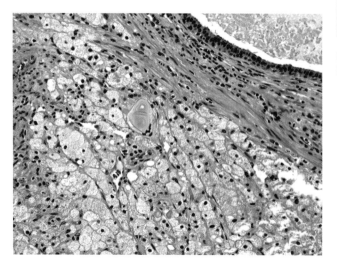

Fig. 5.50 Xanthoma. Sheets of foamy histiocytes with interspersed lymphocytes. These histiocytes are positive for CD68 and negative for keratin and prostate-specific antigen

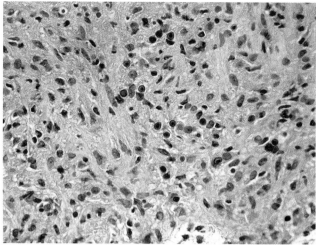

Fig. 5.51 Malakoplakia. This is special form of granulomatous prostatitis associated with defective intracellular lysosomal digestion of bacteria. *Escherichia coli* is commonly isolated from urine culture in these patients. Numerous Michaelis-Gutmann bodies are present among a mixed chronic inflammatory infiltrate. These Michaelis-Gutmann bodies are sharply demarcated spherical structures with an "owl's eye" appearance

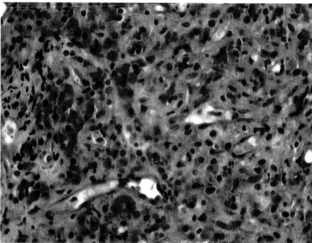

Fig. 5.52 Malakoplakia. Periodic acid-Schiff stain is positive in Michaelis-Gutmann bodies

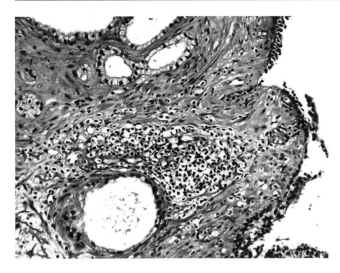

Fig. 5.53 Signet ring-like lymphocytes. Perinuclear clearing of lymphocytes may impart a signet-ring cell appearance

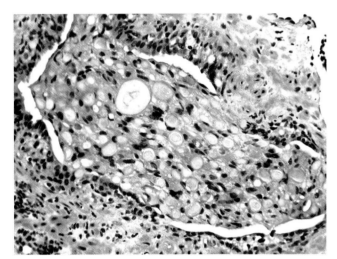

Fig. 5.54 Signet ring-like histocytes. Intraluminal aggregates of signet ring-like histocytes

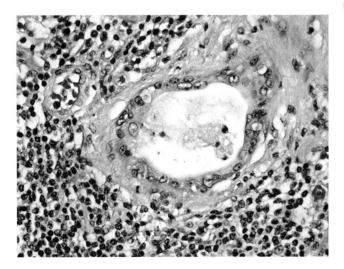

Fig. 5.55 Reactive atypia in acinar epithelium. The epithelial cells have enlarged vesicular nuclei with prominent nucleoli

5.3 Benign Prostatic Entities

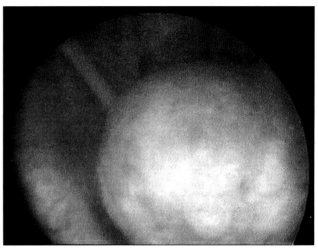

Fig. 5.56 Benign prostatic hyperplasia (BPH). Cystoscopic appearance of BPH

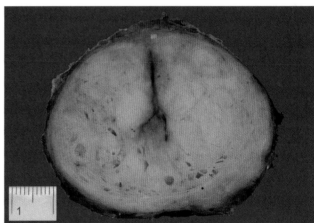

Fig. 5.57 Benign prostatic hyperplasia. Nodular hyperplasia involves transition zone. The lesion has a spongy appearance

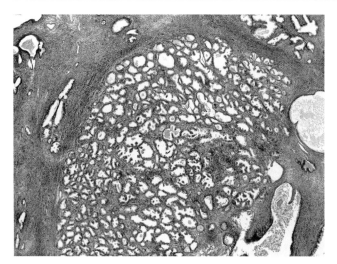

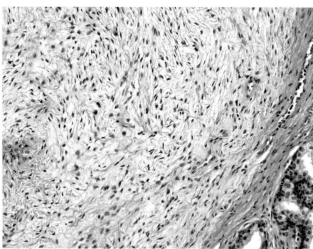

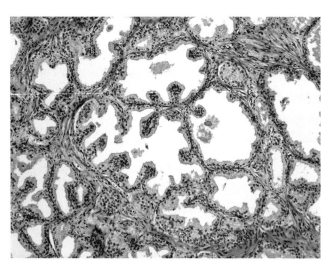

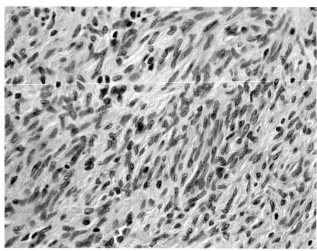

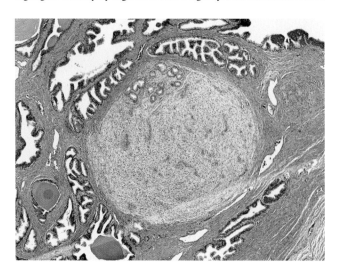

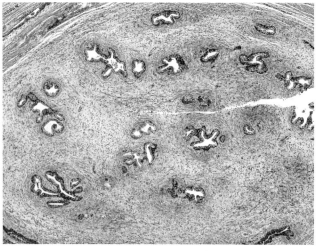

Fig. 5.58 Benign prostatic hyperplasia. The lesion is well circumscribed when viewed at low power. The acini are relatively uniform and evenly spaced

Fig. 5.61 Benign prostatic hyperplasia, stromal nodule. The stromal cells are uniform and spindle-shaped. There is no significant cytologic atypia

Fig. 5.59 Benign prostatic hyperplasia. The acini are lined by columnar secretory cells. The basal cell layers may be inconspicuous, but can be highlighted readily by high molecular weight cytokeratin immunostains

Fig. 5.62 Benign prostatic hyperplasia, stromal nodule. Sheets of spindled stromal cells with interspersed lymphocytes

Fig. 5.60 Benign prostatic hyperplasia, stromal nodule. This nodule is composed of stromal cells with myxoid degeneration

Fig. 5.63 Benign prostatic hyperplasia, fibroadenomatoid type. The special arrangement of epithelial and stromal proliferation is reminiscent of fibroadenoma of the breast

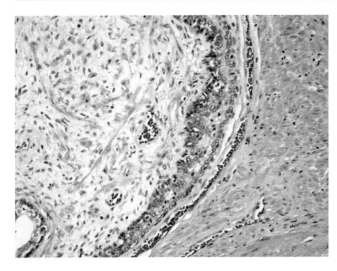

Fig. 5.64 Benign prostatic hyperplasia, fibroadenomatoid type. The glands are compressed. The basal cell layers are visible

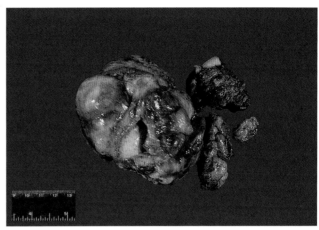

Fig. 5.67 Stromal hyperplasia with atypia. The lesion has a multinodular appearance

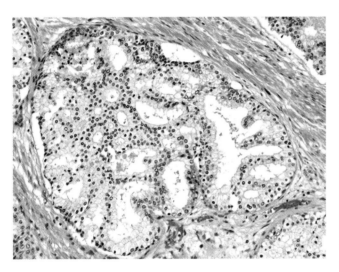

Fig. 5.65 Clear cell cribriform hyperplasia. There is a well-circumscribed epithelial proliferation forming cribriform architecture

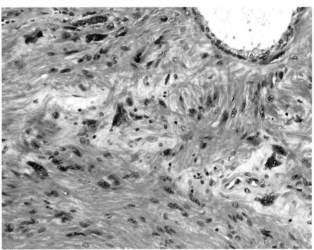

Fig. 5.68 Stromal hyperplasia with atypia. Bizarre stromal cells are noted. The nuclei are hyperchromatic, smudged and degenerative

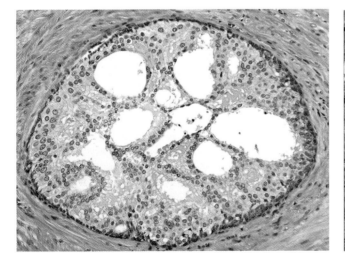

Fig. 5.66 Clear cell cribriform hyperplasia. The cells are relatively uniform lacking prominent nucleoli. Note the presence of basal cell layer

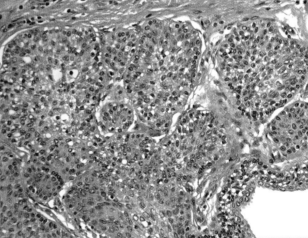

Fig. 5.69 Basal cell hyperplasia. Exuberant proliferation of basal cells forms solid nests. Nuclear grooves are frequently observed

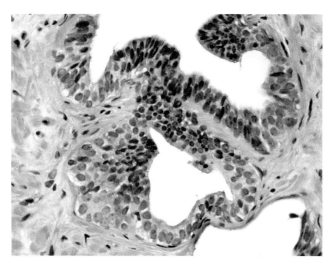

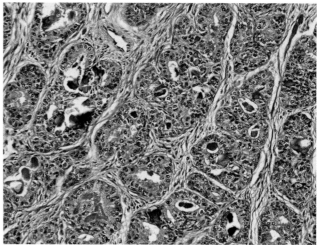

Fig. 5.70 Atypical basal cell hyperplasia. There is an eccentric proliferation of basal cells that display cytologic atypia including prominent nucleoli. The nuclei are uniform with powdery chromatin pattern

Fig. 5.72 Basal cell adenoma. The nodule contains uniformly spaced acini lined by multiple layers of basal cells. Prominent calcific debris is present within acinar lumens

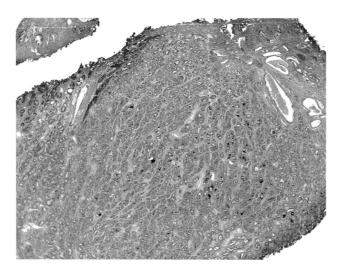

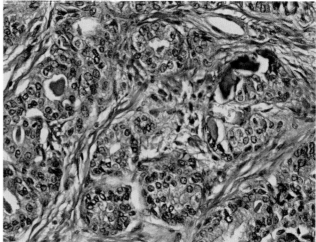

Fig. 5.71 Basal cell adenoma. A large well-circumscribed nodule is evident at low power

Fig. 5.73 Basal cell adenoma. The basal cells lack prominent nucleoli. Nuclei have evenly distributed chromatin

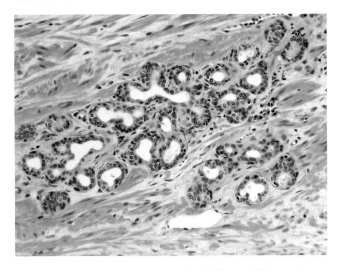
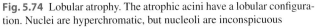

Fig. 5.74 Lobular atrophy. The atrophic acini have a lobular configuration. Nuclei are hyperchromatic, but nucleoli are inconspicuous

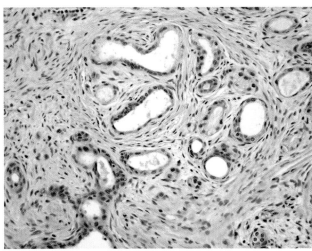

Fig. 5.76 Sclerotic atrophy. The stroma is fibrotic. The glands are dilated and distorted. The flattened epithelium is lined by cells with hyperchromatic nuclei. The stroma is fibrotic and contains scattered chronic inflammatory cells

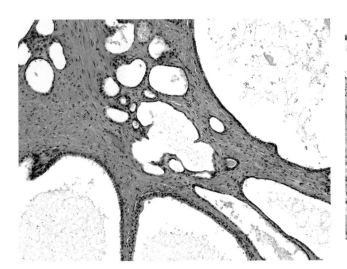

Fig. 5.75 Cystic atrophy. The glands are dilated and distorted. The flattened epithelium is lined by cells with hyperchromatic nuclei. The stroma is fibrotic and contains scattered chronic inflammatory cells

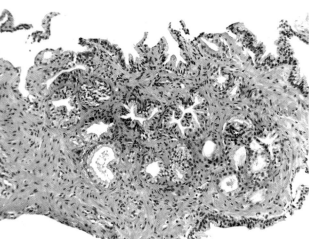

Fig. 5.77 Partial atrophy. The acini are distorted but the lobular architecture is intact. The cells have pale to clear cytoplasm without nuclear hyperchromasia. Nucleoli are inconspicuous

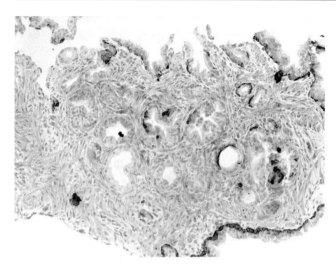

Fig. 5.78 Partial atrophy. Immunostain for high molecular weight cytokeratin 34βE12 shows a fragmented and discontinuous basal cell layer

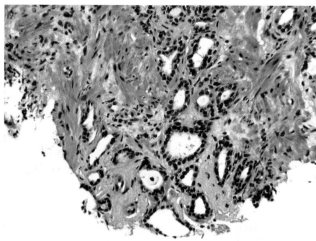

Fig. 5.80 Postatrophic hyperplasia. The acini are lined by a layer of cuboidal secretory cells with enlarged hyperchromatic nuclei. Prominent nucleoli are lacking

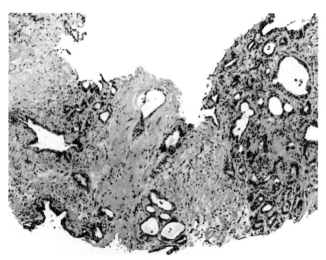

Fig. 5.79 Postatrophic hyperplasia. Lobules of closely packed small atrophic acini appear centered around large central ducts. The stroma is sclerotic

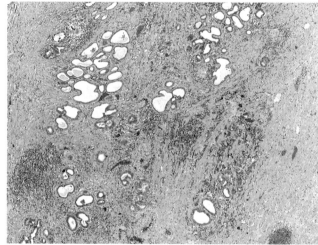

Fig. 5.81 Proliferative inflammatory atrophy. The lesion is characterized by the presence of discrete foci of proliferative glandular epithelium with the morphological appearance of simple atrophy or postatrophic hyperplasia, in a background of chronic inflammation

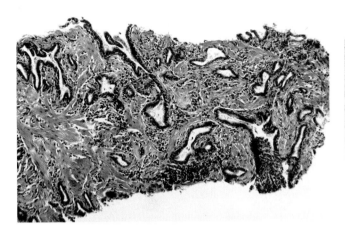

Fig. 5.82 Proliferative inflammatory atrophy. The key features of this lesion are the presence of two distinct epithelial cell layers in the acini, mononuclear and/or polymorphonuclear inflammatory cells in both the epithelial and stromal compartments, and stromal atrophy with variable amounts of fibrosis

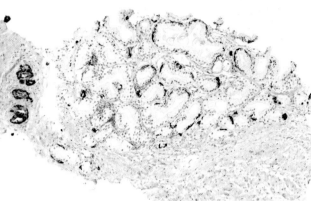

Fig. 5.84 Atypical adenomatous hyperplasia. Some of the crowded acini have patchy fragmented basal cell layers, highlighted by high molecular weight cytokeratin 34βE12 staining

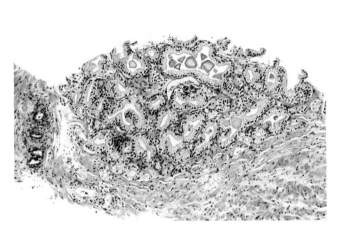

Fig. 5.83 Atypical adenomatous hyperplasia (adenosis). The lesion is well-circumscribed and is composed of closely packed acini with scant intervening stroma. Nucleomegaly and nucleolomegaly are absent

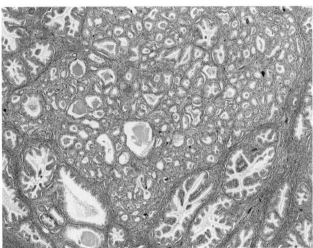

Fig. 5.85 Atypical adenomatous hyperplasia. Low-power view shows proliferation of small acini that vary in size, shape and spacing

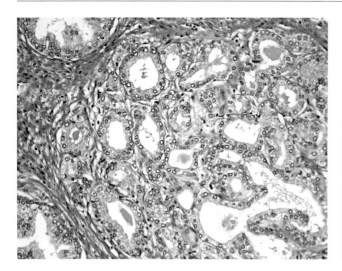

Fig. 5.86 Atypical adenomatous hyperplasia. Higher-magnification view of Fig. 5.85. Prominent nucleoli are absent

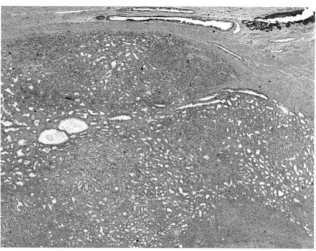

Fig. 5.88 Sclerosing adenosis. The lesion consists of a circumscribed proliferation of small acini in a densely cellular stroma

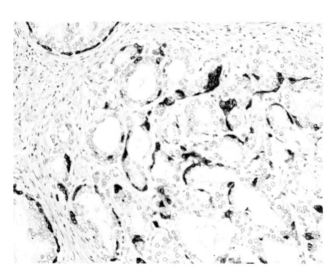

Fig. 5.87 Atypical adenomatous hyperplasia. Immunostain using the PIN4 triple-antibody cocktail (high molecular weight cytokeratin 34βE12, α-methylacyl-CoA racemase, and p63) shows fragmented discontinuous basal cell layers and weak red cytoplasmic granular staining for racemase

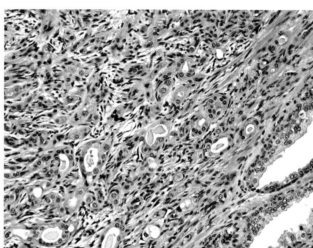

Fig. 5.89 Sclerosing adenosis. The stroma is hyalinized and has a myxoid appearance. The cells lining the acini have clear to eosinophilic cytoplasm and uniform nuclei. There is prominent periacinar basement membrane thickening

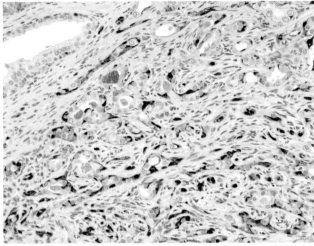

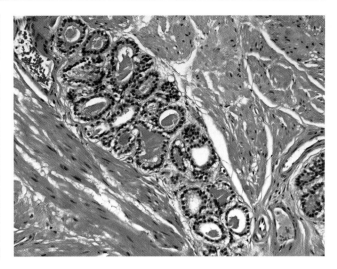

Fig. 5.90 Sclerosing adenosis. S-100 protein immunostaining is positive in the basal cell layer, a unique feature of sclerosing adenosis

Fig. 5.92 Mesonephric remnants. The tubules are closely packed and contain dense eosinophilic colloid-like material

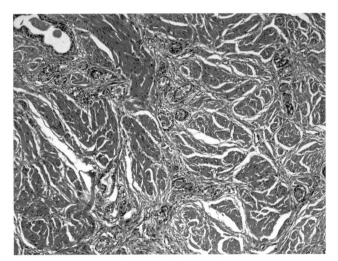

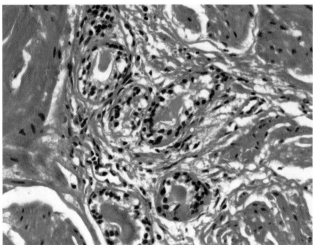

Fig. 5.91 Mesonephric remnants. The lesion consists of a proliferation of small acini and tubules insinuating between muscle bundles without a stromal reaction

Fig. 5.93 Mesonephric remnants. The cells lining the acini are small-to-medium sized and cuboidal, lacking prominent nucleoli. Luminal colloid-like secretions are present

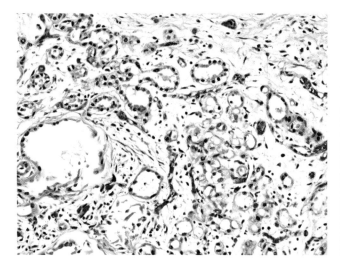

Fig. 5.94 Nephrogenic metaplasia (adenoma). The lesion typically occurs in the prostatic urethra. It consists of a proliferation of small round to oval tubules with eosinophilic luminal secretions. The stroma is edematous and contains scattered chronic inflammatory cells

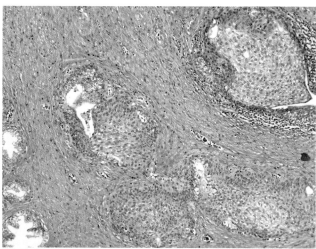

Fig. 5.96 Squamous metaplasia. Squamous metaplasia may be focal or diffuse and appears as intraductal syncytial aggregates of flattened cells with abundant eosinophilic cytoplasm or cohesive aggregates of glycogen-rich clear cells

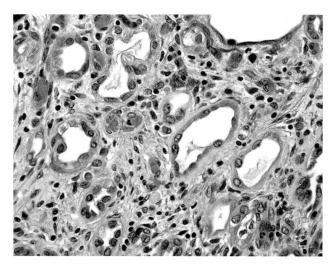

Fig. 5.95 Nephrogenic metaplasia (adenoma). The lining consists of flattened or simple cuboidal cells, often with a distinctive hobnail appearance

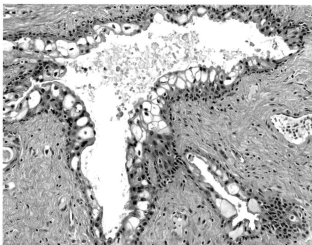

Fig. 5.97 Squamous metaplasia. Acini are lined by glycogen-rich clear cells

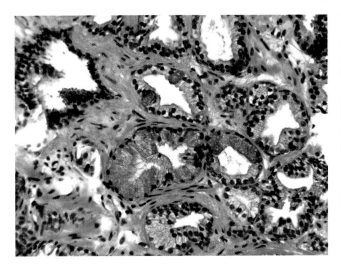

Fig. 5.98 Mucinous metaplasia. The lesion is characterized by numerous tall columnar mucin-producing cells

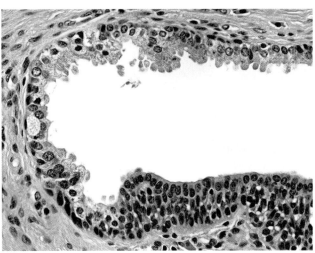

Fig. 5.100 Urothelial (transitional cell) metaplasia. Note transition between normal prostatic epithelium and transitional metaplasia. Urothelial cells have longitudinal arrangement of nuclei and often have prominent nuclear grooves

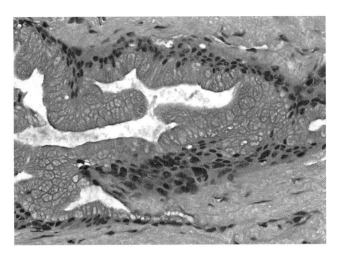

Fig. 5.99 Mucinous metaplasia. Note in addition the presence of numerous benign neuroendocrine cells with intracytoplasmic eosinophilic granules

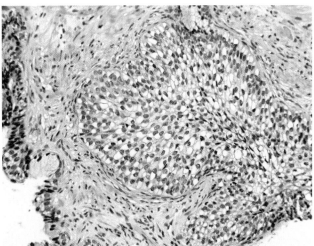

Fig. 5.101 Urothelial (transitional cell) metaplasia. Solid nests of urothelial cells with clear cytoplasm. Prominent nucleoli are absent

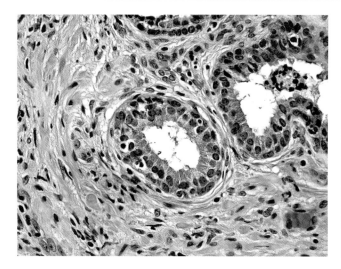

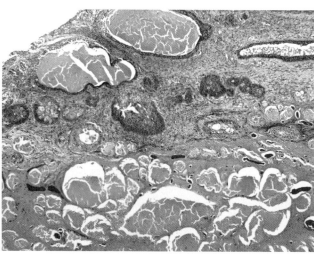

Fig. 5.102 Eosinophilic metaplasia. This form of metaplasia is characterized by the presence of eosinophilic granules in benign prostatic epithelium which also shows reactive changes. Eosinophilic metaplasia is often seen in an inflammatory background

Fig. 5.104 Prostatic infarct with adjacent squamous metaplasia. A sharp demarcation separates viable from nonviable tissue

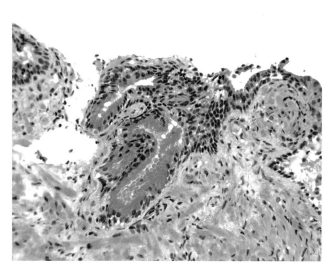

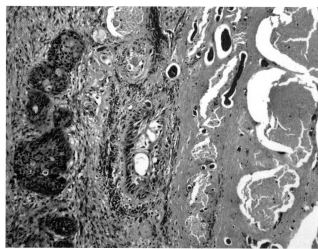

Fig. 5.103 Eosinophilic metaplasia. Note the apically located brightly eosinophilic granules

Fig. 5.105 Prostatic infarct with adjacent squamous metaplasia. Prostatic infarcts are commonly associated with squamous metaplasia in nearby viable prostatic tissue. Basal cell hyperplasia is also present (*left*)

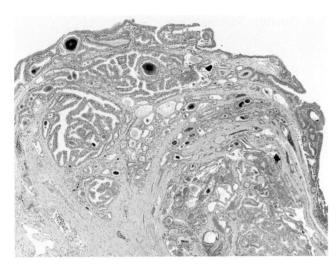

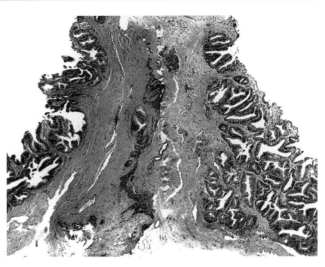

Fig. 5.106 Verumontanum mucosal gland hyperplasia. There is a well-circumscribed proliferation of closely packed small to medium sized acini. Note papillary infoldings in some acini. This entity exhibits distinctive orange-brown luminal concretions, a form of corpora amylacea

Fig. 5.108 Prostatic urethral polyp. A polypoid lesion protrudes into the prostatic urethra

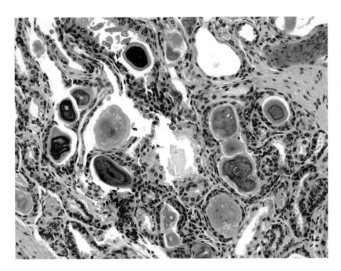

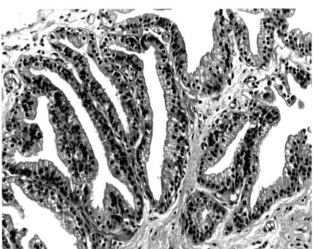

Fig. 5.107 Verumontanum mucosal gland hyperplasia. The acini have typical luminal secretory cell layers with underlying intact basal cells. The cells lack prominent nucleoli

Fig. 5.109 Prostatic urethral polyp. It consists of large prostatic acini in a loose stroma. The cells lining these acini lack prominent nucleoli. The basal cell layer is intact

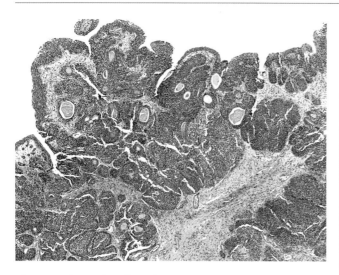

Fig. 5.110 Inverted papilloma in the prostatic urethra. It shows a characteristic downward growth of solid nests and trabeculae of urothelial cells

5.4 Benign Seminal Vesicle Entities

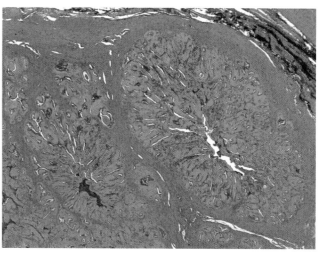

Fig. 5.112 Amyloidosis of the seminal vesicle. Note subepithelial deposition of amorphous eosinophilic fibrillar materials

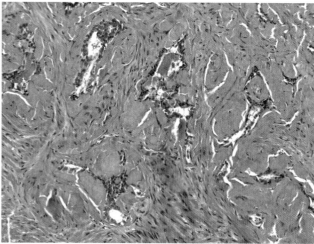

Fig. 5.113 Amyloidosis of the seminal vesicle. The epithelium is compressed and atrophic

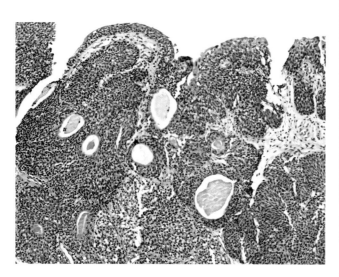

Fig. 5.111 Inverted papilloma in the prostatic urethra. The cells are small and uniform, and lack any significant cytologic atypia. Mitotic figures are inconspicuous. The surface urothelium is intact

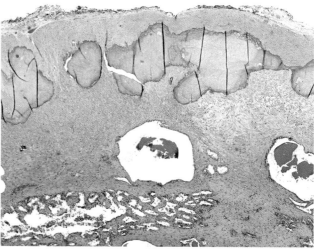

Fig. 5.114 Mural calcifications of the seminal vesicle. Calcifications are present in the muscular wall. Glandular structures are uninvolved

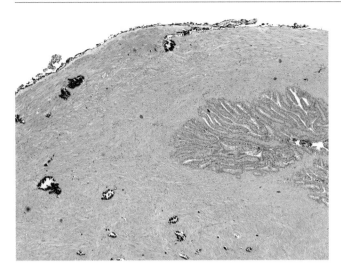

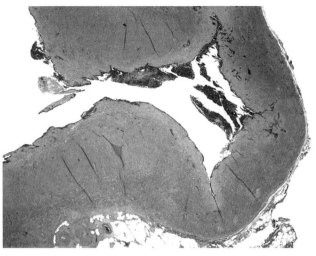

Fig. 5.115 Mural calcifications of the seminal vesicle. The etiology of such calcifications is unknown, but it may be comparable to the occurrence of similar calcifications in the vas deferens in patients with diabetes mellitus, as well as in nondiabetic patients, although it is six times more common in the former. In nondiabetics, vas deferens calcification is regarded as a manifestation of aging; similar mechanisms may account for seminal vesicle microcalcifications

Fig. 5.117 Cyst of the seminal vesicle. Cystic dilation of the seminal vesicle is noted

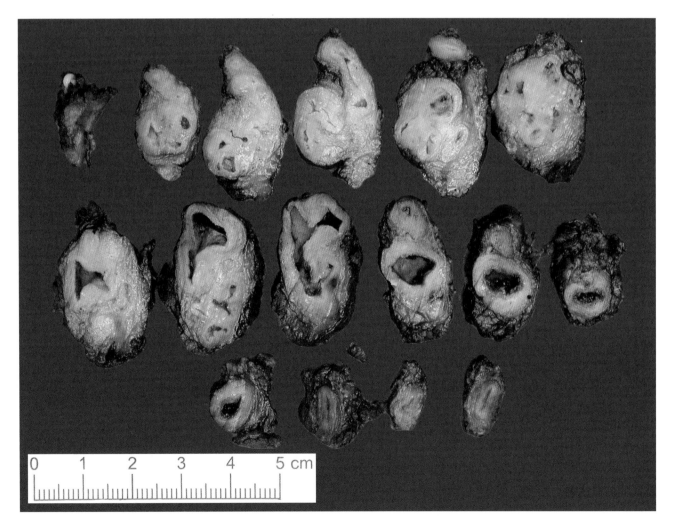

Fig. 5.116 Cyst of the seminal vesicle. Note large unilocular cyst that presented as a mass clinically

5.5 Prostatic Intraepithelial Neoplasia

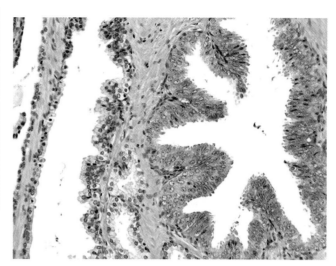

Fig. 5.120 High-grade prostatic intraepithelial neoplasia (PIN), compared with normal glandular epithelium. High-grade PIN is characterized by cellular proliferations within preexisting ducts and acini, with cytologic atypia of the lining epithelium, including nuclear and nucleolar enlargement, nuclear hyperchromasia, and stratification

Fig. 5.118 Cyst of seminal vesicle. The cyst is lined by simple cuboidal cells with cilia

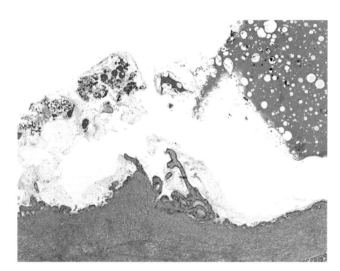

Fig. 5.119 Cystadenoma of the seminal vesicle. Note papillary projects that are lined by simple cuboidal cells. The cyst is surrounded by a muscular wall

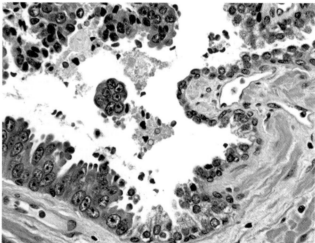

Fig. 5.121 High-grade prostatic intraepithelial neoplasia (PIN), compared with normal glandular epithelium. Note the striking contrast of nuclear features between PIN and benign epithelial cells. Cytoplasm is more amphophilic in the cells of PIN compared with the pale-to-clear cytoplasm of adjacent benign epithelial cells

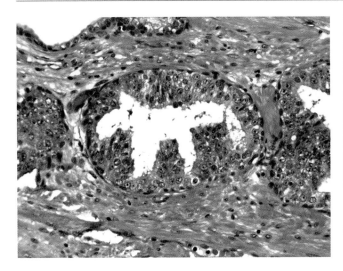

Fig. 5.122 High-grade prostatic intraepithelial neoplasia, tufting type. The majority of secretory cells have prominent nucleoli. The basal cell layer is still present but fragmented

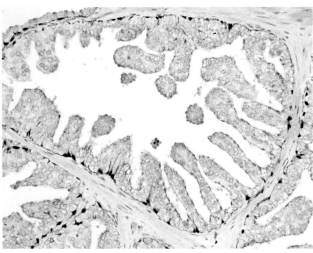

Fig. 5.124 High-grade prostatic intraepithelial neoplasia, micropapillary type. Immunostain using the PIN4 triple-antibody cocktail (high molecular weight cytokeratin 34βE12, α-methylacyl-CoA racemase, and p63) shows fragmented discontinuous basal cell layers and strong red cytoplasmic granular staining of racemase in the secretory cells

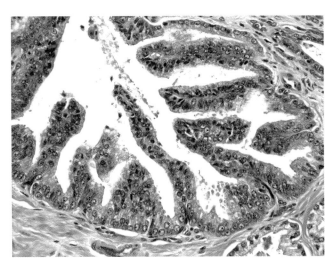

Fig. 5.123 High-grade prostatic intraepithelial neoplasia, micropapillary type

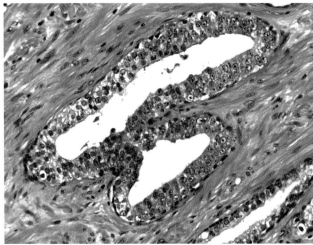

Fig. 5.125 High-grade prostatic intraepithelial neoplasia, flat type

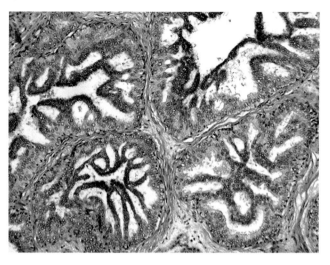

Fig. 5.126 High-grade prostatic intraepithelial neoplasia, cribriform type

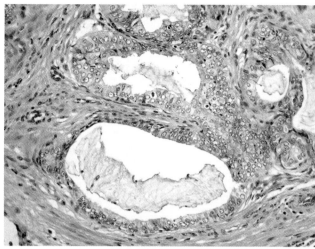

Fig. 5.129 High-grade prostatic intraepithelial neoplasia, mucinous variant. Note luminal mucin secretions

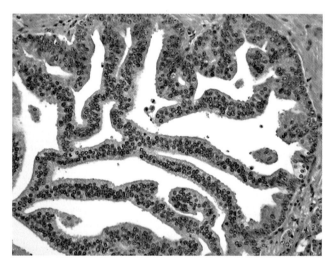

Fig. 5.127 High-grade prostatic intraepithelial neoplasia, cribriform type

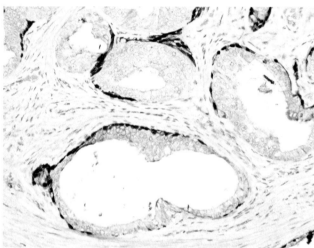

Fig. 5.130 High-grade prostatic intraepithelial neoplasia, mucinous variant. Immunostaining with high molecular weight cytokeratin 34βE12 shows a fragmented basal cell layer

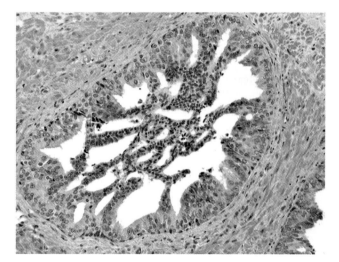

Fig. 5.128 High-grade prostatic intraepithelial neoplasia, small cell variant. Note small neuroendocrine cells in the center

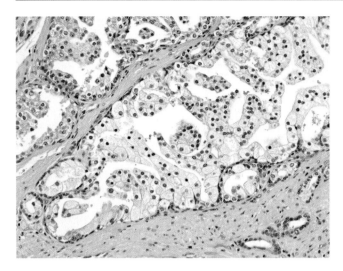

Fig. 5.131 High-grade prostatic intraepithelial neoplasia, foamy gland variant. Neoplastic cells have voluminous cytoplasm expanded by the presence of innumerable minute vacuoles

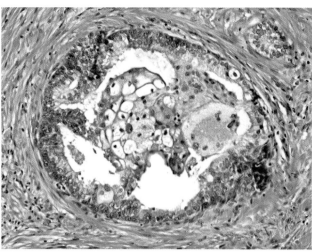

Fig. 5.133 High-grade prostatic intraepithelial neoplasia with squamous differentiation

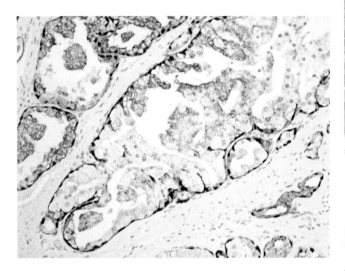

Fig. 5.132 High-grade prostatic intraepithelial neoplasia, foamy gland variant. Immunostain using the PIN4 triple-antibody cocktail (high molecular weight cytokeratin 34βE12, α-methylacyl-CoA racemase, and p63) shows strong red cytoplasmic granular staining of racemase in the secretory cells, and confirms the presence of basal cells

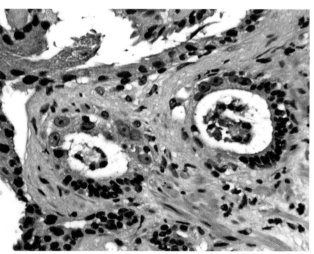

Fig. 5.134 High-grade prostatic intraepithelial neoplasia with pagetoid spread

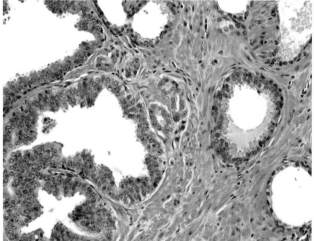

Fig. 5.135 High-grade prostatic intraepithelial neoplasia (PIN) with microinvasion. The invading malignant acini are small compared with adjacent large PIN glands. These acini lack basal cell layers

5.6 Atypical Small Acinar Proliferations

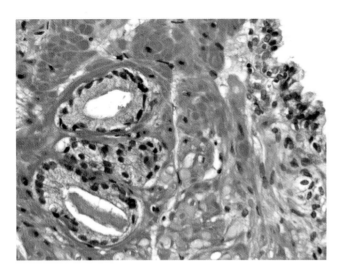

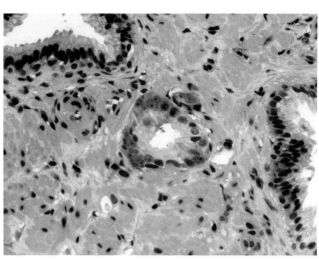

Fig. 5.138 Atypical small acinar proliferation ASAP, suspicious for but not diagnostic of malignancy. Due to the small size of the focus, the most appropriate diagnosis for these highly atypical glands is ASAP

Fig. 5.136 Atypical small acinar proliferation, suspicious for but not diagnostic of malignancy. Three atypical acini are present adjacent to a benign large gland

5.7 Prostatic Adenocarcinoma

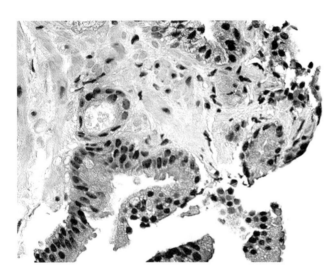

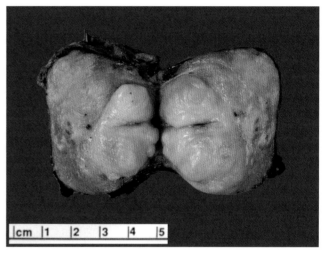

Fig. 5.137 Atypical small acinar proliferation, suspicious for but not diagnostic of malignancy. Several atypical small acini are present adjacent to high-grade prostatic intraepithelial neoplasia

Fig. 5.139 Prostatic adenocarcinoma. Prostatic adenocarcinomas typically arise in the peripheral zone and diffusely infiltrate the gland, sometimes forming grossly visible yellow masses, usually lacking circumscription, as in this case. Note benign prostatic hyperplasia nodules in the transition zone

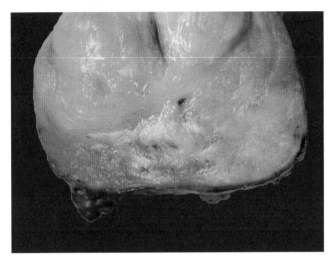

Fig. 5.140 Prostatic adenocarcinoma. A large yellow tumor mass is present in the posterolateral aspect of the prostate

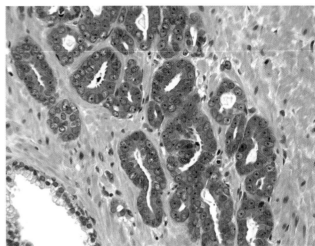

Fig. 5.142 Prostatic adenocarcinoma with amphophilic cytoplasm. Cancer cells often acquire amphophilic cytoplasm. The adjacent benign epithelial cells have clear cytoplasm with small nuclei and inconspicuous nucleoli

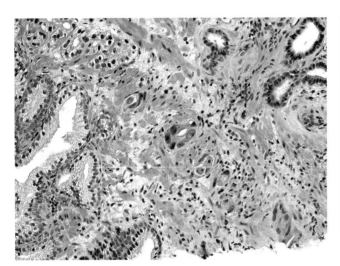

Fig. 5.141 Prostatic adenocarcinoma with enlarged nuclei and prominent nucleoli. Cancer cells have enlarged nuclei and prominent nucleoli. The presence of double nucleoli is a very helpful feature in the diagnosis

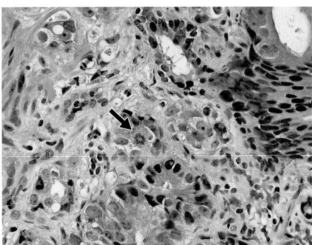

Fig. 5.143 Prostatic adenocarcinoma with mitotic figure Note mitotic figure (*arrow*) and multiple nucleoli in enlarged nuclei

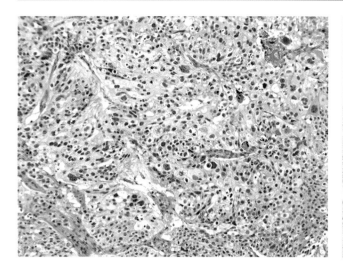

Fig. 5.144 Prostatic adenocarcinoma with apoptotic bodies. Numerous apoptotic bodies are present

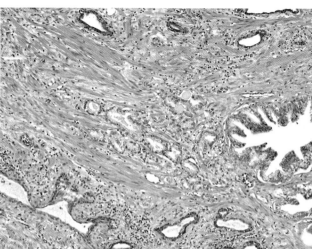

Fig. 5.146 Prostatic adenocarcinoma with loss of basal cells. A small focus of infiltrative acini arising from adjacent high-grade prostatic intraepithelial neoplasia. These malignant acini lack basal cells

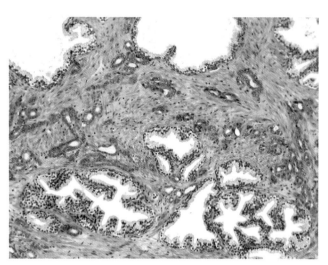

Fig. 5.145 Prostatic adenocarcinoma with infiltrative small acini. Low power view shows a typical appearance of small irregular acini infiltrating between normal glands. Tumor cells have amphophilic cytoplasm, in contrast to the pale or clear cytoplasm in benign glandular cells

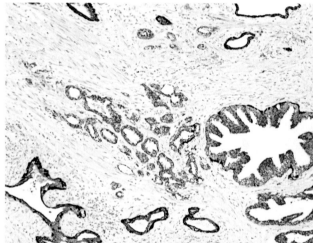

Fig. 5.147 Prostatic adenocarcinoma. From the previous case, immunostain using the PIN4 triple-antibody cocktail (34βE12, racemase, and p63) shows absence of a basal cell layer in the malignant acini and fragmented discontinuous basal cell layers in high-grade prostatic intraepithelial neoplasia (PIN). Both cancer and high-grade PIN display strong red cytoplasmic granular staining of racemase

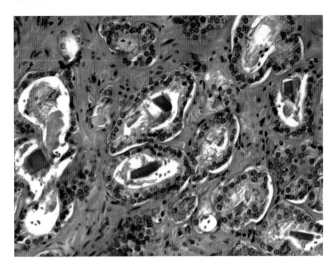

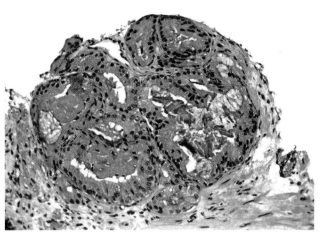

Fig. 5.150 Prostatic adenocarcinoma with crystalloids and mucin. Note prominent crystalloids and mucin secretions. Crystalloids and mucins can also be seen in benign acini, and therefore are not pathognomonic of cancer

Fig. 5.148 Prostatic adenocarcinoma with intraluminal crystalloids and mucin. Crystalloids are sharp needle-like eosinophilic structures that are sometimes present in the lumens of malignant glands. Luminal mucin secretions are also present

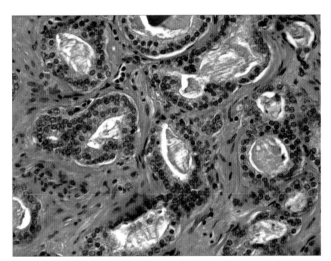

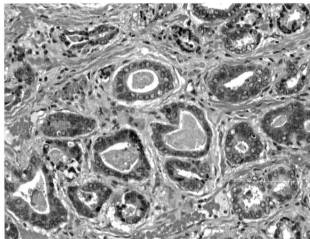

Fig. 5.149 Prostatic adenocarcinoma with intraluminal mucin. Acidic sulfated and nonsulfated mucins are often present in malignant acini, appearing as amorphous or delicate threadlike faintly basophilic intraluminal secretions. Note the haphazard arrangement of acini

Fig. 5.151 Prostatic adenocarcinoma with eosinophilic amorphous secretions. Eosinophilic amorphous secretions are more commonly seen than crystalloids and mucins

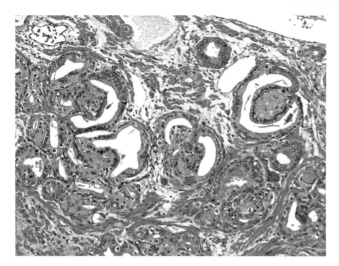

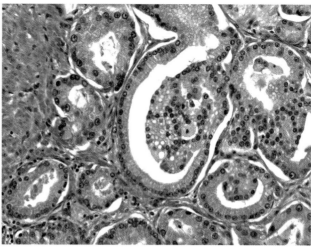

Fig. 5.152 Prostatic adenocarcinoma with collagenous micronodules. Collagenous micronodules consist of microscopic nodular masses of paucicellular eosinophilic fibrillar materials that impinge upon acinar lumens. Collagenous micronodules are found only in prostatic adenocarcinoma; they are not found in benign prostatic tissue

Fig. 5.154 Prostatic adenocarcinoma with glomerulations. Glomerulations consist of intraluminal protrusion of abnormally proliferating epithelium, forming structures morphologically similar to renal glomeruli. Glomerulation is found only in prostatic adenocarcinoma; it is not a feature of benign prostatic tissue

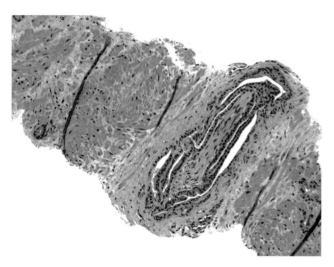

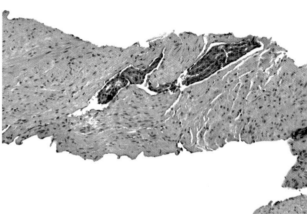

Fig. 5.153 Prostatic adenocarcinoma with perineural invasion. Acinar structures completely encircling nerves, within nerves, or within ganglia are malignant acini

Fig. 5.155 Prostatic adenocarcinoma with lymphovascular invasion. Lymphovascular invasion is another feature that is specific for prostatic adenocarcinoma

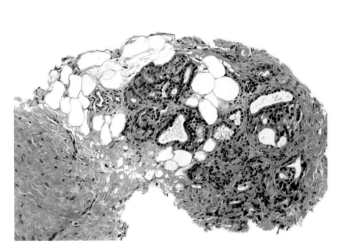

Fig. 5.156 Prostatic adenocarcinoma with extraprostatic extension. Extraprostatic extension, another feature of prostatic adenocarcinoma, may rarely be evident in biopsy specimens

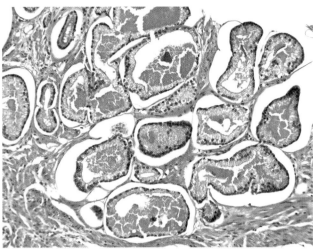

Fig. 5.158 Prostatic adenocarcinoma with retraction artifact. Note retraction artifact and abundant amorphous eosinophilic secretions

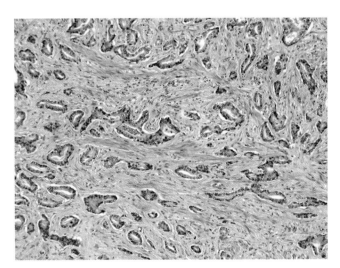

Fig. 5.157 Prostatic adenocarcinoma with desmoplasia. Note prominent dense fibrotic stromal reaction (desmoplasia). Unlike certain other cancers, such as colon cancer, prostatic adenocarcinoma rarely incites a desmoplastic stromal reaction

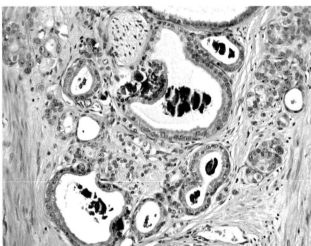

Fig. 5.159 Prostatic adenocarcinoma with microcalcifications. Microcalcifications are uncommon and can be seen in both benign and malignant acini

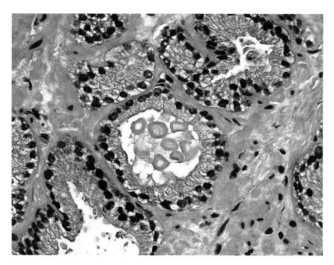

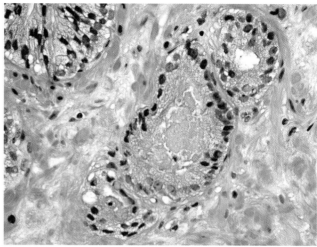

Fig. 5.160 Prostatic adenocarcinoma with corpora amylacea. Corpora amylacea may be rarely seen in malignant glands. Therefore, their presence does not necessarily exclude the diagnosis of cancer

Fig. 5.162 Minimal (limited) adenocarcinoma in needle biopsy. These glands are lined by malignant cells with enlarged nuclei and prominent nucleoli. A few cells have double nucleoli. The glands have intraluminal eosinophilic amorphous secretions and wispy mucin materials

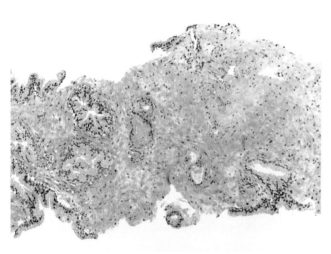

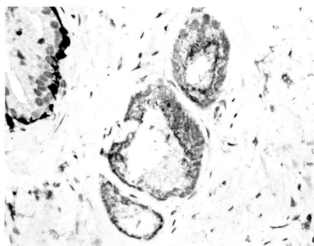

Fig. 5.161 Minimal (limited) adenocarcinoma in needle biopsy. Definite diagnosis of prostatic adenocarcinoma in needle biopsy usually requires the presence of three or more atypical glands

Fig. 5.163 Minimal (limited) adenocarcinoma in needle biopsy. Immunostain using the PIN4 triple-antibody cocktail (high molecular weight cytokeratin 34βE12, α-methylacyl-CoA racemase, and p63) shows strong red cytoplasmic granular staining of malignant cells. The malignant glands lack basal cell layers (same case as Figs. 5.161 and 5.162). The adjacent benign glands show the presence of basal cell layer and lack of racemase staining (*upper left*)

5.8 Gleason Grading

Prostatic adenocarcinoma
(histologic grades)

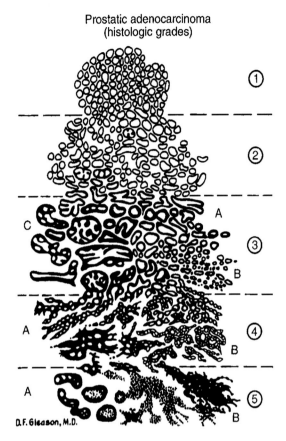

Fig. 5.164 Gleason grading system, schematic drawing of five Gleason patterns. The primary pattern (grade) is the most common or predominant grade; the secondary pattern (grade) is the next most common grade. The Gleason score is a scalar measurement that combines primary and secondary Gleason patterns into a total of nine discrete groups (Gleason scores 2–10)

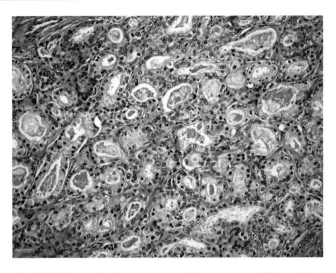

Fig. 5.166 Prostatic adenocarcinoma, Gleason pattern 1. The acini are relatively uniform and closely packed with scant intervening stroma

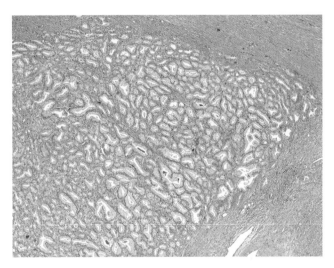

Fig. 5.167 Prostatic adenocarcinoma, Gleason pattern 2. Gleason pattern 2 is less circumscribed with greater stromal separation and has more variation in acinar size and shape as compared to Gleason pattern 1

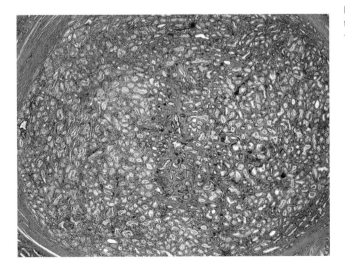

Fig. 5.165 Prostatic adenocarcinoma, Gleason pattern 1. It consists of a circumscribed nodule of simple round acini that are relatively uniform in size, shape, and spacing

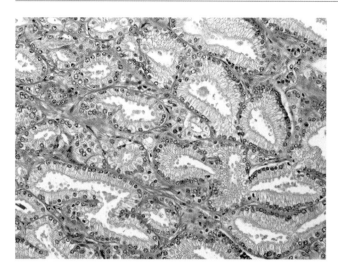

Fig. 5.168 Prostatic adenocarcinoma, Gleason pattern 2. Higher magnification of the same case in Fig. 5.167 shows prominent nucleoli and absence of basal cell layers. The acini are less compact as compared to Gleason pattern 1 tumor

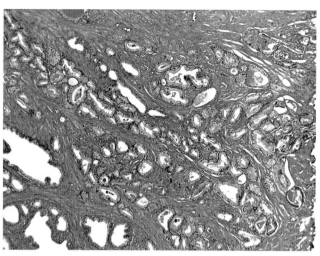

Fig. 5.170 Prostatic adenocarcinoma, Gleason pattern 3. The malignant acini are haphazardly arranged with prominent variation in size, shape, and spacing. Despite this variation, the acini remain discrete and separate, unlike the fused acini in Gleason pattern 4

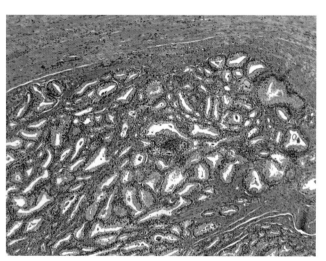

Fig. 5.169 Prostatic adenocarcinoma, Gleason pattern 2. The nodule is less well-circumscribed than Gleason pattern 1 cancer, but not as infiltrative as Gleason pattern 3 tumor

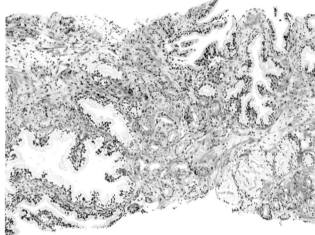

Fig. 5.171 Prostatic adenocarcinoma, Gleason pattern 3. The small irregular acini infiltrate between benign glands which have large luminal spaces and are lined by cells with clear cytoplasm, and stand out in sharp contrast to them. Some malignant glands may appear to be fused due to tangential sectioning

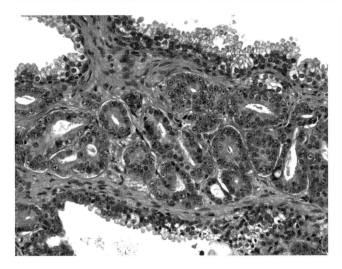

Fig. 5.172 Prostatic adenocarcinoma, Gleason pattern 3. Small malignant acini invade between large benign glands. Note nucleomegaly, nucleolomegaly, and amphophilic cytoplasm in tumor cells

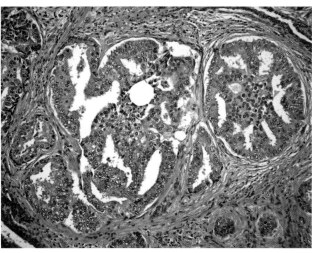

Fig. 5.174 Prostatic adenocarcinoma, Gleason pattern 4. Acinar fusion forms a cribriform pattern. The outline of the structure formed by the fused acini is irregular

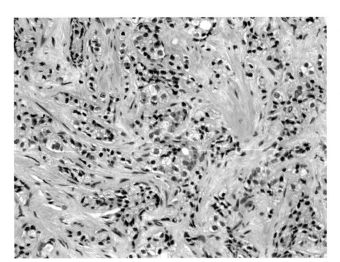

Fig. 5.173 Prostatic adenocarcinoma, Gleason pattern 4. Gleason pattern 4 is characterized by fused acini and raggedly infiltrating cords and nests of tumor cells

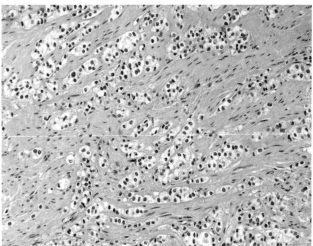

Fig. 5.175 Prostatic adenocarcinoma, Gleason pattern 4. Infiltrating cords and nests are composed of cells with clear or pale cytoplasm, the so-called "hypernephroid" pattern

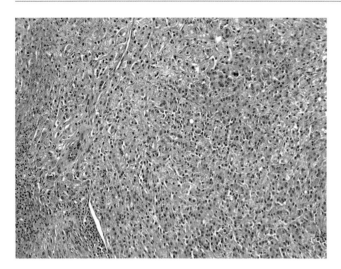

Fig. 5.176 Prostatic adenocarcinoma, Gleason pattern 5. Gleason pattern 5 is characterized by fused sheets and solid masses of tumor cells without apparent glandular formation

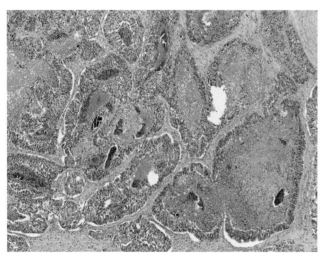

Fig. 5.177 Prostatic adenocarcinoma, Gleason pattern 5. The presence of comedonecrosis in this ductal adenocarcinoma indicates Gleason pattern 5 carcinoma. Ductal adenocarcinoma, in the absence of comedonecrosis, is graded as Gleason pattern 4 cancer

5.9 Variants of Prostatic Adenocarcinoma

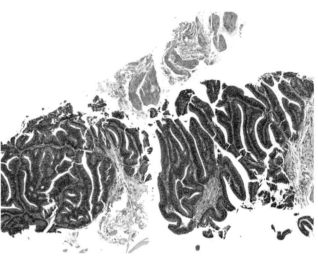

Fig. 5.178 Ductal adenocarcinoma. The tumor shows papillary architecture and should be graded as Gleason pattern 4 cancer (Gleason score 4 + 4)

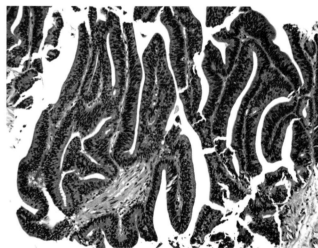

Fig. 5.179 Ductal adenocarcinoma. The tumor cells are tall, columnar and pseudostratified with hyperchromatic nuclei. Prostate-specific antigen and prostate-specific acid phosphatase immunostains are positive in tumor cells

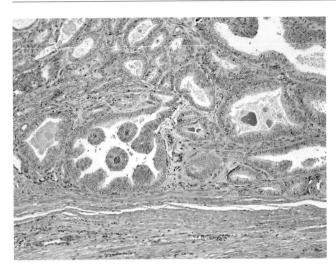

Fig. 5.180 Adenocarcinoma with stratified epithelium (prostatic intraepithelial neoplasia-like ductal adenocarcinoma). Tumor has stratified epithelium with nuclear overlapping, hyperchromasia, and prominent nucleoli

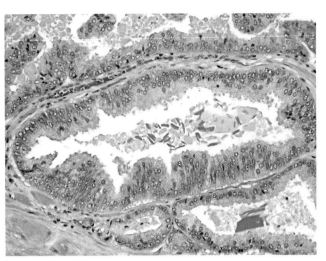

Fig. 5.182 Adenocarcinoma with stratified epithelium (prostatic intraepithelial neoplasia [PIN]-like ductal adenocarcinoma). It may superficially resemble high-grade PIN (tufting pattern)

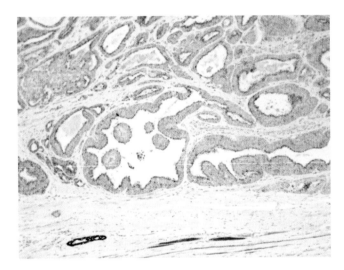

Fig. 5.181 Adenocarcinoma with stratified epithelium (prostatic intraepithelial neoplasia-like ductal adenocarcinoma). Immunostain using the PIN4 triple-antibody cocktail shows complete absence of basal cell layers and strong red cytoplasmic granular staining of racemase. Note dark brown staining in the benign gland (*left* lower corner), indicating the presence of basal cells

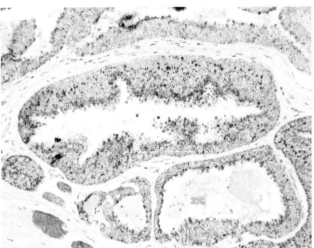

Fig. 5.183 Adenocarcinoma with stratified epithelium (prostatic intraepithelial neoplasia-like ductal adenocarcinoma). Complete lack of basal cells and strong cytoplasmic racemase stainings (PIN4 triple-antibody cocktail) supports the diagnosis of adenocarcinoma

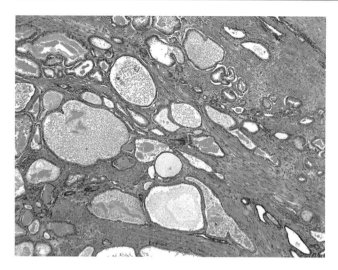

Fig. 5.184 Pseudohyperplastic adenocarcinoma. The dilated glands have smooth luminal borders. These glands are arranged haphazardly and have abundant intraluminal amorphous eosinophilic secretions with scattered crystalloids. Typical small acinar prostatic adenocarcinoma is also present (*right* middle field)

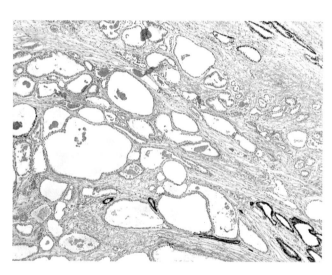

Fig. 5.185 Pseudohyperplastic adenocarcinoma. The absence of basal cells in the malignant acini is confirmed by high molecular weight cytokeratin 34βE12 staining

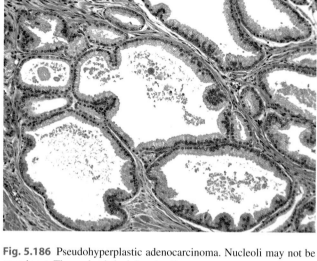

Fig. 5.186 Pseudohyperplastic adenocarcinoma. Nucleoli may not be prominent. These glands lack basal cells

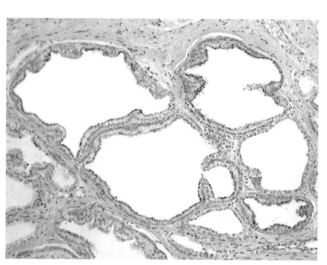

Fig. 5.187 Pseudohyperplastic adenocarcinoma. Immunostain for α-methylacyl-CoA racemase is strongly positive in tumor cells

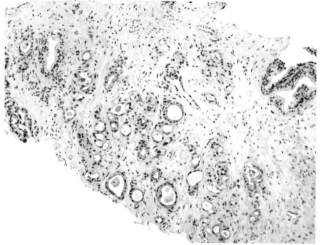

Fig. 5.188 Atrophic adenocarcinoma. The malignant acini exhibit an atrophic appearance but have an infiltrative growth pattern

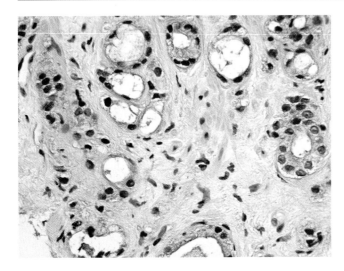

Fig. 5.189 Atrophic adenocarcinoma. Features of prostatic adenocarcinoma such as nuclear enlargement and prominent nucleoli are present

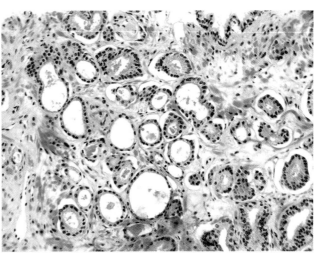

Fig. 5.191 Atrophic adenocarcinoma. Some atrophic acini are dilated with smooth luminal borders

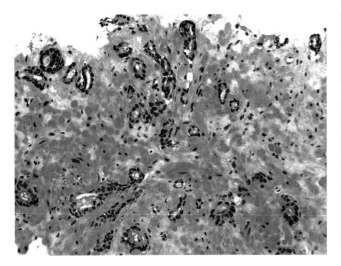

Fig. 5.190 Atrophic adenocarcinoma. Nuclei are hyperchromatic, and a few cells have prominent nucleoli. Intraluminal mucin is present. Distinguishing this special variant from postatrophic hyperplasia can be challenging, and immunostains for high molecular weight cytokeratin 34βE12 and α-methylacyl-CoA racemase can be helpful

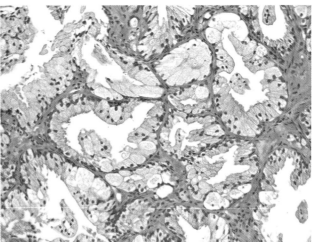

Fig. 5.192 Foamy gland adenocarcinoma. Tumor cells with abundant vacuolated cytoplasm may impart a foamy or xanthomatous appearance

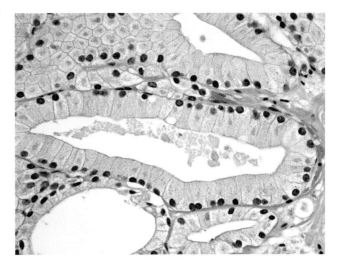

Fig. 5.193 Foamy gland adenocarcinoma. The nuclei are small and only a few have prominent nucleoli

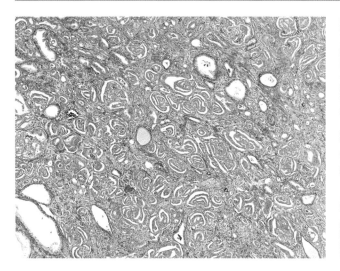

Fig. 5.194 Adenocarcinoma with glomeruloid features. This tumor has extensive intraluminal glomerulus-like epithelial proliferation

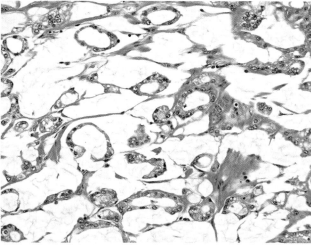

Fig. 5.196 Mucinous (colloid) adenocarcinoma. Tumor cells border the mucin lakes and appear to "float" on a mucin lake. The diagnosis arbitrarily requires that 25% or more of the tumor is composed of pools of extracellular mucin

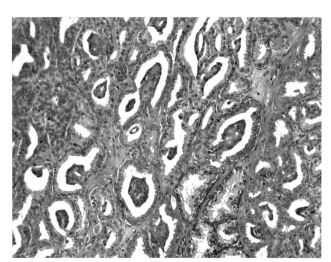

Fig. 5.195 Adenocarcinoma with glomeruloid features. Fine fibrovascular cores are seen in the glomeruloid structures

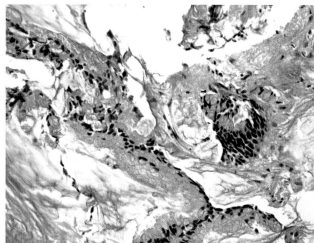

Fig. 5.197 Mucinous (colloid) adenocarcinoma. Nuclei are small and hyperchromatic. Prominent nucleoli may not be seen

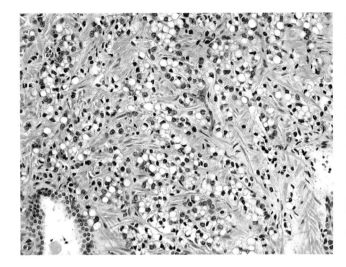

Fig. 5.198 Signet ring cell carcinoma. The accepted definition of signet ring cell adenocarcinoma arbitrarily requires that at least 25% of the cancer is composed of signet ring cells

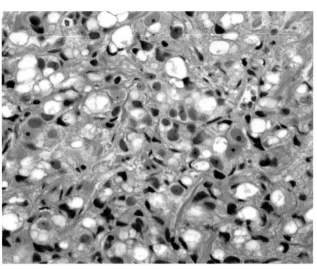

Fig. 5.200 Signet ring cell carcinoma. Note prominent nucleoli

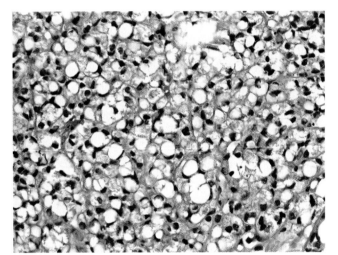

Fig. 5.199 Signet ring cell carcinoma. The tumor is composed of sheets of cells with large cytoplasmic vacuoles that compress the nuclei to the periphery, imparting a "signet ring"appearance. The tumor is graded as Gleason pattern 5 carcinoma

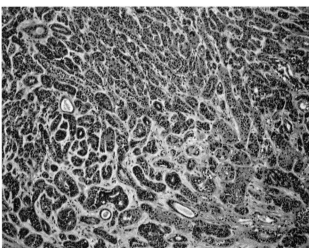

Fig. 5.201 Adenoid cystic/basal cell carcinoma. The tumor is composed of basal cell nests of varying size in a myxoid stroma

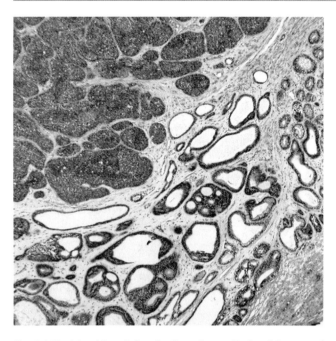

Fig. 5.202 Adenoid cystic/basal cell carcinoma. Both solid nests and adenoid cystic patterns are seen

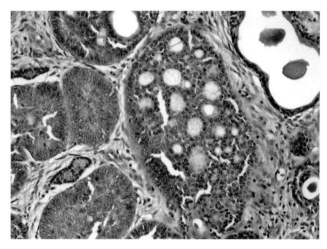

Fig. 5.203 Adenoid cystic/basal cell carcinoma. Solid nests are punctuated by round fenestrations containing basophilic mucinous materials. Nuclei are typical of basal cells with fine chromatin

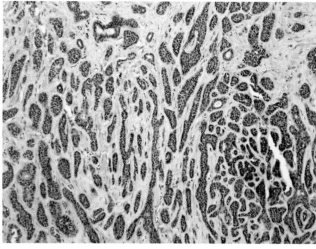

Fig. 5.204 Adenoid cystic/basal cell carcinoma. Infiltrating cords, nests, and tubules of basal cells in myxoid stroma

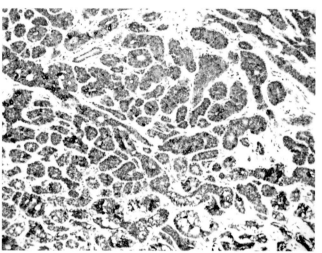

Fig. 5.205 Adenoid cystic/basal cell carcinoma. Tumor cells are strongly positive for high molecular weight cytokeratin 34βE12

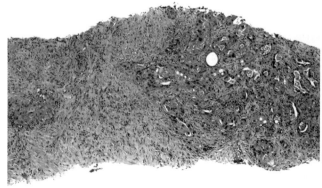

Fig. 5.206 Adenosquamous carcinoma. The tumor has mixed squamous cell carcinoma and adenocarcinoma components

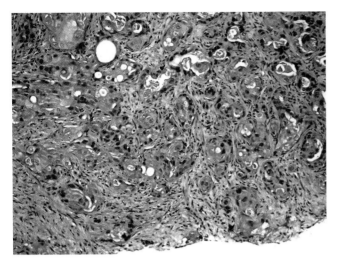

Fig. 5.207 Adenosquamous carcinoma. Both glandular and squamous differentiation is present

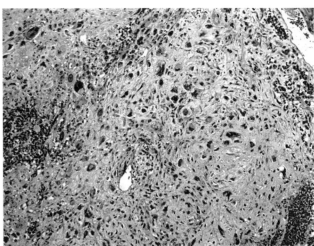

Fig. 5.210 Carcinosarcoma. Note cartilaginous differentiation

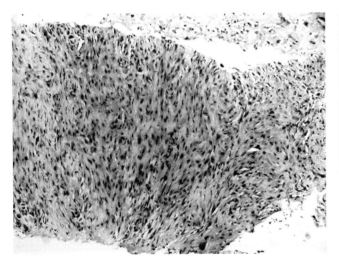

Fig. 5.208 Sarcomatoid carcinoma. The tumor is composed of sheets of spindle cells with a high degree of cytologic atypia. Immunostains for cytokeratin are strongly positive in sarcomatoid prostate cancer

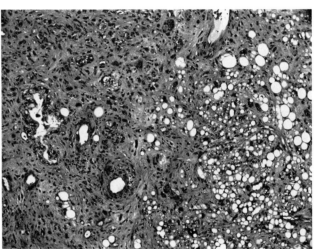

Fig. 5.211 Carcinosarcoma. The tumor is composed of both high-grade malignant spindle cells and a liposarcoma component

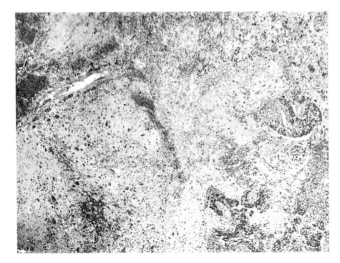

Fig. 5.209 Carcinosarcoma. Both chondrosarcoma and malignant epithelial elements are present

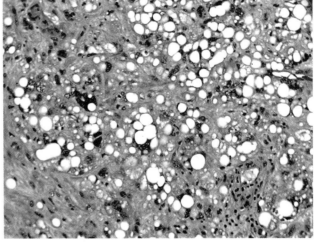

Fig. 5.212 Carcinosarcoma. Note the presence of numerous lipoblasts

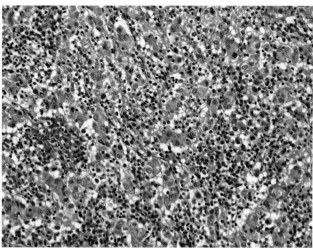

Fig. 5.213 Lymphoepithelioma-like carcinoma. The tumor resembles lymphoepithelioma of the nasopharynx. It is composed of a syncytial growth of malignant epithelial cells in an inflammatory background that includes abundant eosinophils

5.10 Other Prostatic Epithelial and Neuroendocrine Neoplasms

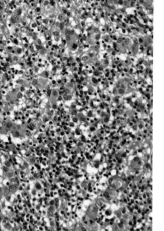

Fig. 5.215 Urothelial (transitional cell) carcinoma. The tumor is composed of solid nests in a desmoplastic and inflammatory background

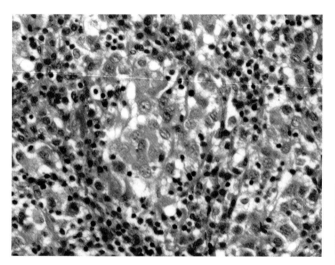

Fig. 5.214 Lymphoepithelioma-like carcinoma. Tumor cells have large round to oval vesicular nuclei with smooth nuclear membranes. Nucleoli are inconspicuous. Cell borders are indistinct. Note the presence of numerous eosinophils in the inflammatory background

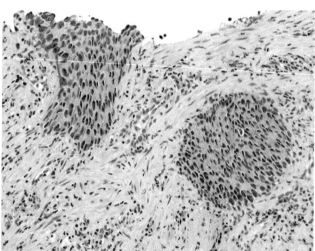

Fig. 5.216 Urothelial carcinoma (transitional cell carcinoma). The cells have eosinophilic cytoplasm and hyperchromatic nuclei with nuclear and nucleolar enlargement

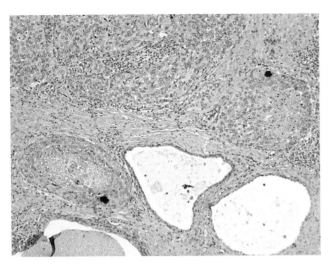

Fig. 5.217 Urothelial carcinoma (transitional cell carcinoma). Significant nuclear pleomorphism is uncommon in typical prostatic adenocarcinoma. Comedonecrosis is often present in urothelial carcinoma. Note the presence of a few dilated benign prostatic ducts

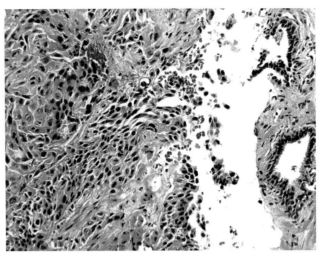

Fig. 5.219 Squamous cell carcinoma. Note significant nuclear pleomorphism and hyperchromasia and numerous apoptotic bodies and mitotic figures

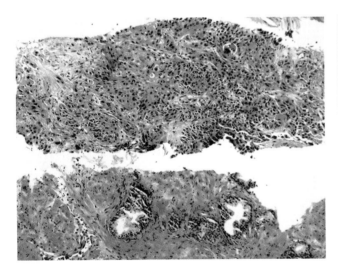

Fig. 5.218 Squamous cell carcinoma. Note syncytial growth of cells with eosinophilic cytoplasm and keratin pearls. Prominent nucleoli may not been seen

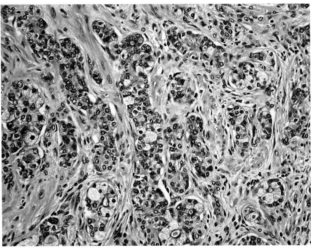

Fig. 5.220 Adenocarcinoma with neuroendocrine differentiation (Paneth cell-like change [PCLC]). Malignant neuroendocrine cells with large eosinophilic granules, designated as PCLC are uncommonly seen. This special form of neuroendocrine differentiation is not known to have any particular clinical significance

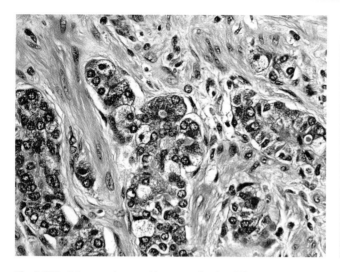

Fig. 5.221 Adenocarcinoma with neuroendocrine differentiation (Paneth cell-like change). Note large intracytoplasmic eosinophilic granules

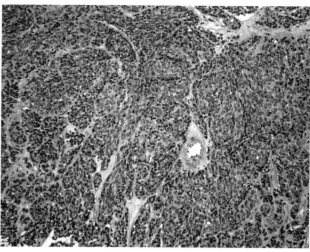

Fig. 5.223 Small cell carcinoma. Tumor cells have scant cytoplasm and hyperchromic nuclei with nuclear molding and inconspicuous nucleoli

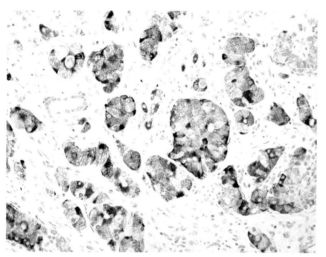

Fig. 5.222 Adenocarcinoma with neuroendocrine differentiation (Paneth cell-like change). Immunostains for neuroendocrine markers, such as synaptophysin, are strongly positive in tumor cells

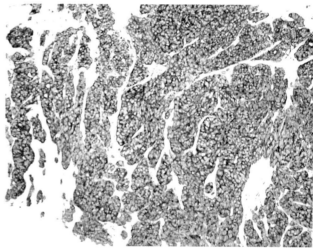

Fig. 5.224 Small cell carcinoma. Immunostain for synaptophysin is strongly positive

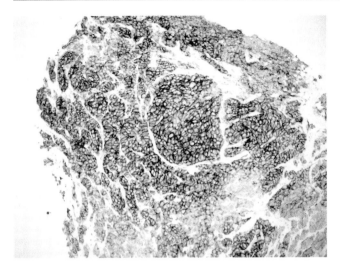

Fig. 5.225 Small cell carcinoma. Immunostain for CD56 is also strongly positive

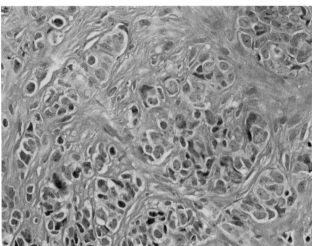

Fig. 5.227 Large cell neuroendocrine carcinoma. The tumor is composed of cells with moderate amounts of cytoplasm and irregular nuclei with prominent nucleoli. Note the presence of nuclear molding as well

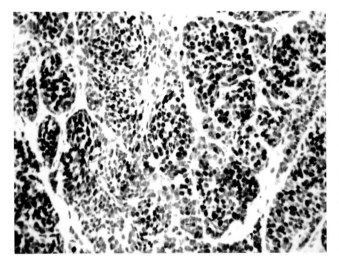

Fig. 5.226 Small cell carcinoma. Nuclear immunoreactivity for thyroid transcription factor-1 is frequently noted in prostatic small cell carcinoma. It does not necessarily indicate a lung primary, although this possibility must be considered clinically

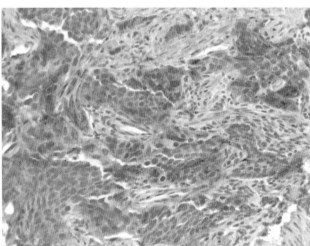

Fig. 5.228 Large cell neuroendocrine carcinoma. The neuroendocrine nature of the malignant cells is confirmed by positive synaptophysin immunostaining

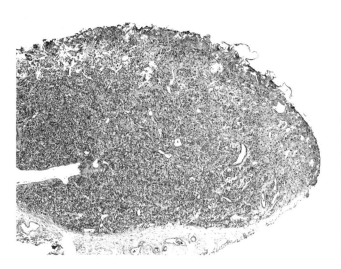

Fig. 5.229 Paraganglioma. This well-circumscribed tumor was discovered incidentally in a patient who underwent transurethral resection for benign prostatic hyperplasia. The patient eventually developed bone metastases

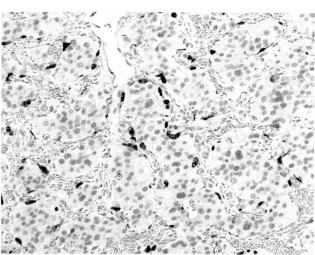

Fig. 5.231 Paraganglioma. Immunostaining for S-100 protein highlights sustentacular cells

5.11 Staging Prostate Cancer

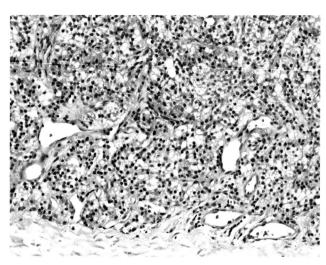

Fig. 5.230 Paraganglioma. The tumor has a Zellballen pattern arrangement of cell nests in fine fibrovascular stroma. Tumor cells have clear cytoplasm and small nuclei

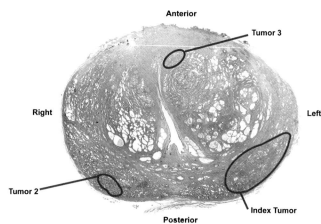

Fig. 5.232 Prostate cancer, pathologic stage pT2c. This is a whole-mount section of a prostate with three separate tumors. In the 2010 American Joint Committee on Cancer TNM staging system, T2 cancer is subclassified as pT2a, pT2b, and pT2c. pT2a cancer is a unilateral tumor involving less than one-half of one side; pT2b cancer is defined by unilateral tumor involving more than one half of one side; pT2c tumor involves both sides of the prostate (bilateral involvement). The majority of prostate cancers are multifocal and bilateral. Stage pT2b cancers are extraordinarily uncommon because tumors occupying more than half of one lobe usually are accompanied by tumor on the other side of midline

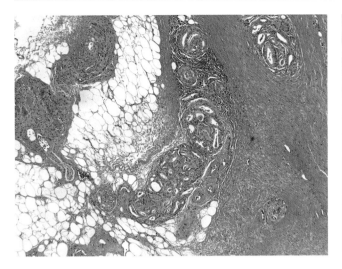

Fig. 5.233 Extraprostatic extension (pT3a). Pathologic stage pT3a cancer is defined by the presence of extraprostatic extension or microscopic invasion of the bladder neck. There are three criteria for extraprostatic extension: (1) cancer in adipose tissue; (2) cancer in perineural space of large neurovascular bundles; and (3) cancer in anterior skeletal muscle. Illustrated here is an example of extraprostatic extension by fat invasion. The tumor has infiltrated beyond the regular contour of the prostate

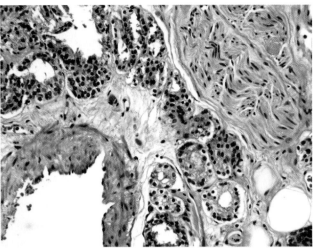

Fig. 5.235 Extraprostatic extension (pT3a). Cancer in perineural space of large neurovascular bundles

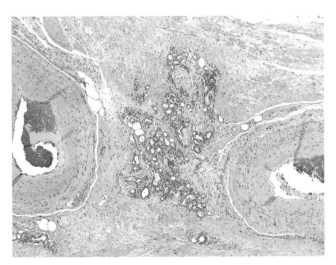

Fig. 5.234 Extraprostatic extension (pT3a). Cancer is present in the perineural space of large posterolateral neurovascular bundles

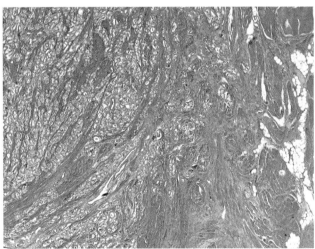

Fig. 5.236 Extraprostatic extension (pT3a). Cancer in anterior skeletal muscle

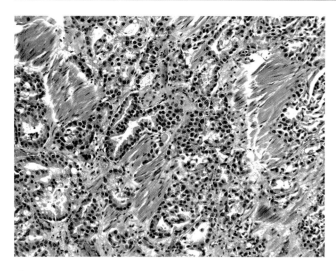

Fig. 5.237 Microscopic invasion of bladder neck (pT3a). Invasion of bladder neck is defined as pT3a cancer in the 2010 TNM classification system

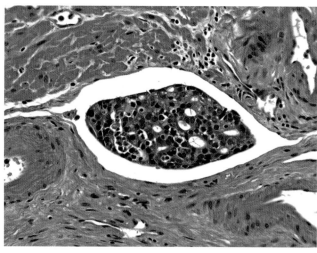

Fig. 5.239 Lymphovascular invasion. Lymphovascular invasion is associated with poor prognosis of prostate cancer

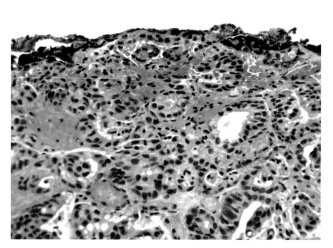

Fig. 5.238 Positive surgical margins. Tumor is present at the inked black margin

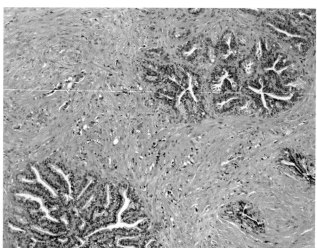

Fig. 5.240 Seminal vesicle invasion (pT3b). Tumor invades into the muscular wall of the seminal vesicle

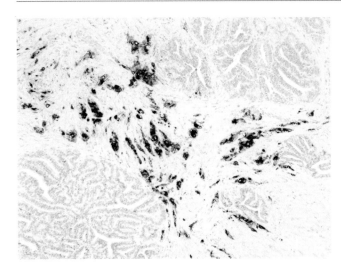

Fig. 5.241 Seminal vesicle invasion (pT3b). Prostate-specific antigen immunostaining show positive immunoreactivity in prostatic cancer and negative staining in seminal vesicle epithelium

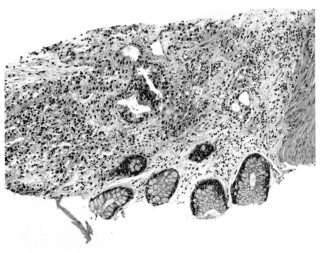

Fig. 5.243 Invasion of rectum (pT4). pT4 cancer is defined by the invasion of rectum, levator muscle, and/or pelvic wall

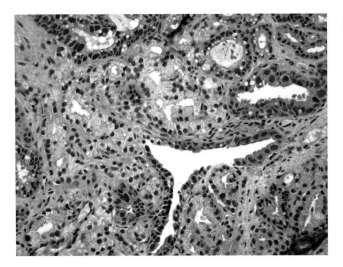

Fig. 5.242 Seminal vesicle invasion (pT3b). Prostatic adenocarcinoma infiltrates between benign seminal vesicle glands. Note golden brown lipofuscin pigments in the epithelium of seminal vesicle

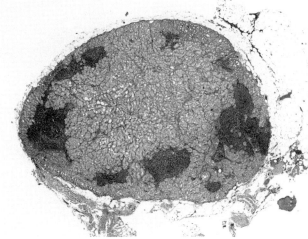

Fig. 5.244 Lymph node metastasis. The lymph node is almost entirely replaced by prostate cancer

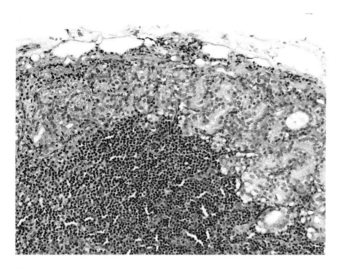

Fig. 5.245 Lymph node metastasis. The metastatic cancer is morpho-logically similar to primary prostatic adenocarcinoma

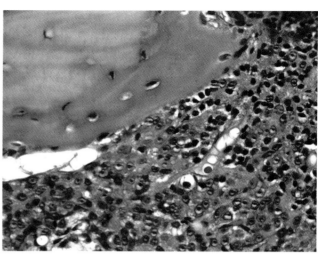

Fig. 5.247 Bone metastasis. Bone is the frequent site of distant metas-tasis for prostate cancer. Tumor often presents as osteolytic lesion

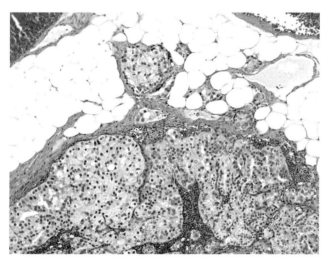

Fig. 5.246 Lymph node metastasis. Extranodal extension of tumor is present

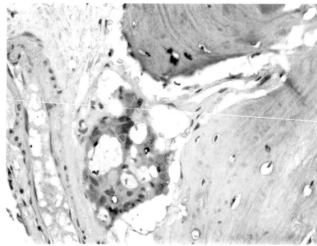

Fig. 5.248 Bone metastasis. Bone biopsy shows marrow involvement by acinar glands that show positive immunostaining for prostate-specific antigen

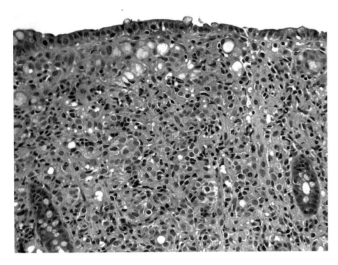

Fig. 5.249 Distant metastasis. In this case, metastatic prostate cancer presented as a cecal mass, visualized at colonoscopy. Biopsy shows diffuse sheets and cords of malignant cells infiltrating the colonic mucosa

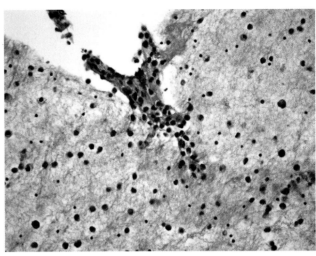

Fig. 5.251 Metastatic prostatic adenocarcinoma cells in ascites. An acinar structure is evident in a cell block of the fluid shown in Fig. 5.250

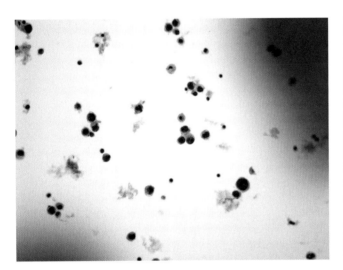

Fig. 5.250 Metastatic prostatic adenocarcinoma cells in ascites. Scattered tumors are present. These tumor cells have high nuclear to cytoplasmic ratio, hyperchromatic nuclei and prominent nucleoli. This patient presented with abdominal pain and swelling due to ascites. At the time of presentation, he had no established diagnosis of cancer

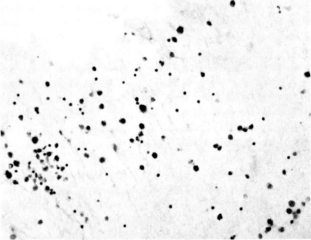

Fig. 5.252 Metastatic prostatic adenocarcinoma cells in ascites. Immunostaining for prostate specific antigen is positive in malignant cells in the cell block

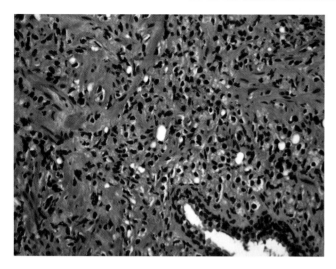

Fig. 5.253 Metastatic prostatic adenocarcinoma. Prostate needle biopsy was performed subsequently in the patient who presented with malignant ascites and showed high-grade adenocarcinoma

5.12 Histologic Findings After Radiation Therapy

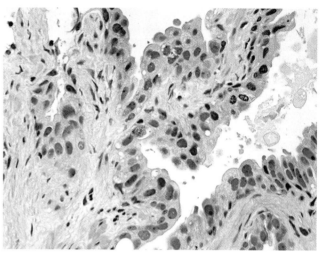

Fig. 5.255 Radiation atypia in benign prostate. The acini are distorted and are lined by cells with marked nuclear abnormalities. The cells have eosinophilic and vacuolated cytoplasm

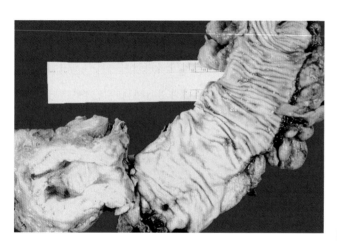

Fig. 5.254 Fistula formation connecting the prostate to the rectum. This patient received radiation therapy for prostate cancer, and developed a fistula

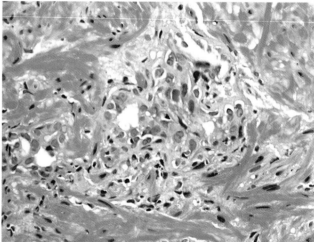

Fig. 5.256 Benign prostate after radiation therapy. Atypical basal cell hyperplasia is very frequent after radiation therapy. The cells have enlarged nuclei with fine powdery chromatin and prominent nucleoli. Note prominent stromal fibrosis and hyalinization

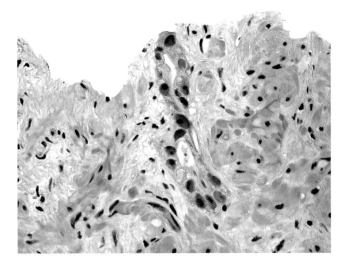

Fig. 5.257 Prostatic adenocarcinoma after radiation therapy. There are marked cytologic abnormalities with prominent nucleoli and occasional double nucleoli. The cytoplasm is amphophilic and finely vacuolated

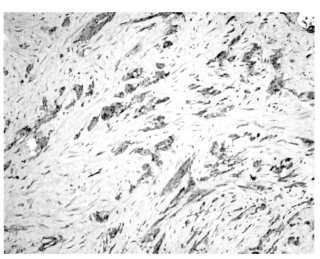

Fig. 5.259 Prostatic adenocarcinoma after radiation therapy. Immunostain using the PIN4 triple-antibody cocktail (high molecular weight cytokeratin 34βE12, α-methylacyl-CoA racemase, and p63) shows complete absence of basal cell layers and weak red cytoplasmic granular staining of racemase in malignant glands

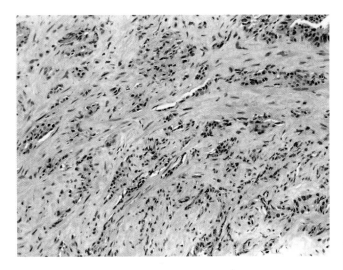

Fig. 5.258 Prostatic adenocarcinoma after radiation therapy. Infiltrative cords and single cells are seen in a fibrotic stroma. Nucleoli appear inconspicuous

5.13 Histologic Findings After Hormonal Therapy

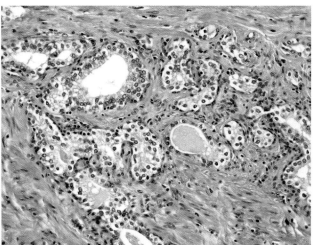

Fig. 5.260 Benign prostate after hormonal therapy. Lobular architecture is retained. Note clearing of the cytoplasm

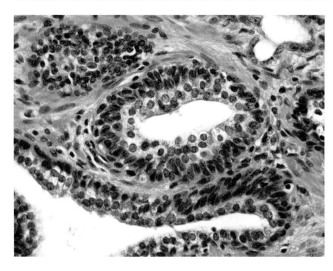

Fig. 5.261 Benign prostate after hormonal therapy. Note basal cell prominence in the benign prostatic glands

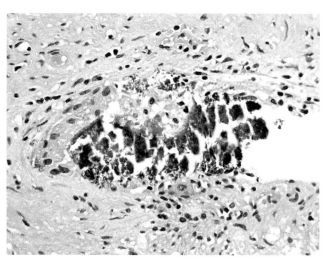

Fig. 5.263 Benign prostate after hormonal therapy. The acini become atrophic, distorted, and calcified

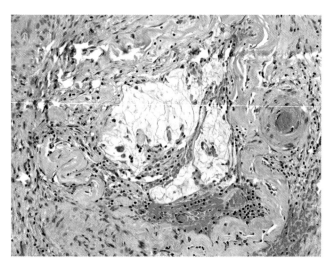

Fig. 5.262 Benign prostate after hormonal therapy. Note mucin and red blood cell extravasation. The stroma is fibrotic with scattered inflammatory cell infiltrate

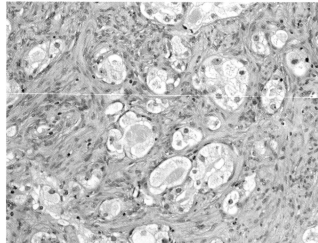

Fig. 5.264 Prostatic adenocarcinoma after hormonal therapy. Cytoplasmic vacuolization and clearing are common after hormonal therapy. Note the infiltrative growth of malignant acini. Prominent nucleoli are seen

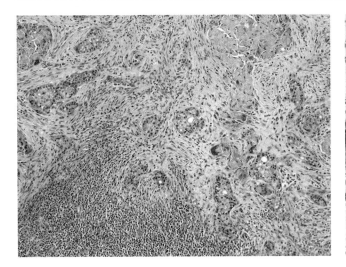

Fig. 5.265 Prostatic adenocarcinoma after hormonal therapy. Infiltrating acini are present in a densely fibrotic stroma. Chronic inflammatory infiltrate is also present (*lower left*). Tumor nuclei may be small and hyperchromatic without prominent nucleoli. Scattered multinucleated giant cells are present

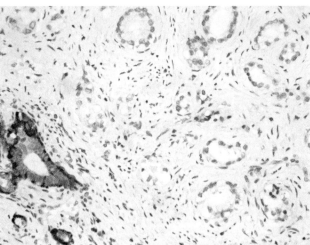

Fig. 5.267 Prostatic adenocarcinoma after hormonal therapy. Immunostain using the PIN4 triple-antibody cocktail (34βE12, racemase, and p63) shows complete loss of basal cell layers in malignant acini, in contrast to intact basal cell layers in the benign glands (*lower left*)

5.14 Mesenchymal Neoplasms of Prostate

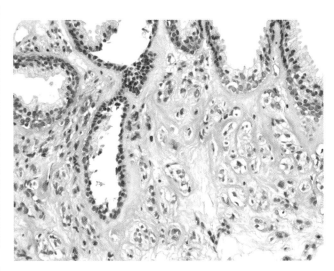

Fig. 5.266 Prostatic adenocarcinoma after hormonal therapy. The malignant cells have enlarged nuclei and prominent cytoplasmic clearing. A few cells have prominent nucleoli

Fig. 5.268 Benign smooth muscle proliferation with epithelioid features. This is an unusual form of smooth muscle proliferation. These epithelioid cells have amphophilic cytoplasm with vacuolization and enlarged nuclei. Immunostain for smooth muscle actin was strongly positive

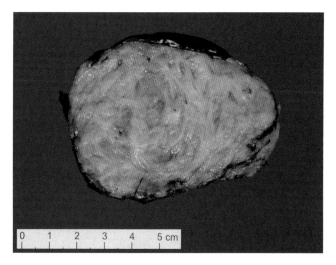

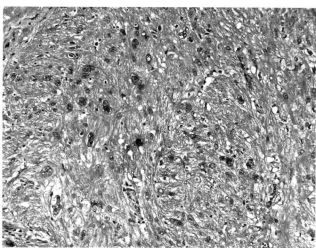

Fig. 5.269 Leiomyoma. The tumor is gray-white and its cut surface has a whorled appearance. This lesion was identified immediately adjacent to the prostate, and was clinically indistinguishable from malignancy, prompting excision

Fig. 5.271 Leiomyoma. Nuclear atypia is present. However, features of malignancy such as necrosis and mitotic Fig.s are not present. Some nuclei are vacuolated and tend to have degenerative appearance

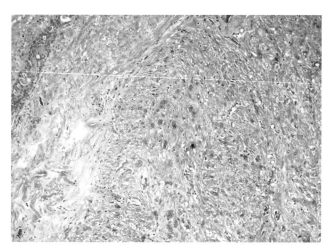

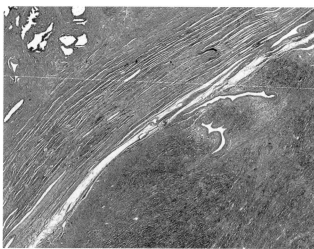

Fig. 5.270 Leiomyoma. The tumor cells are arranged in sheets and fascicles. A benign prostatic acinus is present (*upper left*)

Fig. 5.272 Solitary fibrous tumor. The tumor is well-circumscribed and is composed of proliferating spindle cells. Immunostain for CD34 was strongly positive

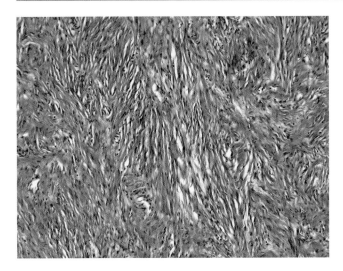

Fig. 5.273 Solitary fibrous tumor. The tumor cells have a fibroblast-like appearance. Note fascicular growth pattern and prominently hyalinized stroma

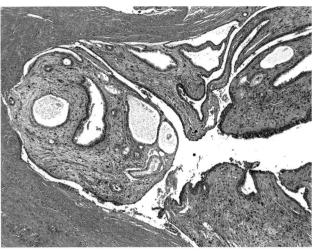

Fig. 5.275 Phyllodes tumor. The tumor has a leaf-like configuration and a high stromal to epithelial ratio, prominent stromal cellularity and overgrowth. Prominent cytologic atypia and increased mitotic activity is often seen in the stromal component. These tumors are not benign and tend to develop recurrence and metastases

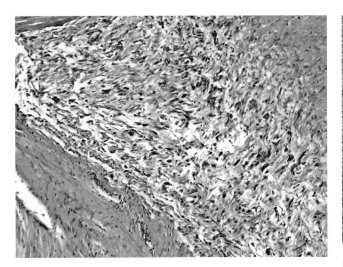

Fig. 5.274 Solitary fibrous tumor. Increased cellularity and nuclear atypia may be seen

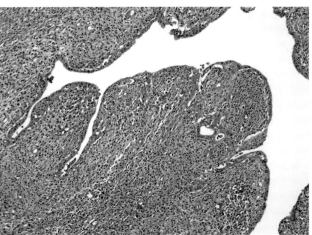

Fig. 5.276 Phyllodes tumor. Marked stromal proliferation produces leaflike structures that appear to project into a cystic space. The overlying epithelium is unremarkable

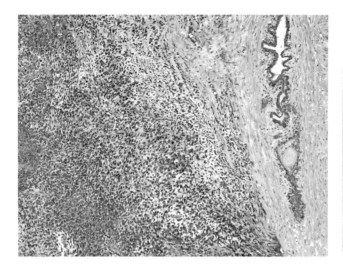

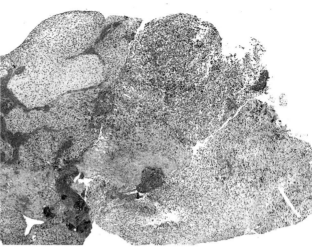

Fig. 5.277 Stromal sarcoma. There is significantly increased cellularity in stromal sarcoma. The neoplastic cells are pleomorphic and spindle shaped with increased nuclear to cytoplasmic ratio. Stromal sarcoma is a diagnosis of exclusion. A panel of immunostains should be performed to rule out other diagnostic entities such as rhabdomyosarcoma, leiomyosarcoma, and tumors of neural origin. Metastasis from other organ sites should also be ruled out

Fig. 5.279 Embryonal rhabdomyosarcoma. Low-power view shows alternating cellular and myxoid areas. Tumor is composed of primitive "small round blue cells"

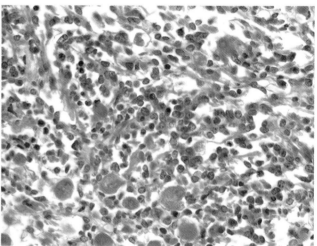

Fig. 5.278 Stromal sarcoma. There is substantial cytologic atypia in this highly cellular stromal tumor. Increased vascularity is noted

Fig. 5.280 Embryonal rhabdomyosarcoma. Tumor cells are arranged in sheets of immature small round cell in a myxoid stroma. Note the presence of rhabdomyoblasts with abundant densely eosinophilic cytoplasm

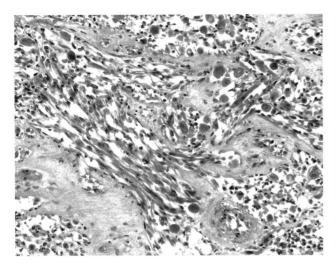

Fig. 5.281 Embryonal rhabdomyosarcoma. Numerous rhabdomyoblasts and strap cells with eosinophilic cytoplasmic processes are present

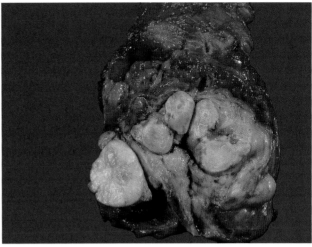

Fig. 5.283 Leiomyosarcoma. The tumor appears multinodular grossly. It obliterates the prostate and protrudes upwards into the lumen of the bladder

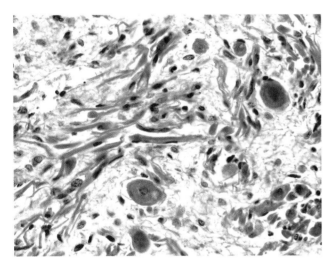

Fig. 5.282 Embryonal rhabdomyosarcoma. Higher magnification of the previous case shows cross-striation in strap cells

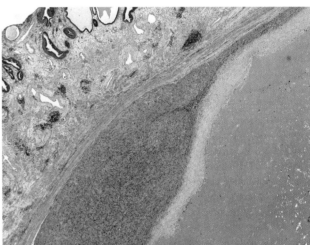

Fig. 5.284 Leiomyosarcoma. Tumor necrosis is present

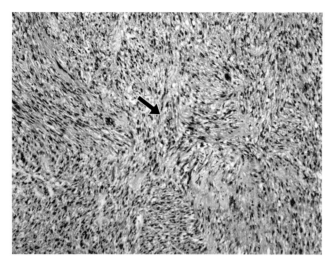

Fig. 5.285 Leiomyosarcoma. It is composed of intersecting fascicles of tumor cells with eosinophilic cytoplasm and blunt-ended nuclei. Atypical mitotic figure can be seen (*arrow*)

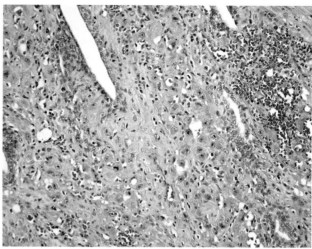

Fig. 5.287 Angiosarcoma. The tumor is composed of pleomorphic epithelioid cells forming cleft-like and sinusoidal spaces filled with red blood cells. The prostatic glands are unremarkable

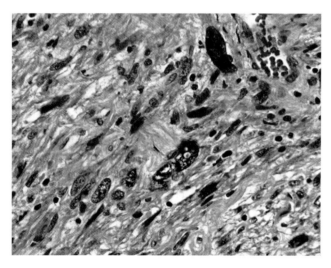

Fig. 5.286 Leiomyosarcoma. Note nuclear anaplasia

5.15 Hematopoietic and Lymphoid Neoplasms

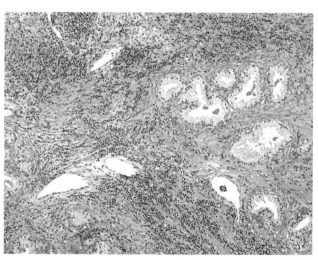

Fig. 5.288 Lymphoma. The stroma is diffusely infiltrated by small lymphocytic B-cell lymphoma

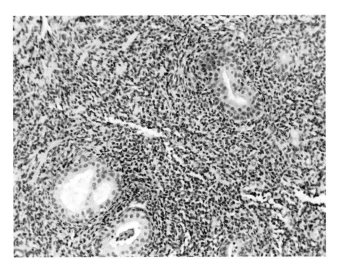

Fig. 5.289 Lymphoma. The stroma is expanded by monotonous small lymphocytes (low grade B-cell lymphoma)

5.16 Cancers Involving Prostate by Direct Extension or Metastasis

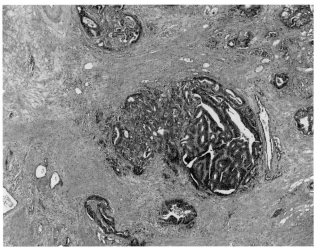

Fig. 5.291 Metastatic colonic adenocarcinoma in the prostate. Note nuclear pleomorphism, desmoplasia and "dirty" comedonecrosis

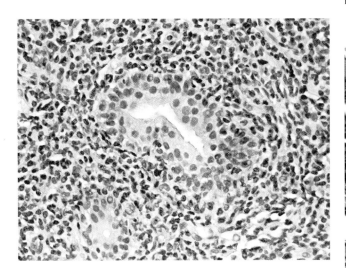

Fig. 5.290 Lymphoma. Note intraepithelial infiltrate by small lymphocytic B-cell lymphoma

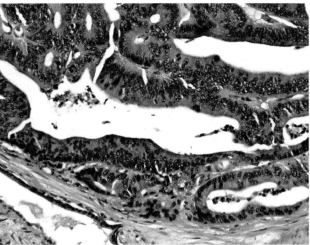

Fig. 5.292 Metastatic colonic adenocarcinoma in the prostate. One of the differential diagnostic considerations is ductal adenocarcinoma. Immunostain for prostate-specific antigen is helpful in making this distinction

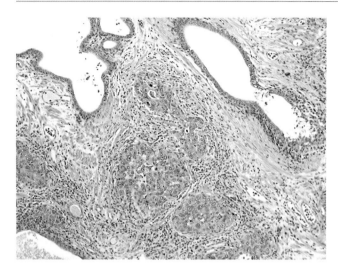

Fig. 5.293 Urothelial carcinoma involving the prostate. Note prominent nuclear pleomorphism, apoptotic bodies, and inflammatory stroma. These features are not common in typical prostatic adenocarcinoma

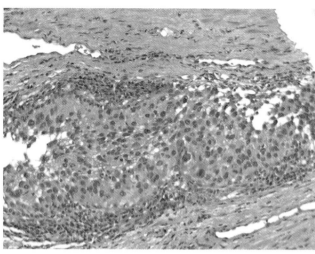

Fig. 5.295 Urothelial carcinoma involving the prostate. The prostatic duct is filled with malignant urothelial cells which have substantial nuclear pleomorphism and prominent eosinophilic cytoplasm, but lack nucleolar prominence. Prior to this biopsy, there was no clinical suspicion for urothelial cancer in this patient, but the diagnosis of bladder cancer was subsequently confirmed

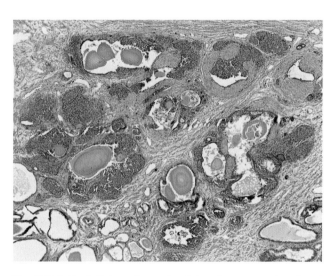

Fig. 5.294 Urothelial carcinoma involving the prostate, intraductal spread. The acini are expanded by malignant urothelial cells. Note the presence of numerous corpora amylacea

5.17 Cancers Involving Seminal Vesicle by Direct Extension or Metastasis

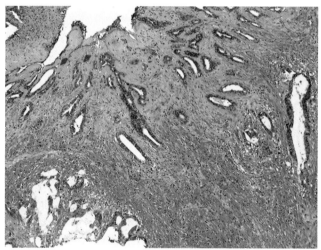

Fig. 5.296 Seminal vesicle invasion by colonic adenocarcinoma. The muscular wall is infiltrated by colonic adenocarcinoma. There is minimal stromal reaction

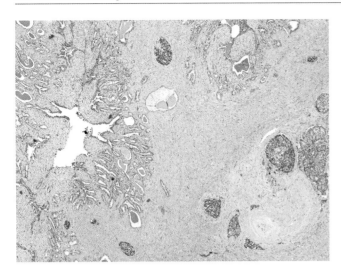

Fig. 5.297 Seminal vesicle invasion by urothelial carcinoma. Urothelial carcinoma directly invades into the muscular wall of the seminal vesicle. Immunostains are useful in distinguishing urothelial carcinoma from prostatic adenocarcinoma. Urothelial carcinoma is usually positive for cytokeratin 20, p63 and high molecular weight cytokeratin 34βE12, and negative for prostate-specific antigen and prostatic-specific acid phosphatase

Testis

6

The testis is the site of many diverse pathologic conditions in males of all ages. In children, nondescent is a common problem. After the onset of puberty, males become more susceptible to the development of germ cell tumors and some are troubled by infertility problems. All postpubertal males are at risk for various infectious and noninfectious inflammatory conditions affecting the testis. Older men, although less likely to develop germ cell tumors, experience a gradually increasing incidence of testicular lymphoma

6.1 Normal Histology

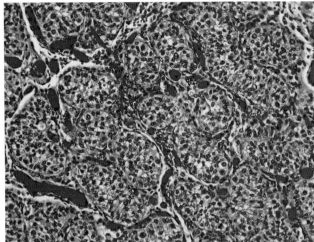

Fig. 6.2 Testis at birth. No lumens are apparent in the seminiferous tubules. The tubules are populated predominantly by Sertoli cells. Also present at this stage of development are two types of germ cells: gonocytes and spermatogonia

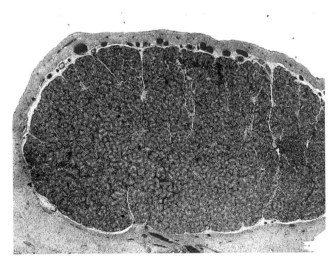

Fig. 6.1 Testis at birth. This is a section is from an 8-day-old neonate. The thin tunica albuginea gives rise to intratesticular septa which separate the testis into lobules

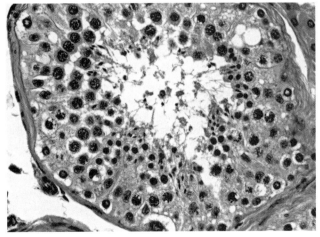

Fig. 6.3 Normal testis, postpuberty. The seminiferous tubule is enclosed by a basement membrane, myofibroblasts, fibroblasts, collagen, elastic fibers, and extracellular matrix, which together comprise the 6 μm thick tunica propria. Spermatogonia are basal cells with pale cytoplasm, round nuclei, and eccentric nucleoli. Above these are Sertoli cells with large central nucleoli. The inner layers include primary and secondary spermatocytes, spermatids, and mature spermatozoa

G. MacLennan and L. Cheng, *Atlas of Genitourinary Pathology*, DOI: 10.1007/978-1-84882-395-2_6,
© Springer-Verlag London Limited 2011

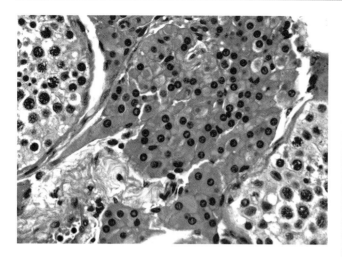

Fig. 6.4 Normal testis, postpuberty. Leydig cells occupy the interstitium of the testis, singly and in clusters. They have abundant eosinophilic cytoplasm and round eccentric nuclei with one or two nucleoli. Their cytoplasm sometimes contains lipofuscin pigment or Reinke's crystalloids

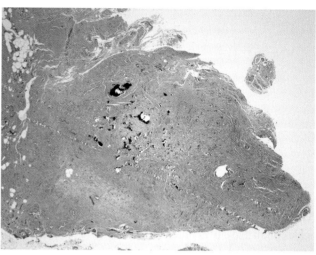

Fig. 6.6 Vanishing testis syndrome. The nodule at the terminus of the vas deferens in this case consists only of fibrous tissue, with abundant microcalcifications and scattered hemosiderin-laden macrophages

6.2 Congenital Lesions

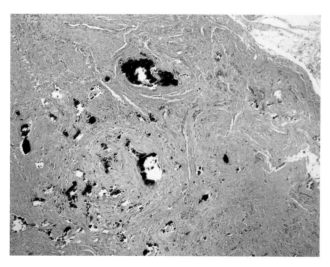

Fig. 6.5 Vanishing testis syndrome. This is considered to represent the remnants of in utero testicular infarction. Exploration for an impalpable testis discloses the presence of a vas deferens that ends in a small fibrotic nodule. In some cases, remnants of epididymis are present; in others, such as the case shown here, neither epididymis nor testicular tissue are found

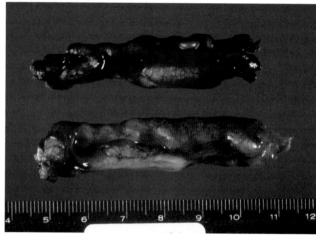

Fig. 6.7 Gonadal dysgenesis. Streak gonads are a component of several different gonadal dysgenesis syndromes, in which affected patients are phenotypic females with amenorrhea, uterine and fallopian tube hypoplasia and streak gonads, exemplified in this image of the gonads from a 16-year-old girl with amenorrhea. Gonadal dysgenesis in a patient with a Y chromosome imparts a substantial risk of development of germ cell tumors. Both ovaries in this patient were streak ovaries; a microscopic focus of gonadoblastoma was present in one of them (*see* MacLennan GT, Resnick MI, Bostwick DG, 2003. With permission)

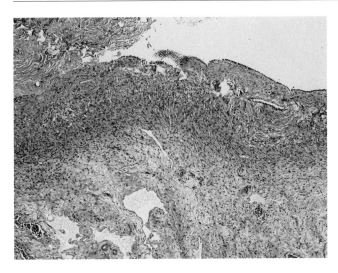

Fig. 6.8 Gonadal dysgenesis. This is a streak ovary from a 12-year-old phenotypic female with gonadal dysgenesis. It is predominantly fibrous tissue, but beneath the surface is a zone of tissue resembling ovarian stroma. No germ cell elements are present

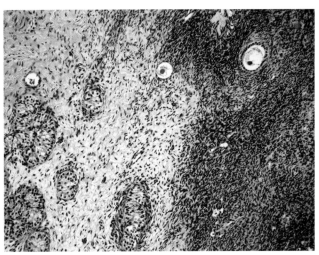

Fig. 6.10 True hermaphroditism. Higher power view of the section shown in Fig. 6.9. Immature seminiferous tubules on the left, ovarian stroma with a few primordial follicles on the right

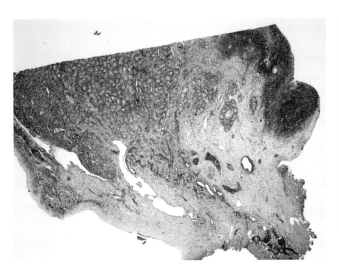

Fig. 6.9 True hermaphroditism. This term implies the presence of both testicular and ovarian tissue in the same individual. In this ovotestis, seminiferous tubules and rete testis are present at left; at right, ovarian tissue is present

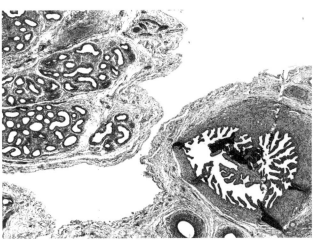

Fig. 6.11 True hermaphroditism. This gonad had components of epididymis (*left*) and fallopian tube (*right*)

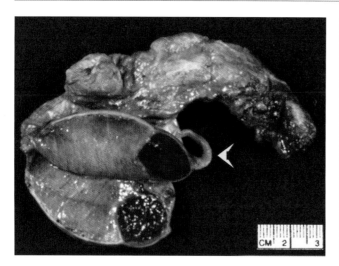

Fig. 6.12 Splenogonadal fusion. Splenic and gonadal tissue sometimes fuse during fetal development, and after birth, the splenic tissue is apparent as a circumscribed red nodule, usually less than 1.0 cm in size and adjacent to or, less frequently, within the testis. In some cases, a fibrous cord (*arrowhead*) may maintain some continuity between the spleen and the testis as it descends; the cord may contain elements of splenic tissue (*see* MacLennan GT, Resnick MI, Bostwick DG, 2003. With permission)

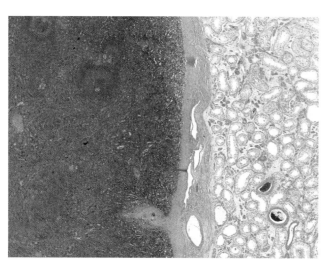

Fig. 6.13 Splenogonadal fusion. The nodule consists of normal splenic tissue (*left*) separated from the normal testicular tissue by a fibrous interface

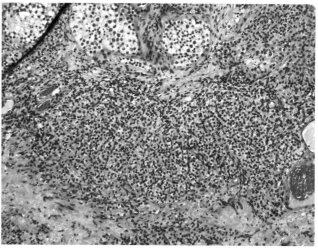

Fig. 6.14 Ectopic adrenal tissue in testis. Nodules of intratesticular ectopic adrenal tissue are usually less than 0.5 cm in size; the small aggregate of ectopic adrenal cortical cells shown here was an incidental finding in a testis excised for unrelated reasons

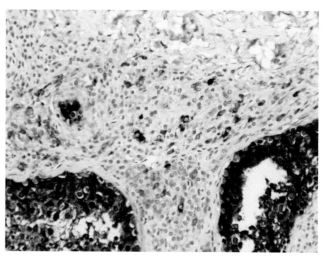

Fig. 6.15 Ectopic adrenal tissue in testis. The ectopic adrenal cells in the interstitium show positive immunostaining for inhibin

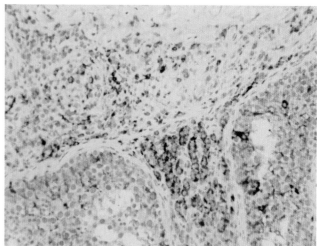

Fig. 6.16 Ectopic adrenal tissue in testis. The ectopic adrenal cells in the interstitium show positive immunostaining for Melan A

6.3 Inflammatory Conditions

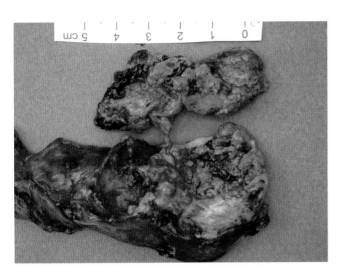

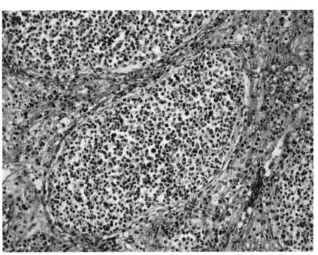

Fig. 6.19 Mumps orchitis. The testis becomes painful and swollen 4–6 days after symptoms of parotitis. The testis is involved by widespread foci of acute inflammation of the seminiferous tubules and interstitial tissues. Acute and chronic inflammatory cells destroy the normal intraluminal cellular components of the seminiferous tubules, which ultimately become hyalinized, and the testis becomes atrophic. Bilateral involvement commonly results in infertility

Fig. 6.17 Acute and chronic epididymoorchitis. Most cases of bacterial orchitis arise in conjunction with bacterial epididymitis. The orchiectomy specimen shown here was from a man who presented initially with purulent material draining from a sinus in his scrotum connected to an intratesticular abscess with extensive necrosis. Cultures grew several different types of bacteria *(Image courtesy of* Pedro Ciarlini, MD)

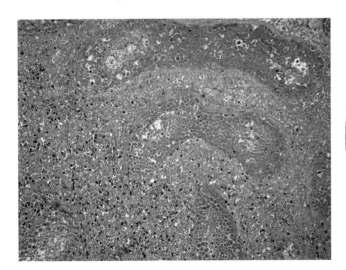

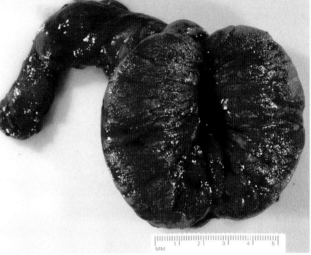

Fig. 6.18 Acute and chronic epididymoorchitis. A section from the specimen in Fig. 6.17 shows the ghostly outlines of infarcted seminiferous tubules, surrounded by purulent exudate containing neutrophils and other inflammatory cells

Fig. 6.20 Idiopathic granulomatous orchitis. Typically, this enigmatic lesion arises in older adult males, often with associated symptoms of urinary infection, trauma, or flu-like illness. The testis becomes swollen, painful, and tender initially but later may have a residual mass indistinguishable from a neoplasm, prompting orchiectomy. The testis shown here had no distinct mass lesion, but was swollen and edematous with a bulging cut surface *(see* MacLennan GT, Resnick MI, Bostwick DG, 2003. With permission)

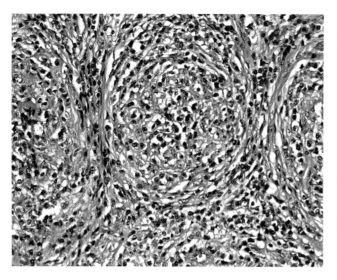

Fig. 6.21 Idiopathic granulomatous orchitis. No granulomas are present, but the interstitial and intratubular aggregation of epithelioid histiocytes, lymphocytes, and plasma cells imparts a granulomatous appearance. Sertoli cells and germ cells are absent from the seminiferous tubules

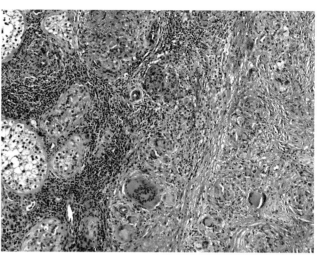

Fig. 6.23 Sarcoidosis of the testis. Sarcoidosis can affect the testis, and can mimic malignancy, particularly if accompanied by radiologic pulmonary abnormalities. This images shows nonnecrotizing granulomas involving testicular parenchyma. Special stains for fungal organisms and acid-fast bacilli were negative, and other clinical parameters were found to be consistent with sarcoidosis

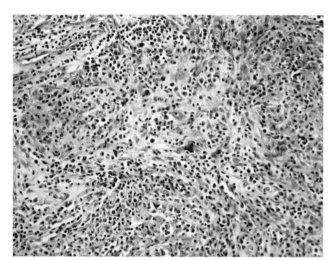

Fig. 6.22 Idiopathic granulomatous orchitis. The diffuse infiltration of testicular parenchyma by a polymorphous assortment of chronic inflammatory cells, including lymphocytes, plasma cells, eosinophils, macrophages, and multinucleated giant cells, has left no structural resemblance to normal testicular tissue

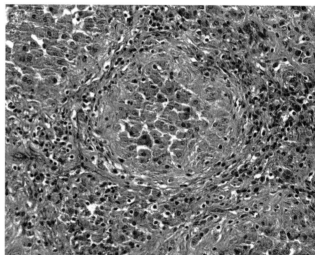

Fig. 6.24 Malakoplakia of testis. Malakoplakia may affect only the testis, or less commonly, both testis and epididymis, resulting in formation of soft yellow, tan, or brown nodules that replace normal testicular parenchyma. The tubules and interstitium are extensively infiltrated by large histiocytes that have abundant eosinophilic granular cytoplasm (von Hansemann histiocytes)

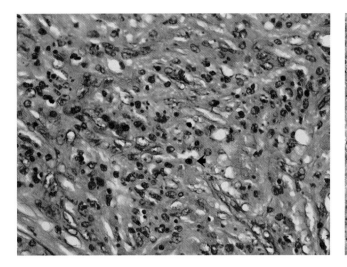

Fig. 6.25 Malakoplakia of testis. Careful search reveals the presence of solid and targetoid basophilic inclusions (Michaelis-Gutmann bodies, *arrow*) supporting the diagnosis of malakoplakia

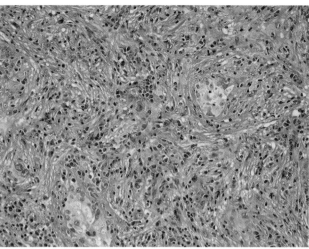

Fig. 6.27 Myofibroblastic pseudotumor of testis. Section from the nodule shown in Fig. 6.26 showing an atypical inflammatory and myofibroblastic reaction with fasciitis-like large cells. Features of malignancy were absent. The process was regarded as a benign reactive and proliferative process of uncertain etiology

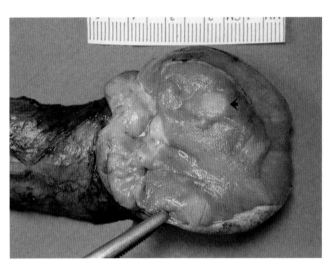

Fig. 6.26 Myofibroblastic pseudotumor of testis. Lesion in the testis of a patient with quadriplegia, recurrent urinary infection, and a bout of epididymoorchitis; lesion was noted on ultrasound, and was followed for 1 year without changing significantly. Orchiectomy was done due to uncertainty regarding neoplasia (*Image courtesy of* Stacy Kim, MD)

6.4 Vascular Insults

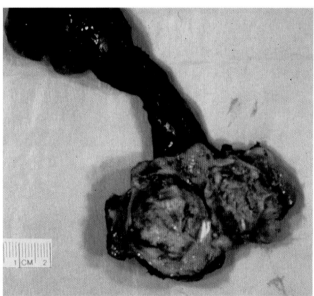

Fig. 6.28 Testicular infarction, chemically induced. An unusual case, in which a man's sexual partner injected lactic acid directly into both of his testes, as part of sex play. The testes became painful and both were excised several days later; both appeared gangrenous

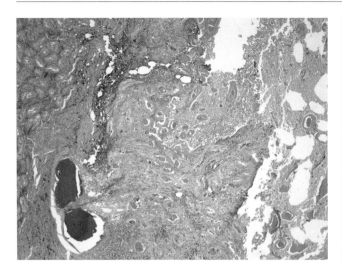

Fig. 6.29 Testicular infarction, chemically induced. Section from the testis shown in Fig. 6.28, showing thrombosed blood vessels and extensive ischemic necrosis of testicular parenchyma

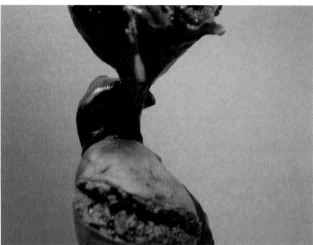

Fig. 6.32 Testicular torsion. This image illustrates the "bell-clapper deformity," in which the tunica vaginalis completely encircles the distal spermatic cord, the epididymis, and testis, rather than reflecting off the posterolateral aspect of the testis. Consequently, the testis is free to swing and rotate within the tunica sac, much like a clapper inside a bell

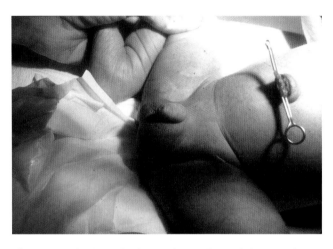

Fig. 6.30 Testicular torsion in a newborn male. The left scrotum is reddened and swollen

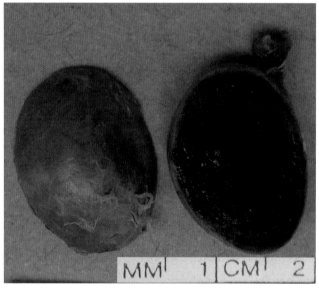

Fig. 6.33 Testicular torsion. Sectioned testis from the patient shown in Fig. 6.30. The testis is hemorrhagic and ischemic

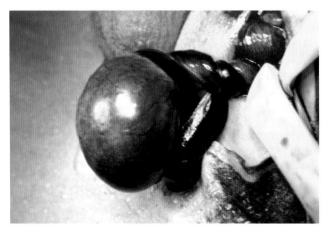

Fig. 6.31 Testicular torsion. The testis has undergone at least two complete revolutions and is obviously ischemic (*see* MacLennan GT, Resnick MI, Bostwick DG, 2003. With permission)

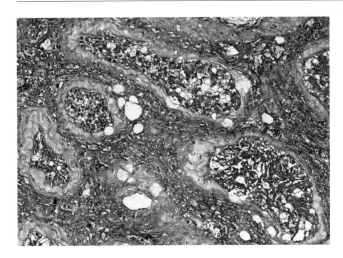

Fig. 6.34 Testicular torsion. Only the ghostly outlines of testicular parenchyma are present; tissue is nonviable

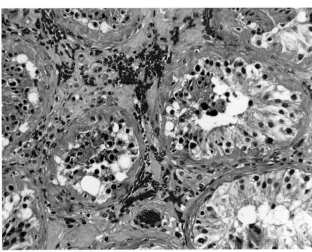

Fig. 6.36 Testicular infarction, segmental, due to vasculitis. Some cells within the seminiferous tubules appear viable; others appear nonviable

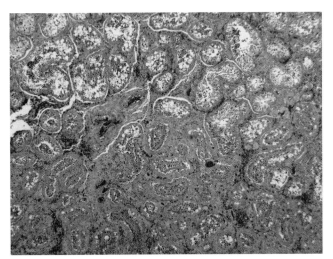

Fig. 6.35 Testicular infarction, segmental, due to vasculitis. Patient was a 35-year-old man with systemic lupus erythematosus who developed rather abrupt onset of severe testicular pain and underwent orchiectomy. Testis was grossly unremarkable on sectioning but microscopy revealed areas of segmental testicular infarction

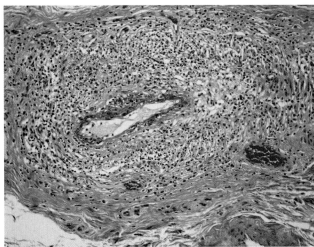

Fig. 6.37 Testicular infarction, segmental, due to vasculitis. Section of a spermatic cord blood vessel from patient illustrated in Figs. 6.42 and 6.43. The blood vessel wall shows fibrinoid material in the luminal surface and full thickness infiltration by inflammatory cells, morphologically consistent with lymphocytic vasculitis. Within 2 months after loss of this testis, patient developed necrosis in the opposite testis, with abscess formation, necessitating orchiectomy

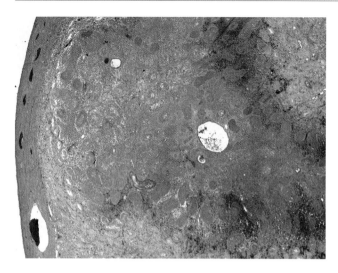

Fig. 6.38 Testicular infarction, segmental, associated with organizing thrombi in spermatic cord vessels. This 44-year-old man presented with testicular discomfort. Ultrasound showed a mass indeterminate for neoplasia, prompting radical orchiectomy. On sectioning, the testis had a 1.3 cm poorly circumscribed hemorrhagic mass. Section from the mass, shown here, shows segmental infarction of the testis

6.5 Entities Contributing to Infertility

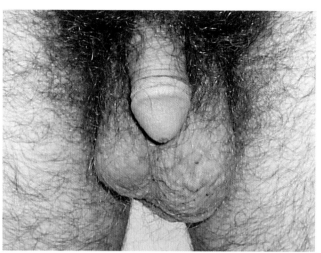

Fig. 6.40 Varicocele. Patient with oligospermia. When upright, the left side of the patient's scrotum is visibly larger than the right, due to the presence of large varicosities of the pampiniform plexus of the spermatic cord. The majority of varicoceles are left-sided (*Image courtesy of* Allen Seftel, MD)

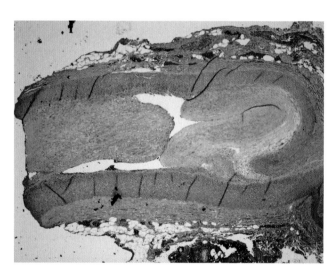

Fig. 6.39 Testicular infarction, segmental. Section from cord blood vessel in the case shown in Fig. 6.38 shows an organizing thrombus, which may have contributed to the testicular infarct. Cause of the vascular disturbance was not apparent; patient was otherwise well

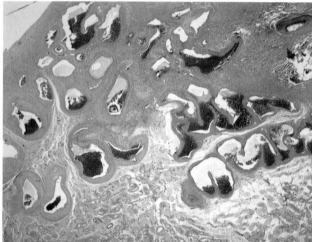

Fig. 6.41 Varicocele. Markedly dilated veins with eccentric mural fibrosis abut the testis

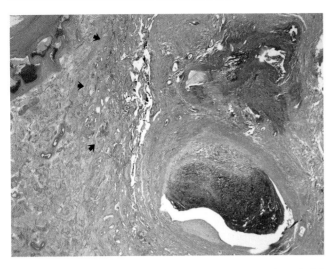

Fig. 6.42 Varicocele. The rete testis, indicated by arrows, is encircled by dilated thick-walled veins, one of which contains a thrombus. One theory of the relationship between varicocele and oligospermia holds that the tortuous veins disrupt and compress the rete testis cavities and partially obstruct the tubuli recti; the adverse effects initially involve the ipsilateral testis, but with time, pressure effects develop in the contralateral testis as well

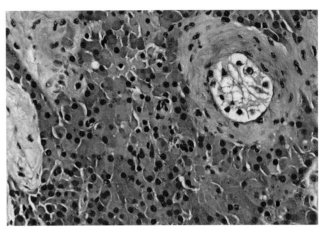

Fig. 6.44 Klinefelter's syndrome. There is pseudoadenomatous clustering of Leydig cells. The apparent hyperplasia reflects a normal population of Leydig cells in a reduced testicular volume due to relative paucity of other elements such as seminiferous tubules and their contents

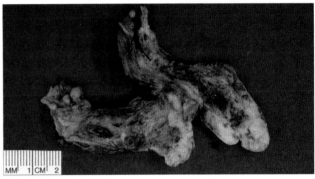

Fig. 6.45 Undescended testis. The specimen is from a 20-year-old man; the testis was in the inguinal canal and was associated with an inguinal hernia. Specimen is predominantly composed of blood vessels, fibromuscular tissue, and portions of epididymis. Very little testicular parenchyma is present (*arrow*)

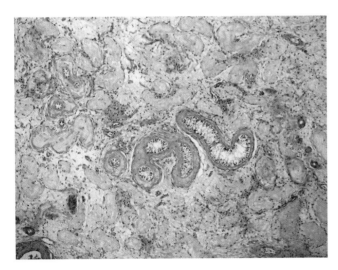

Fig. 6.43 Klinefelter's syndrome. Testis shows tubular dysgenesis. Seminiferous tubules are small, and most are completely hyalinized. Scattered patent tubules with markedly thickened walls are present, but contain only Sertoli cells; no germ cell elements are present

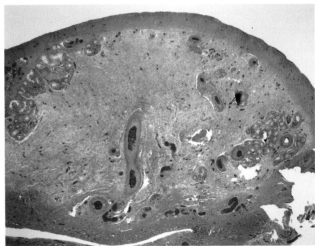

Fig. 6.46 Undescended testis. Seminiferous tubules are greatly diminished in number

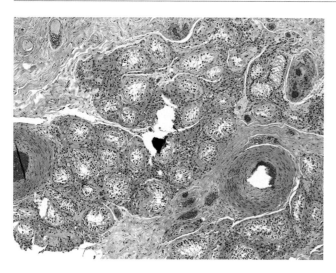

Fig. 6.47 Undescended testis. Tubules are small and have some mural hyalinization. No spermatogenesis is evident

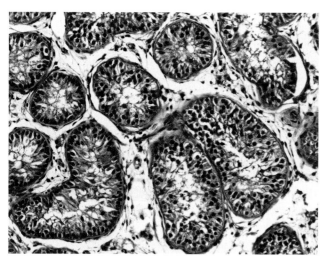

Fig. 6.48 Undescended testis. Tubules are small and are populated by rare spermatogonia and by Sertoli cells that appear immature

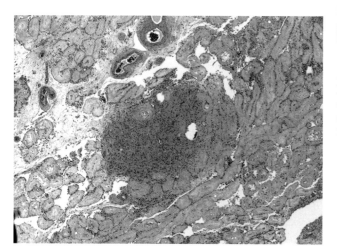

Fig. 6.49 Undescended testis. Extensive tubular hyalinization and one of many Leydig cell nodules, which are also commonly abundant in cases of Klinefelter's syndrome (compare with Fig. 6.44)

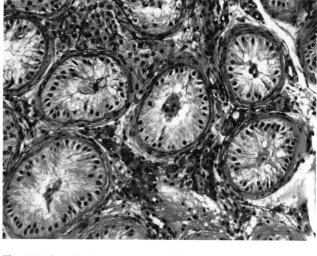

Fig. 6.50 Sertoli cell-only syndrome. This is a descriptive term, applied in all cases of azoospermia in which the seminiferous epithelium consists only of Sertoli cells, as in the image shown here. It is not a single syndrome; it is the common finding in a variety of syndromes that may be primary or secondary in origin

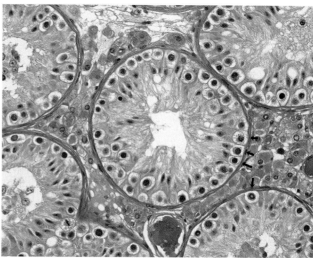

Fig. 6.51 Spermatogonial maturation arrest. A layer of spermatogonia (*arrows*) lies adjacent to the wall of the tubule, beneath the Sertoli cells. No other germ cell types are present. Abundant Leydig cells are present in the interstitium. Spermatogonial maturation arrest and the two variants of hypospermatogenesis are the most frequent histologic findings in testicular biopsies from men with infertility

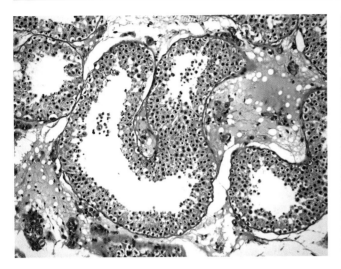

Fig. 6.52 Pure hypospermatogenesis. This is one of the two quantifiable variants of hypospermatogenesis; the other is hypospermatogenesis associated with primary spermatocyte sloughing (*see* Fig. 6.54). In pure hypospermatogenesis, there is a proportionate diminution in the numbers of all germ cell types; few or no mature spermatozoa are present

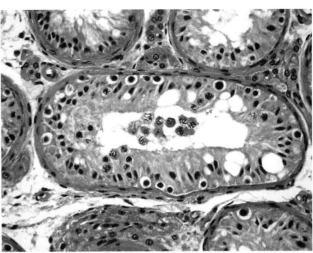

Fig. 6.54 Hypospermatogenesis associated with primary spermatocyte sloughing. Spermatogonia and primary spermatocytes are the only types of germ cells present

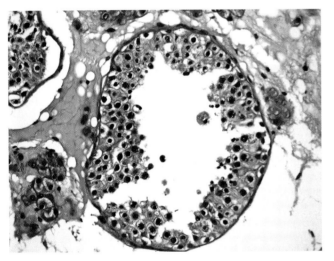

Fig. 6.53 Pure hypospermatogenesis. All germ cell layers are limited in number. No spermatozoa are present

6.6 Intratubular Germ Cell Neoplasia

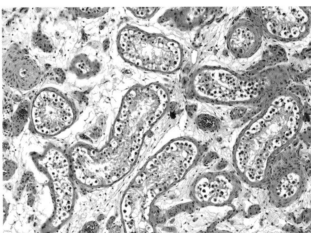

Fig. 6.55 Intratubular germ cell neoplasia, unclassified (IGCNU). Cells with large dark nuclei and abundant optically clear cytoplasm are arrayed basally in the seminiferous tubules, and have displaced the residual Sertoli cells towards the lumen. No spermatogenesis is evident

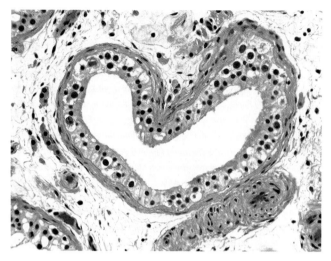

Fig. 6.56 Intratubular germ cell neoplasia, unclassified (IGCNU). In some cases, the cells of IGCNU have one or two prominent nucleoli. In some cases, such as this one, the diagnosis of IGCNU is not as readily apparent as in Fig. 6.55. Compare this image with Fig. 6.51, which illustrates spermatogonial maturation arrest. In such cases, immunostains are often helpful in making the distinction

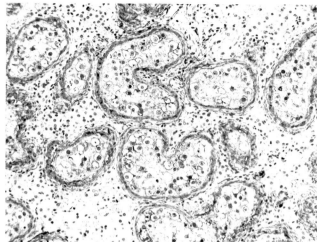

Fig. 6.58 Intratubular germ cell neoplasia, unclassified (IGCNU). Immunostaining using antibodies directed against placental alkaline phosphatase shows predominantly cytoplasmic membrane positivity in cells of IGCNU

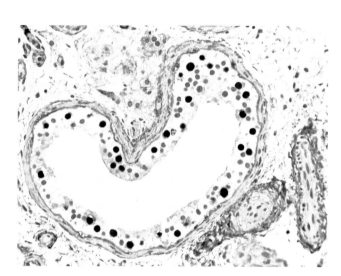

Fig. 6.57 Intratubular germ cell neoplasia, unclassified (IGCNU). Cells of IGCNU typically show strong nuclear immunostaining for OCT4. Normal intratubular spermatogenic cells show no OCT4 immunostaining

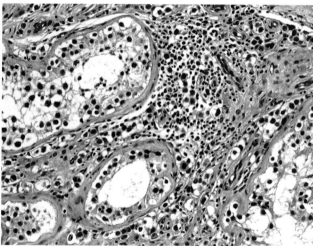

Fig. 6.59 Intratubular germ cell neoplasia, unclassified (IGCNU), with extratubular extension. A few malignant germ cells are present in the stroma of tubules involved by IGCNU. The tumor cells do not form an expansile mass

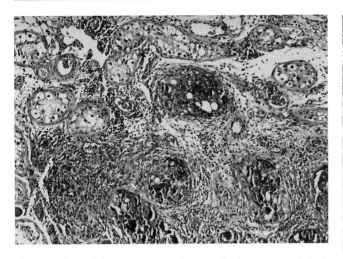

Fig. 6.60 Intratubular germ cell neoplasia, unclassified (IGCNU). This is an example of IGCNU, at top, admixed with intratubular embryonal carcinoma (*center* and *lower right*)

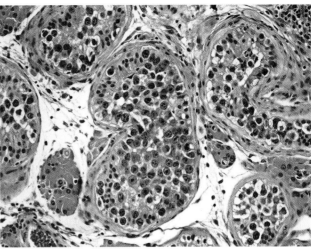

Fig. 6.62 Intratubular seminoma. The seminiferous tubules are entirely filled with seminoma cells. In most instances, invasive seminoma is also present in the specimen

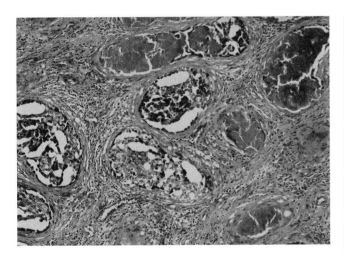

Fig. 6.61 Intratubular embryonal carcinoma. The tubules are filled with neoplastic cells that are morphologically similar to those of invasive embryonal carcinoma. There is extensive necrosis, which is often accompanied by microcalcifications

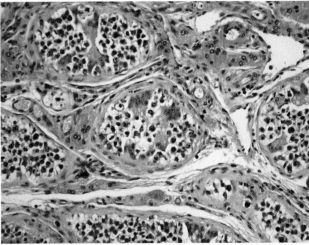

Fig. 6.63 Intratubular seminoma with syncytiotrophoblastic cells. This is an uncommon finding, but not surprising in view of the frequency with which similar cells are noted in invasive seminomas

6.7 Germ Cell Tumors

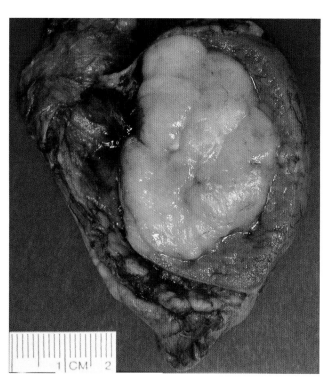

Fig. 6.64 Seminoma. Seminoma is usually well circumscribed, bulging, and lobulated, and clearly demarcated from adjacent normal testicular tissue. Cut surface may be light cream-colored, yellow, tan, or pink. Hemorrhage and necrosis are limited in most, but occasionally necrosis may be extensive *(Image courtesy of Kelly Nigro, MD)*

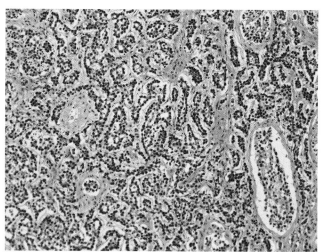

Fig. 6.66 Seminoma. The growth patterns of seminoma are diverse, depending upon the degree of stromal edema and fibrosis. In addition to growing in diffuse sheets, tumor cells may form small nests, cords, pseudotubules, microcysts, pseudoglands, and cribriform spaces. Shown here is an example of pseudotubular pattern of growth

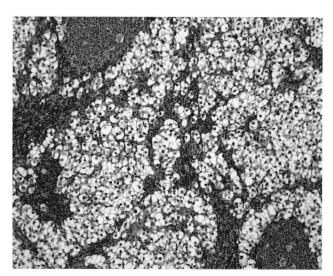

Fig. 6.65 Seminoma. Tumor cells grow in sheets separated by fibrous septa containing blood vessels. Lymphoid infiltrates are virtually always present, sometimes imparting a florid reactive appearance with germinal centers

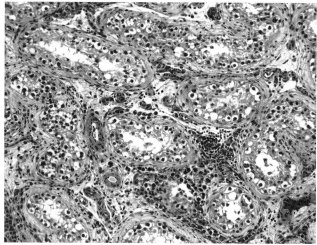

Fig. 6.67 Seminoma. This image illustrates interstitial growth of seminoma, leaving native tubules intact. In most instances, this is seen at the periphery of an obvious expansile seminoma; rarely, however, this may be the predominant pattern or even the only pattern of growth apparent in the specimen

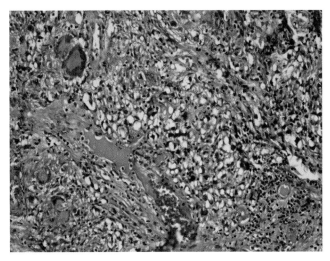

Fig. 6.68 Seminoma. About half of seminomas show varying degrees of granulomatous inflammation. This image shows numerous multinucleated giant cells and epithelioid histiocytes mixed with and almost obscuring the seminoma cells

Fig. 6.70 Seminoma. Tumor cells have a plasmacytoid appearance, with eccentric nuclei and dark eosinophilic to amphophilic cytoplasm

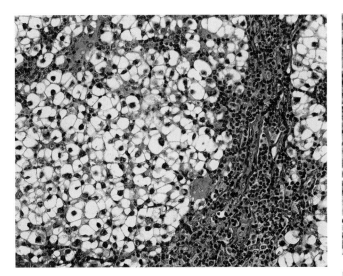

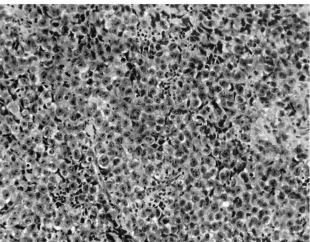

Fig. 6.69 Seminoma. Tumor cells are typically optically clear to lightly eosinophilic. Nuclear membranes are slightly thickened and are quite distinct. Nuclei do not overlap; they are round to oval, fairly uniform in size, with dispersed chromatin and one or two prominent nucleoli. Lymphoid infiltrates tend to clusters in the region of the fibrovascular septa

Fig. 6.71 Seminoma. Many seminomas display abundant mitotic figures. The degree of mitotic activity in seminoma has not been convincingly linked to prognosis

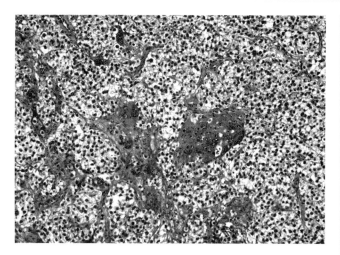

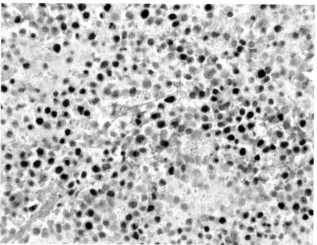

Fig. 6.72 Seminoma. Syncytiotrophoblasts are found in 4–7% of semi-nomas, usually randomly scattered. They may be accompanied by small collections of blood, but the extensive bleeding and necrosis typically seen in choriocarcinoma are absent, and the tumor cells mingled with the syncytiotrophoblasts are seminoma cells, not cytotrophoblasts, as would be seen in choriocarcinoma

Fig. 6.74 Seminoma. Despite being nonviable, seminoma cells often display nuclear immunoreactivity to antibodies against OCT4, as shown here, as well as against CD117. The use of immunostains for OCT4, CD117, pankeratin, and CD30, and assessment for the presence of coarse intratubular calcifications, can be helpful in placing most totally necrotic testicular tumors into clinically important groups

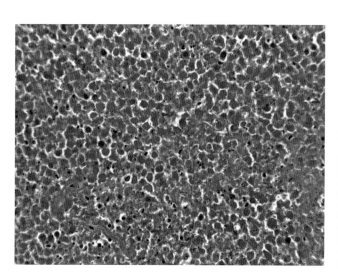

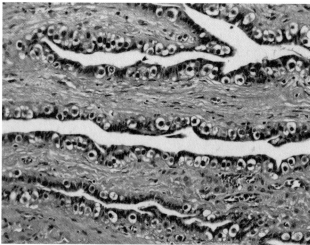

Fig. 6.73 Seminoma. Necrosis in seminoma is typically focal, but is extensive in 12% of cases. Usually, the ghostly outlines of necrotic tumor cells are recognizable. This can be diagnostically problematic when assessing small biopsies of retroperitoneal or mediastinal mass lesions

Fig. 6.75 Seminoma. Tumor cells involve the rete testis by pagetoid spread. This process can occur in cases of IGCNU as well as in invasive seminoma. Invasion of the stroma of the rete testis does not alter prognosis and is not a staging parameter

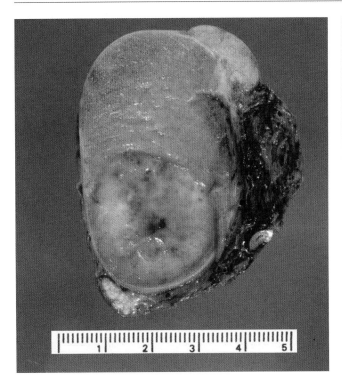

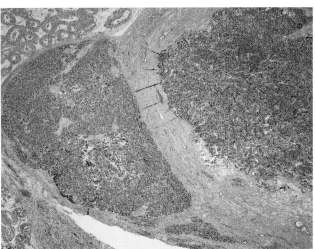

Fig. 6.78 Spermatocytic seminoma. Tumor cells are arranged in diffuse sheets. In some spermatocytic seminomas, the sheets are intersected by bands of fibrous stroma, which are usually delicate but occasionally are broad, as in this case

Fig. 6.76 Spermatocytic seminoma. Spermatocytic seminoma ranges from 3 to 15 cm in diameter; it is usually well-circumscribed, soft, and gray-tan. It may be multilobulated or multicentric. The cut surface may be mucoid or friable, and cysts may be present. Hemorrhage and necrosis are limited in extent (*see* MacLennan GT, Resnick MI, Bostwick DG, 2003. With permission)

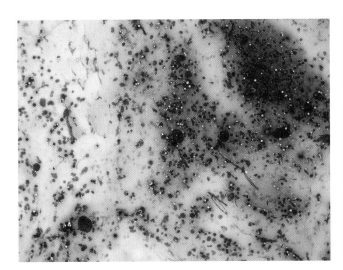

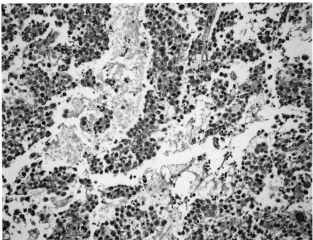

Fig. 6.77 Spermatocytic seminoma. This tumor arose in an older man, and a Diff-Quik stain was done on cells scraped from the fresh specimen to assess for the possibility of lymphoma. The cytologic preparation shows a polymorphous cell population, with a remarkable disparity in the size of the tumor cells, which is not typical of lymphoma

Fig. 6.79 Spermatocytic seminoma. Areas of intercellular edema are often present, artifactually creating architectural complexity. The tumor cells may appear to be forming glandular structures, nests, or trabeculae

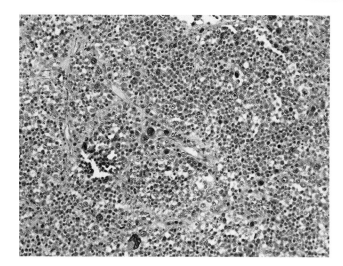

Fig. 6.80 Spermatocytic seminoma. Tumors cells are typically arranged in large sheets. Unlike classic seminoma, lymphoid infiltrates are rare and granulomatous reactions are absent. Even at low power, it is evident that the tumor is composed of a polymorphous cell population

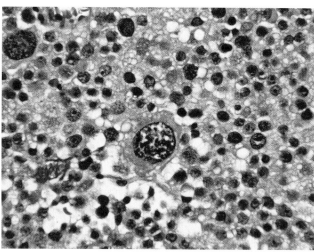

Fig. 6.82 Spermatocytic seminoma. The nuclei of the giant cells may exhibit a filamentous or "spireme" chromatin distribution that mimics the appearance of primary spermatocytes in meiotic prophase. Medium and giant cell nuclei often have one or more nucleoli

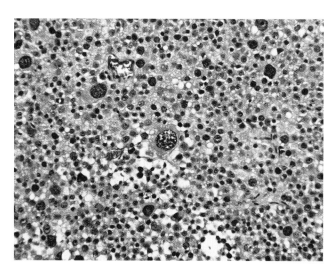

Fig. 6.81 Spermatocytic seminoma. The tumor cells are of three types. Small cells are about 6–8 μm in diameter, with scant cytoplasm and very dark nuclei, and may be degenerate cells. Medium-sized (intermediate) cells are about 15–20 μm in diameter. Giant cells range from 50 to 100 μm in diameter. Cell membranes are indistinct. Mitotic activity varies, but may be quite brisk

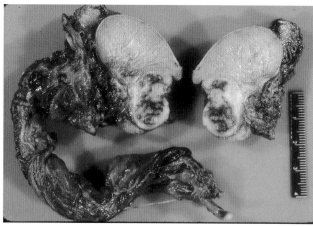

Fig. 6.83 Embryonal carcinoma. This purely embryonal carcinoma, associated with a varicocele, was excised from a 14-year-old male. The cut surface of embryonal carcinoma is often somewhat granular in consistency; necrosis and hemorrhage are common and may be extensive. It is typically smaller than seminoma and its interface with adjacent normal parenchyma may be somewhat indistinct

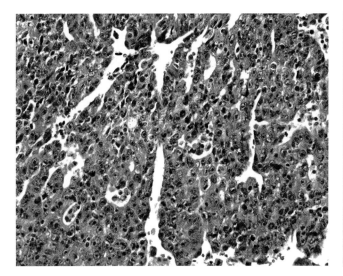

Fig. 6.84 Embryonal carcinoma. Tumor architecture is variable. Tumor cells often grow in diffuse sheets and may be arranged to resemble poorly formed glands. Tumor cells are large and tend to overlap one another, and cell membranes are difficult to discern, lending a syncytial appearance to the tumor. Tumor cell nuclei are vesicular with irregular outlines, coarse chromatin, and prominent nucleoli. Mitotic figures and apoptotic cells are abundant

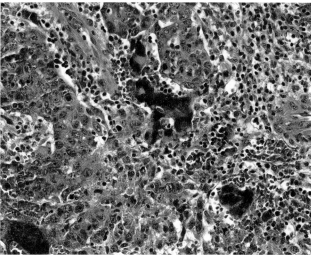

Fig. 6.86 Embryonal carcinoma. Syncytiotrophoblasts are commonly identifiable in embryonal carcinoma. As is the case in seminoma (Fig. 6.72), absence of large blood lakes and absence of cytotrophoblasts negates the likelihood of choriocarcinoma (*see* MacLennan GT, Resnick MI, Bostwick DG, 2003. With permission)

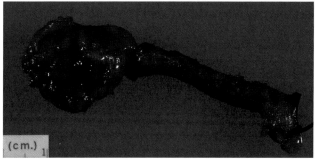

Fig. 6.87 Yolk sac tumor. This is the commonest testicular tumor in children, the majority of whom are less than 2 years old. The tumor in this image was from a young child. In children, yolk sac tumor is typically pure in its makeup. It tends to be bulging, shiny, or mucoid, and may show areas of cystic degeneration (*Image courtesy of* Beverly Dahms, MD)

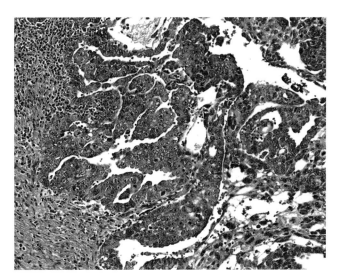

Fig. 6.85 Embryonal carcinoma. Papillary structures are commonly present; some contain a fibrovascular core, whereas others lack a stromal core and consist simply of piled-up malignant cells

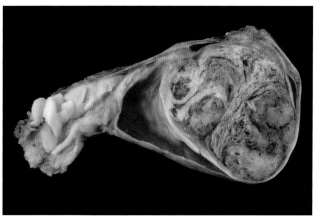

Fig. 6.88 Yolk sac tumor. In adults, yolk sac tumor is almost invariably a component of a mixed germ cell tumor. The tumor shown in this image had only rare microscopic foci of teratoma; the remainder was yolk sac tumor. Hemorrhage, necrosis, cystic degeneration, mucoid consistency, and poor circumscription are findings typical of yolk sac tumor

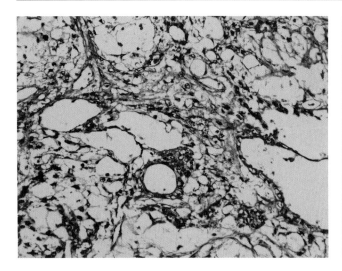

Fig. 6.89 Yolk sac tumor. There are several recognized growth patterns of yolk sac tumor. The commonest is the reticular pattern, shown here. Thin cords of tumor cells or thin cytoplasmic processes anastomose to form a sieve-like appearance. The microcystic appearance of the reticular pattern is in part related to the presence of prominent cytoplasmic vacuoles within tumor cells. The vacuolated tumor cells may resemble lipoblasts

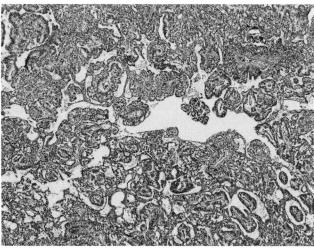

Fig. 6.91 Yolk sac tumor. The endodermal sinus pattern of yolk sac tumor is characterized by the presence of irregular interconnecting labyrinthine-like spaces and Schiller-Duval bodies, several of which are nicely illustrated (*lower right*)

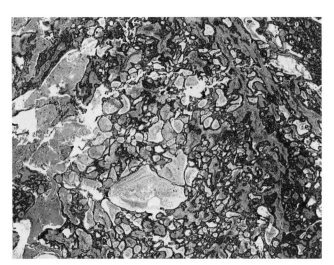

Fig. 6.90 Yolk sac tumor. Microcysts and macrocysts intermingle. The background stroma appears myxoid

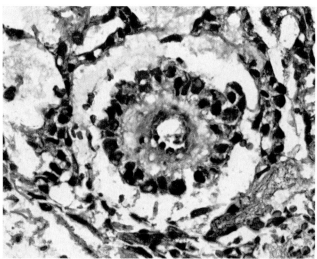

Fig. 6.92 Yolk sac tumor. Schiller-Duval bodies consist of a transversely or longitudinally sectioned fibrovascular papillary structure, lined by malignant cells, encircled within a small cystic space that is also lined by flattened malignant cells. This architectural arrangement was originally recognized as being similar to the endodermal sinuses of the rat placenta, accounting for the alternative designation of "endodermal sinus tumor" (*see* MacLennan GT, Resnick MI, Bostwick DG, 2003. With permission)

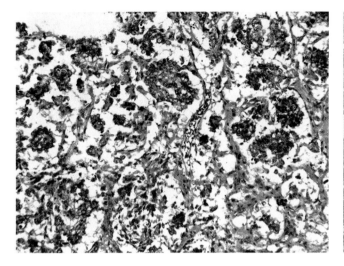

Fig. 6.93 Yolk sac tumor. This tumor exhibits papillary structures of nonspecific type

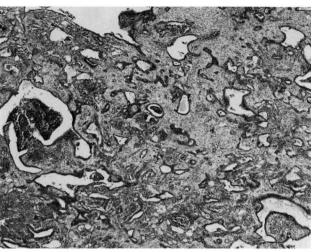

Fig. 6.95 Yolk sac tumor. The glandular variant of yolk sac tumor is characterized by irregularly shaped glandular structures. The epithelium lining the glands is variable in appearance; it often resembles enteric epithelium

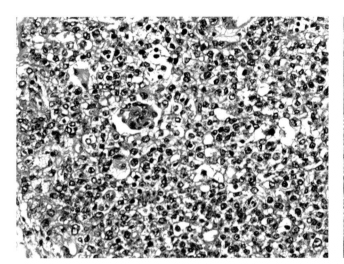

Fig. 6.94 Yolk sac tumor. The solid variant of yolk sac tumor is shown here, composed of a sheet-like arrangement of polygonal tumor cells with distinct cell membranes and abundant clear to lightly eosinophilic cytoplasm. Tumor cells do not overlap, and their nuclei are fairly uniform in size, with small but distinct nucleoli. This pattern may mimic seminoma, but lacks the fibrovascular septae and the inflammatory cell component typically seen in seminoma

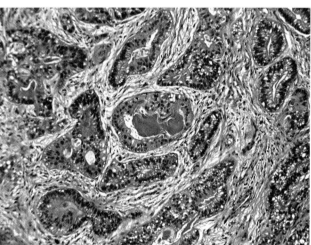

Fig. 6.96 Yolk sac tumor. Infrequently, the epithelium lining the glands in yolk sac tumors with glandular architecture resembles early secretory endometrium

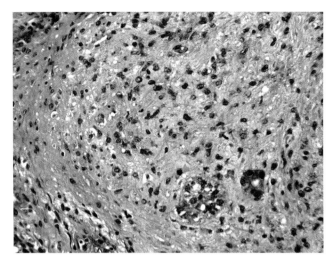

Fig. 6.97 Yolk sac tumor. The myxomatous variant of yolk sac tumor is somewhat hypocellular; it is composed of stellate, spindled, and in this case, some small epithelioid cells, dispersed in abundant myxoid stroma

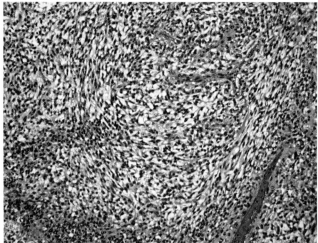

Fig. 6.99 Yolk sac tumor. Sarcomatoid morphology is uncommon; it is usually seen in a background of another pattern. In this case, the tumor was predominantly solid, with areas of myxoid change, but showed foci of proliferating spindle cells

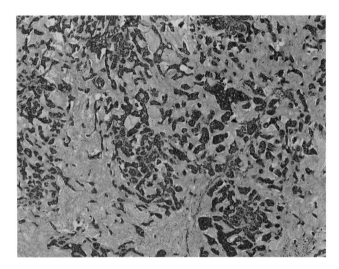

Fig. 6.98 Yolk sac tumor. A myxomatous component is common in yolk sac tumors of various morphologic types; in this case, the tumor is predominantly of solid type

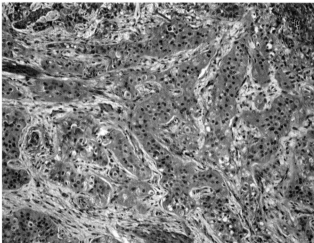

Fig. 6.100 Yolk sac tumor. This is an example of the hepatoid variant of yolk sac tumor. This pattern is seen in about 20% of yolk sac tumors, usually only focally. It consists of clusters of tumor cells resembling hepatocytes, arranged in nests or trabeculae, which show positive immunostaining for α-fetoprotein. In some, small canaliculi may be apparent

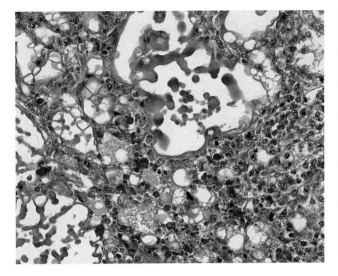

Fig. 6.101 Yolk sac tumor. The abundant brightly eosinophilic structures are aggregates of basement membrane material in the extracellular space, and are considered indicative of parietal differentiation in yolk sac tumor (see MacLennan GT, Resnick MI, Bostwick DG, 2003. With permission)

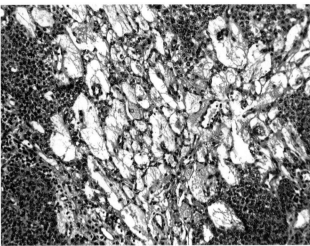

Fig. 6.103 Yolk sac tumor. Another example of mixed architectural patterns in yolk sac tumor: this is a mixture of microcystic and solid patterns

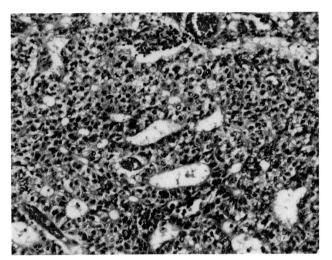

Fig. 6.102 Yolk sac tumor. Mixed patterns of tumor cell growth are common in yolk sac tumor. This image shows a mixture of solid and glandular architecture

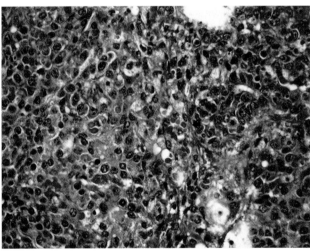

Fig. 6.104 Yolk sac tumor. Yolk sac tumors often contain clusters of hyaline eosinophilic globules (arrow) which are in the cytoplasm of tumor cells but may be extracellular after tumor cell death. They occur in tumors other than yolk sac tumor, but are not usually seen in other types of testicular germ cell tumors

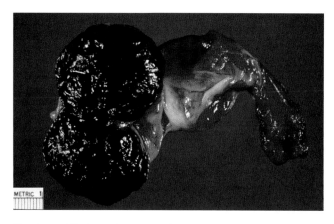

Fig. 6.105 Choriocarcinoma. In this instance, the testis is replaced by a bloody bulging mass. More typically, choriocarcinoma tends to be somewhat smaller, and may not significantly distort the testis (*see* MacLennan GT, Resnick MI, Bostwick DG, 2003. With permission)

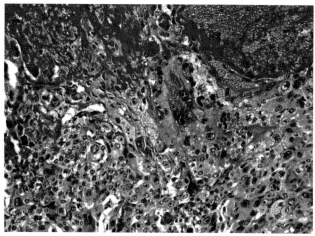

Fig. 6.108 Choriocarcinoma. The multinucleated syncytiotrophoblasts have voluminous eosinophilic cytoplasm and large darkly staining irregular nuclei with prominent nucleoli. The smaller mononuclear cytotrophoblasts are fairly uniform in size. They have modest amounts of clear to amphophilic cytoplasm; they bear some resemblance to the tumor cells of solid yolk sac tumor

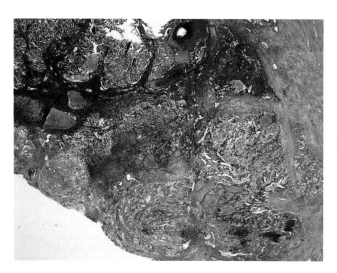

Fig. 6.106 Choriocarcinoma. At very low power, the most striking feature is a large zone of blood and necrosis with viable tumor surrounding it

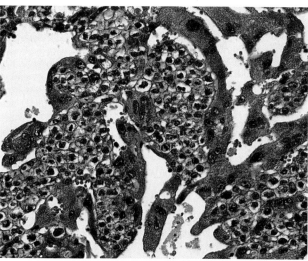

Fig. 6.109 Choriocarcinoma. Tumor consists of sheets of pale cytotrophoblast cells encircled or "capped" by syncytiotrophoblasts, somewhat resembling the appearance of immature placental villi. The cell membranes of the cytotrophoblasts are distinctly outlined (*see* MacLennan GT, Resnick MI, Bostwick DG, 2003. With permission)

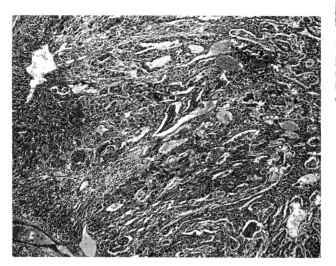

Fig. 6.107 Choriocarcinoma. The tumor is composed of a mixture of large multinucleated cells and smaller mononuclear cytotrophoblast cells

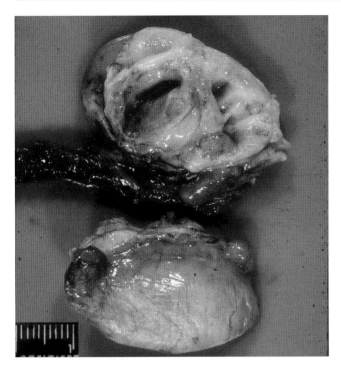

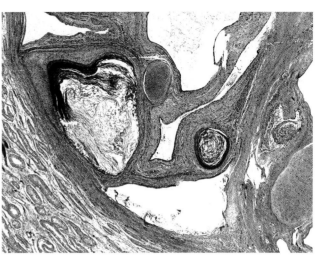

Fig. 6.112 Teratoma. At low power, the presence of somatic-type tissues is evident: squamous-lined cysts containing keratin (ectodermal), cartilage (mesodermal), and large glandular structures lined by columnar epithelium (endodermal)

Fig. 6.110 Teratoma. Teratomas typically have both solid and cystic components. The solid component is sometimes recognizable as cartilage. The material within the cysts may be serous, mucoid, or keratinous. This tumor arose in the testis of a 2-year-old boy, and as such was considered benign (*Image courtesy of* Beverly Dahms, MD)

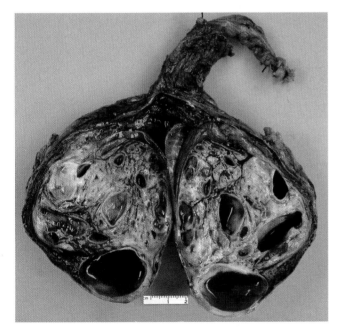

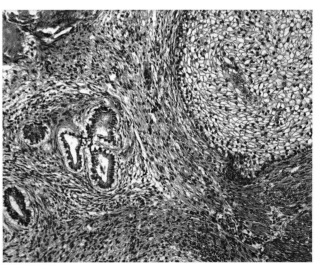

Fig. 6.113 Teratoma. Glands and an island of squamous epithelium set in a fibrous stroma

Fig. 6.111 Teratoma. This was a pure teratoma in a 26-year-old man. Teratomas are often large and nodular and distort the tunica albuginea, but rarely extend locally beyond the confines of the testis

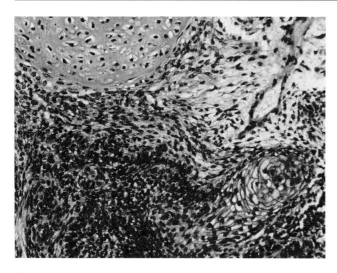

Fig. 6.114 Teratoma. Cartilage and an island of squamous epithelium set in a fibrous stroma

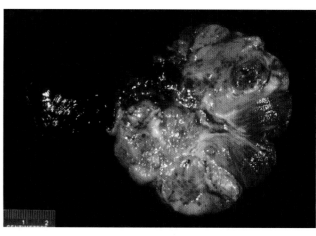

Fig. 6.116 Teratoma with immature elements. This teratoma had a very extensive component of immature elements in the form of primitive neuroectodermal tumor, perhaps accounting for its fleshy bulging encephaloid appearance and the areas of hemorrhage (*see* MacLennan GT, Resnick MI, Bostwick DG, 2003. With permission)

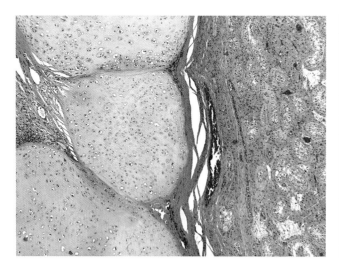

Fig. 6.115 Teratoma. Nodules of cartilage at the interface between a teratoma and the adjacent benign testicular tissue. Rarely, a teratoma is composed only of cartilage

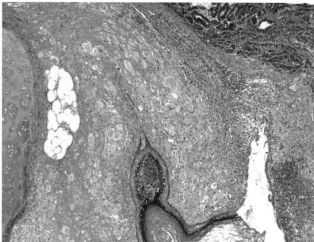

Fig. 6.117 Teratoma with immature elements. This teratoma with mature adipose, cartilage and squamous elements has an area of immature tissue at upper right. Immature elements, if limited, appear to have no influence on prognosis

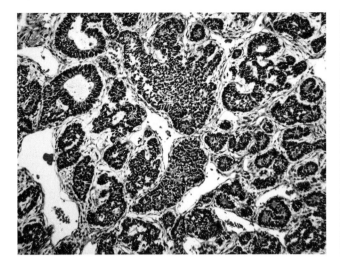

Fig. 6.118 Teratoma with immature elements. Much of the tumor shown in Fig. 6.116 was composed of primitive neuroepithelial elements forming tubules and rosettes, shown here. When teratomas have a substantial pure overgrowth of neuroepithelium, such as in this case, it is probably reasonable to regard that process as a secondary malignant component within a teratoma. Other examples of secondary malignancies are discussed in a later section. The tumor in this case behaved very aggressively, with metastases of the neuroepithelial component evident 2 years after the initial orchiectomy

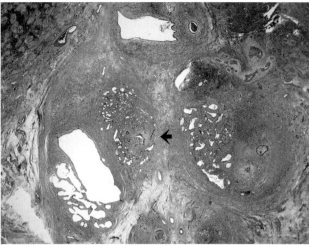

Fig. 6.120 Teratoma with secondary malignancy. This is an example of secondary malignancy in a teratoma, in the form of adenocarcinoma. *Arrow* indicates an aggregate of variably sized irregular glands set in a reactive stroma, in a background of typical teratoma

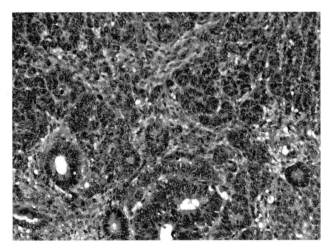

Fig. 6.119 Teratoma with immature elements. Immature elements in teratoma may include blastema and embryonic tubules, shown here. The blastema consists of aggregates of small dark cells with hyperchromatic nuclei and scant cytoplasm. The overall appearance may simulate that of nephroblastoma or pulmonary blastoma

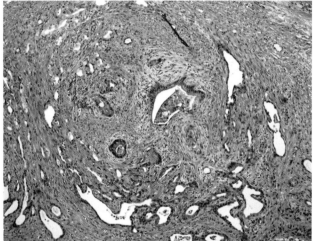

Fig. 6.121 Teratoma with secondary malignancy. Closer inspection of the abnormal glands highlighted in Fig. 6.122 reveals that they are lined by markedly atypical columnar epithelium, with intraluminal necrotic debris, and have incited a desmoplastic stromal response; the overall appearance is similar to that of colonic adenocarcinoma

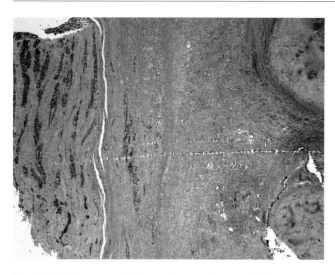

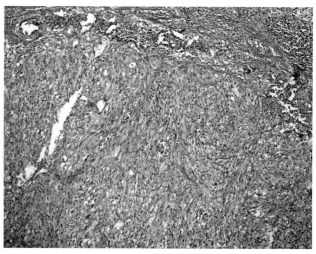

Fig. 6.122 Teratoma with secondary malignancy. This teratoma, shown at right, had an unusual component composed of small blue cells, at left

Fig. 6.124 Teratoma with secondary malignancy. A secondary malignancy in the form of rhabdomyosarcoma arose in the teratomatous component of a mixed germ cell tumor composed of teratoma and embryonal carcinoma. The large expansile mass of spindled cells impinges on an adjacent area of embryonal carcinoma. Many of the spindled cells resembled rhabdomyoblasts and strap cells

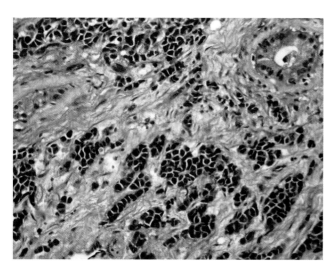

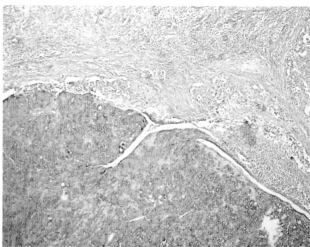

Fig. 6.123 Teratoma with secondary malignancy. The secondary malignancy in this instance consisted of small blue cells that exhibited nuclear molding, and bore some resemblance to small cell carcinoma. Tumor cells showed strong diffuse immunostaining for CD56, synaptophysin and neuron-specific enolase, and focally positive immunostaining for TTF-1 and MOC31, but no immunoreactivity to a large battery of other relevant antibodies. It was considered to be a secondary poorly differentiated malignancy, most consistent with neuroendocrine carcinoma with small cell features, arising in a teratoma

Fig. 6.125 Teratoma with secondary malignancy. The tumor cells of the secondary rhabdomyosarcoma shown in Fig. 6.124 show positive immunostaining for muscle-specific actin (*lower left*). Various types of sarcoma comprise the majority of non-germ cell malignancies in testicular germ cell tumors, and the commonest of them is rhabdomyosarcoma

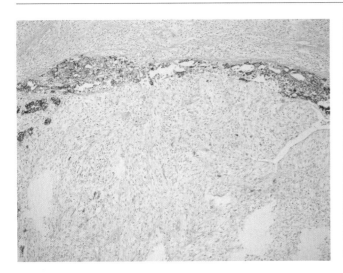

Fig. 6.126 Teratoma with secondary malignancy. Immunostain for keratin AE1/AE3 highlights the tumor cells of the embryonal carcinoma adjacent to the rhabdomyosarcoma shown in Figs. 6.124 and 6.125. Tumor cells of the rhabdomyosarcoma component show no immunoreactivity for this marker

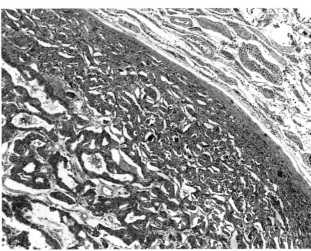

Fig. 6.128 Carcinoid tumor of testis. Tumor cells are arranged in small nests and ribbons and also form glandular structures. This particular carcinoid tumor was present in pure form; no teratomatous elements were identified

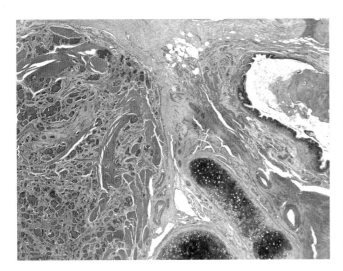

Fig. 6.127 Carcinoid tumor of testis. Carcinoid tumor of the testis is regarded as a form of monodermal teratoma. About 20% of testicular carcinoid tumors are found in a setting that includes other teratomatous elements. This image shows a teratoma that has a component of carcinoid tumor, arranged in nests (*left*)

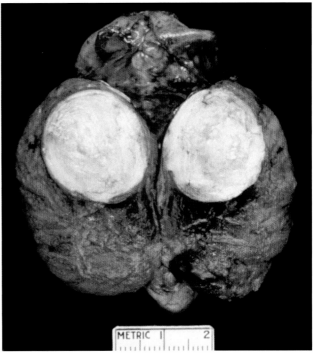

Fig. 6.129 Epidermoid cyst. Epidermoid cysts of the testis are well-circumscribed, soft, round-to-oval intraparenchymal lesions that range in size from 0.5 to 10.5 cm; the average size is about 2 cm. They typically consist of a fibrous capsule of variable thickness, enclosing laminated white or yellowish friable debris. Most tend to be peripheral and close to the tunica albuginea. Whether they represent a monodermal teratoma or are derived from metaplasia of a mesothelial inclusion is unknown (*see* MacLennan GT, Resnick MI, Bostwick DG, 2003. With permission)

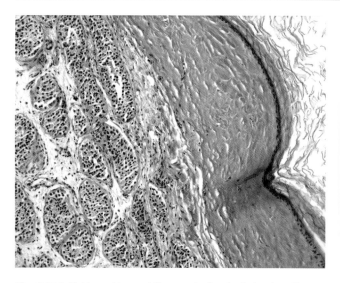

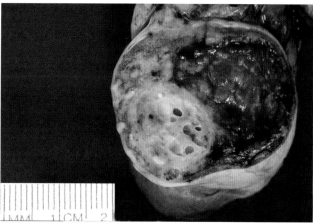

Fig. 6.132 Mixed germ cell tumor. Another mixed germ cell tumor that appears to have several separate grossly different nodules. The solid portion, punctuated by small cysts, is most consistent with teratoma. The tumor had elements of teratoma, embryonal carcinoma and yolk sac tumor

Fig. 6.130 Epidermoid cyst. Microscopically, the lesion is a fibrous-walled cyst lined by keratinizing squamous epithelium. The cyst wall lacks skin adnexal structures such as eccrine glands, hair follicles, or sebaceous units. Epidermoid cyst lacks cytologic atypia and mitotic activity, and intratubular germ cell neoplasia of the unclassified type is not observed in adjacent seminiferous tubules

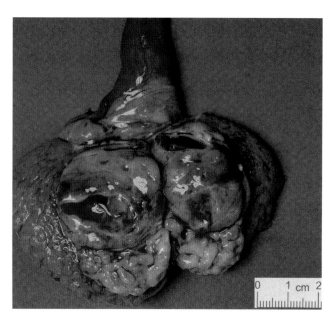

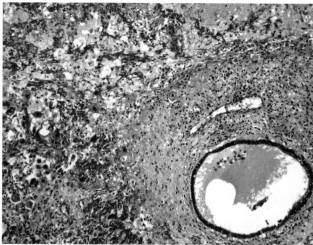

Fig. 6.133 Mixed germ cell tumor. The tumor had elements of teratoma, characterized by the glandular structure (*right*) and choriocarcinoma (*left*)

Fig. 6.131 Mixed germ cell tumor. These tumors are made up of at least two types of germ cell tumor elements. All fall into the category of nonseminomatous germ cell tumors. Virtually any combination of seminoma, embryonal carcinoma, yolk sac tumor, choriocarcinoma, or teratoma may be present. The tumor in the testis shown here was a mixture of yolk sac tumor and teratoma. The two main nodules are grossly quite distinctly different and sharply separated

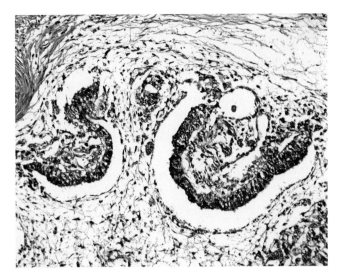

Fig. 6.134 Polyembryoma. This is an example of an "embryoid body," which characterizes a distinctive mixed germ cell tumor designated as polyembryoma. A central core of dark embryonal carcinoma cells overlies an aggregate of yolk sac tumor cells; this structure projects into an empty cystic amniotic-like space. The structure is surrounded by loose myxomatous tissue

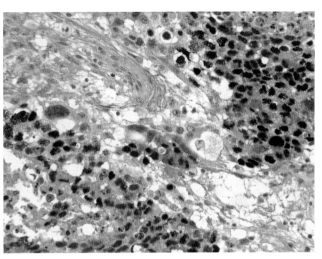

Fig. 6.136 Diffuse embryoma. The embryonal carcinoma cells show positive immunostaining for OCT4. Yolk sac tumor cells show no immunoreactivity for this marker

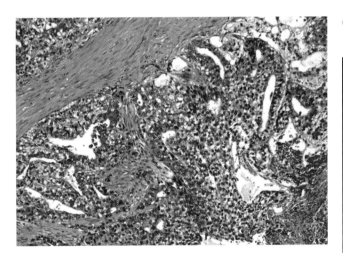

Fig. 6.135 Diffuse embryoma. This is a mixed germ cell tumor composed of approximately equal portions of embryonal carcinoma and yolk sac tumor. It has a "double-layered" pattern: ribbons of embryonal cells are accompanied by parallel ribbons of yolk sac tumor

6.8 Staging Testicular Germ Cell Tumors

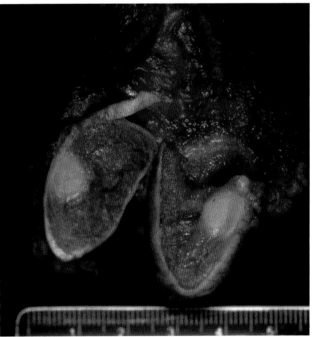

Fig. 6.137 Burnt-out (regressed) germ cell tumor (pT0). The phenomenon of spontaneous primary germ cell tumor regression in a setting of metastatic cancer is well documented. This testis was removed after metastatic seminoma was diagnosed in a retroperitoneal mass. The testis was palpably normal but was abnormal on ultrasound. A circumscribed fibrous nodule was present in the testis (*see* MacLennan GT, Resnick MI, Bostwick DG, 2003. With permission)

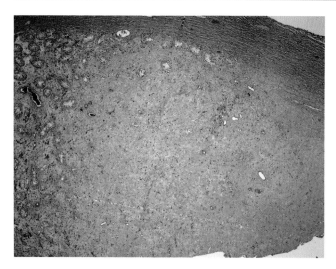

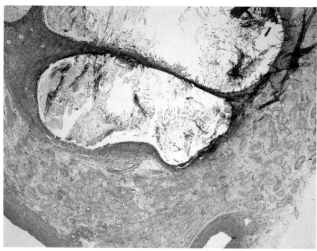

Fig. 6.138 Burnt-out (regressed) germ cell tumor (pT0). Section from the nodule shown in Fig. 6.137. A fibrous scar lies beneath the tunica albuginea, adjacent to atrophic testicular parenchyma

Fig. 6.140 Burnt-out (regressed) germ cell tumor (pT0). Incomplete regression means that small foci of residual invasive germ cell tumor are still identifiable in the testis, most commonly of teratomatous type, as shown here. Residual testicular germ cell tumor in cases of incomplete regression may be histologically different from the metastatic cancer, possibly reflecting selective regression of only discrete elements of a primary testicular mixed germ cell tumor, or else reflecting transformation of tumor types in the metastatic malignancy

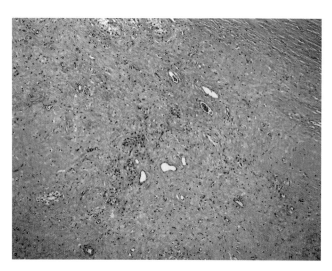

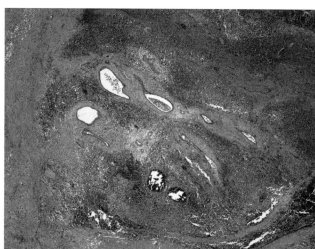

Fig. 6.139 Burnt-out (regressed) germ cell tumor (pT0). Within the fibrous scar are aggregates of Leydig cells and a few tubules lined only by Sertoli cells. No evidence of germ cell tumor was identified in any part of the completely submitted fibrous nodule

Fig. 6.141 Stage pT1 germ cell tumor. Tumor is limited to the testis and epididymis without vascular/lymphatic invasion. This image shows seminoma invading the epididymis

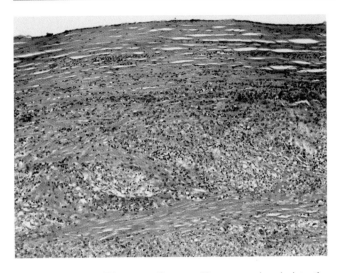

Fig. 6.142 Stage pT1 germ cell tumor. Tumor may invade into the tunica albuginea (as shown here) but not the tunica vaginalis

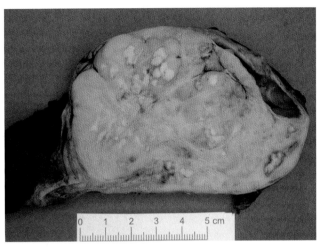

Fig. 6.144 Stage pT3 germ cell tumor. Tumor invades the spermatic cord with or without vascular/lymphatic invasion. This image shows a locally advanced seminoma invading adjacent soft tissues and spermatic cord structures (*Image courtesy of* Hollie Reeves, MD)

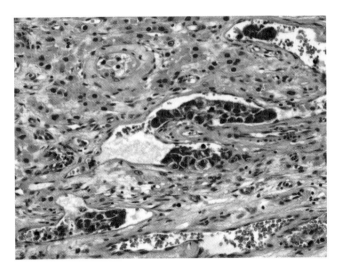

Fig. 6.143 Stage pT2 germ cell tumor. Tumor limited to the testis and epididymis with vascular/lymphatic invasion (as shown here, with embryonal carcinoma in vascular spaces), or tumor extending through the tunica albuginea with involvement of the tunica vaginalis

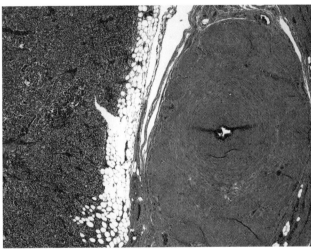

Fig. 6.145 Stage pT3 germ cell tumor. Section from the tumor shown in Fig. 6.144, showing seminoma adjacent to the vas deferens

6.9 Sex Cord-Stromal Tumors

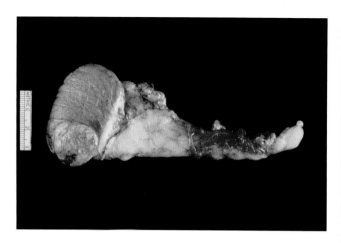

Fig. 6.146 Leydig cell tumor. Leydig cell tumors are usually confined to the testis, solid, well-circumscribed, and yellow, tan, or brown (*see* MacLennan GT, Resnick MI, Bostwick DG, 2003. With permission)

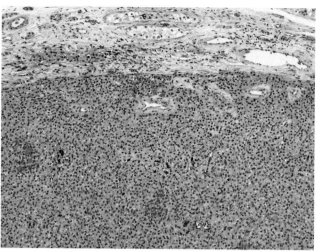

Fig. 6.148 Leydig cell tumor. Sheets of tumor cells form a sharp interface with the adjacent normal testicular parenchyma. Fine granules of lipofuscin pigment are visible

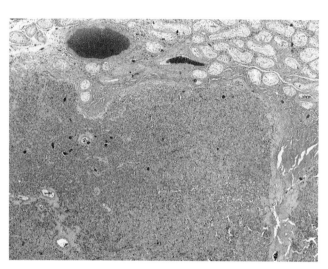

Fig. 6.147 Leydig cell tumor. Formation of diffuse solid sheets of tumor cells is the commonest growth pattern

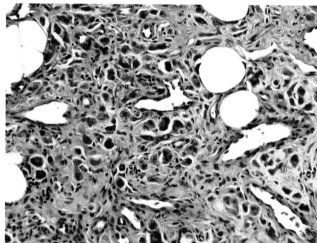

Fig. 6.149 Leydig cell tumor. The finely granular lipofuscin pigment in the cytoplasm of many of the tumor cells contributes to the typical tan or brown color of the gross specimen

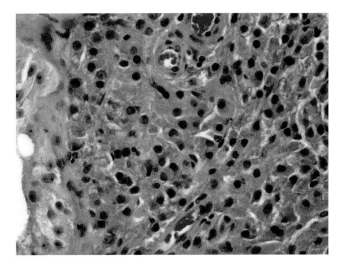

Fig. 6.150 Leydig cell tumor. Tumor cells are polygonal and possess abundant eosinophilic cytoplasm. Their nuclei are round and fairly uniform in size, and most nuclei possess a prominent central nucleolus. Mitotic figures are usually absent or rare

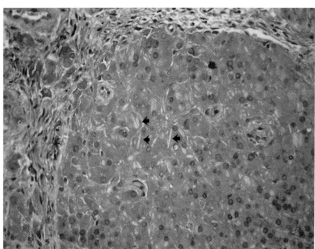

Fig. 6.152 Leydig cell tumor. In contrast to the Reinke's crystals shown in Fig. 6.151, the crystals may be rather indistinct and difficult to identify. Masson's trichrome stain can be used to highlight them (*arrows*)

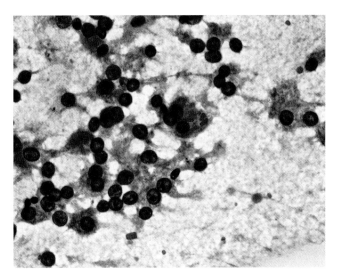

Fig. 6.151 Leydig cell tumor. Reinke's Crystals are identifiable in up to 40% of Leydig cell tumors. They are rod-shaped and lie within the cytoplasm of tumor cells (*see* MacLennan GT, Resnick MI, Bostwick DG, 2003. With permission)

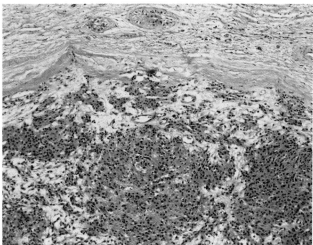

Fig. 6.153 Leydig cell tumor. In some cases, the stroma is edematous or myxoid, and the tumor cells are arranged in irregularly shaped nests or nodules

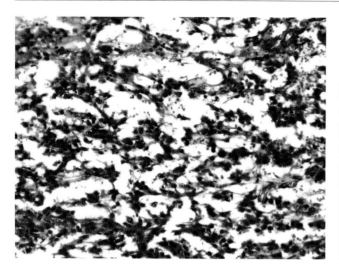

Fig. 6.154 Leydig cell tumor. Stromal variations may sometimes impart a microcystic appearance to the tumor

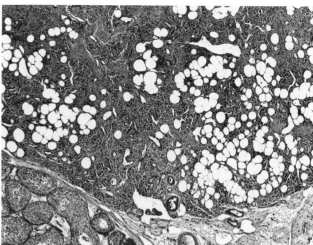

Fig. 6.156 Leydig cell tumor. Fat cells are found in a small proportion of Leydig cell tumors, representing either lipid accumulation within tumor cells or adipose differentiation in stromal cells

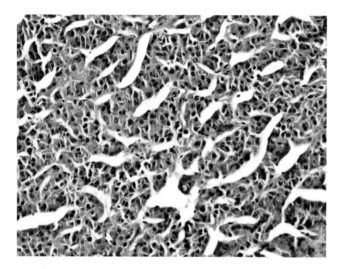

Fig. 6.155 Leydig cell tumor. Rarely, a pseudoglandular appearance is noted

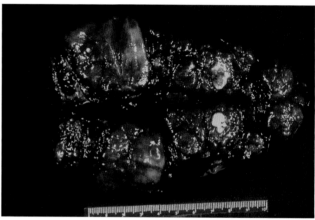

Fig. 6.157 Leydig cell tumor. This lobulated multinodular Leydig cell tumor was clinically malignant. It is very large, and has an area of geographic necrosis. Malignancy in Leydig cell tumor is defined by the occurrence of metastases. However, a number of pathologic findings correlate with malignant behavior, including necrosis and tumor size exceeding 5 cm, as evident in this tumor (*see* MacLennan GT, Resnick MI, Bostwick DG, 2003. With permission)

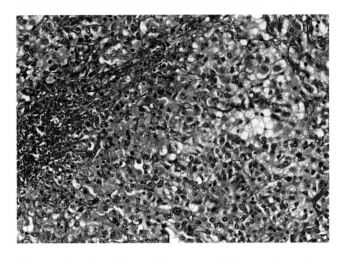

Fig. 6.158 Leydig cell tumor. The tumor exhibits necrosis, moderate cytologic atypia, and mitotic activity

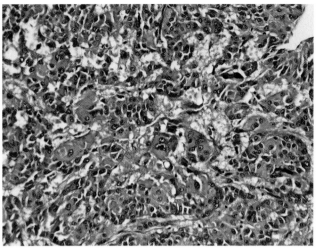

Fig. 6.160 Leydig cell tumor. Significant nuclear atypia in Leydig cell tumors, shown here, and other parameters including mitotic rate exceeding three to five mitotic figures per ten high-power fields, atypical mitotic figures, vascular space invasion, and invasion of the rete testis or epididymis are all associated with malignant behavior, although none of these findings is pathognomonic of malignancy

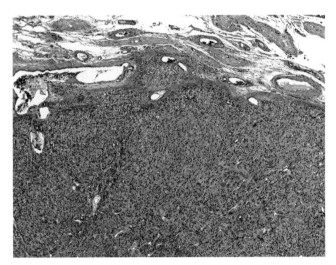

Fig. 6.159 Leydig cell tumor. The presence of an infiltrative border, as shown at top, correlates with malignant behavior in Leydig cell tumors

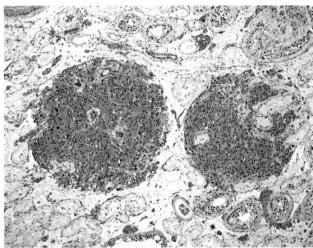

Fig. 6.161 Leydig cell hyperplasia. A number of conditions may enter the differential diagnosis of Leydig cell tumor. Nodular aggregates of Leydig cells may be seen in a variety of conditions, particularly those involving testicular atrophy. In atrophic conditions, such as cryptorchidism or Klinefelter's syndrome, the residual normal Leydig cells stand out more prominently in a background of reduced testicular volume

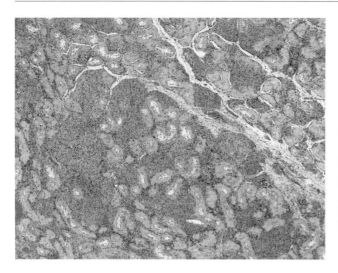

Fig. 6.162 Leydig cell hyperplasia. Pronounced Leydig cell hyperplasia in a setting of severe tubular atrophy may sometimes suggest the possibility of Leydig cell tumor; however, it is notable that seminiferous tubules are preserved within the nodules

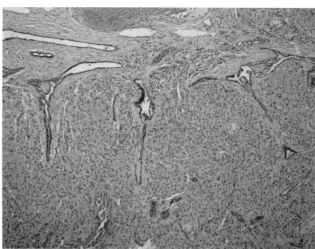

Fig. 6.164 Testicular tumor of the adrenogenital syndrome. The hyperplastic nodules are composed of large steroid-type cells with abundant eosinophilic cytoplasm. The tumor cells surround, rather than effacing, the tubules of the rete testis in this image. The clinical history is critically important in such cases

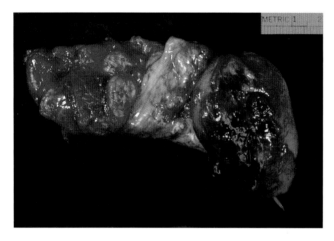

Fig. 6.163 Testicular tumor of the adrenogenital syndrome. Patients with persistently elevated levels of adrenocorticotropic hormone (ACTH), as in adrenogenital syndrome or Nelson's syndrome, sometimes develop multiple bilateral tumor nodules composed of steroid-type cells in the testis and in the hilum. Such nodules, evident in the testis (*right*), differ from Leydig cell tumors by their color, multiplicity, and bilaterality (*see* MacLennan GT, Resnick MI, Bostwick DG, 2003. With permission)

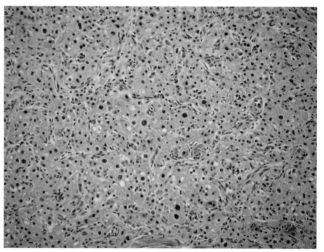

Fig. 6.165 Testicular tumor of the adrenogenital syndrome. The tumor cells are morphologically somewhat similar to those of Leydig cell tumor, but they tend to have more abundant cytoplasm and more lipochrome pigment than cells of the latter, and they lack Reinke's crystals. They often exhibit a modest degree of variability in nuclear size, as shown here, but mitotic figures are absent or rare

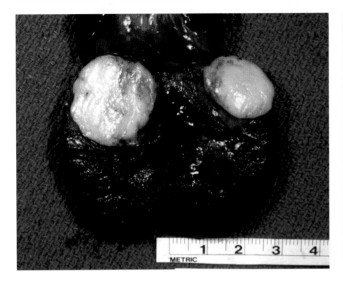

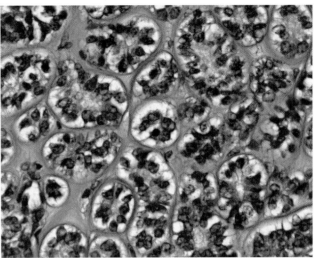

Fig. 6.166 Sertoli cell tumor. Sertoli cell tumors are usually white, tan, or yellow, and are well circumscribed, sometimes cystic, and sometimes have focal hemorrhage (*see* MacLennan GT, Resnick MI, Bostwick DG, 2003. With permission)

Fig. 6.168 Sertoli cell tumor, not otherwise specified. Tumor cells have scant or modest amounts of clear or pale pink cytoplasm. Their nuclei are fairly uniform and round to oval; nucleoli are absent or inconspicuous. The cytoplasmic clarity is due to the presence of lipid

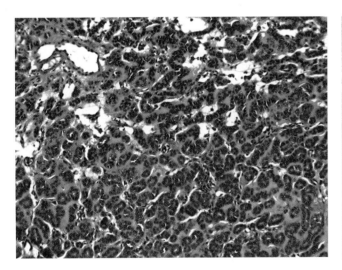

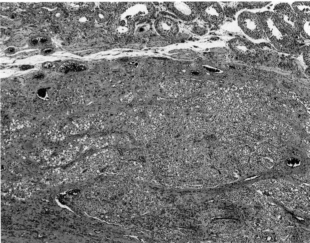

Fig. 6.167 Sertoli cell tumor, not otherwise specified (NOS). There are three subtypes of Sertoli cell tumor. The commonest is the usual or NOS group; the others are sclerosing and large cell calcifying types. The classic finding in Sertoli cell tumors is the presence of tubular structures, with or without visible lumens. The tubular structures are commonly in a fibrous stroma that may show varying degrees of hyalinization or myxoid change

Fig. 6.169 Sertoli cell tumor, not otherwise specified. Solid elongated tubules sometimes coalesce to form sheets of tumor cells; this pattern may be difficult to distinguish from seminoma, particularly a seminoma with pseudotubular architecture (*see* Fig. 6.66)

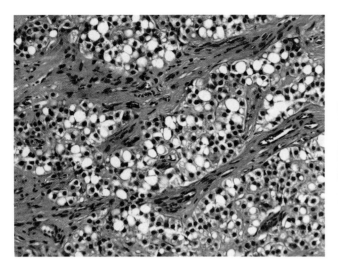

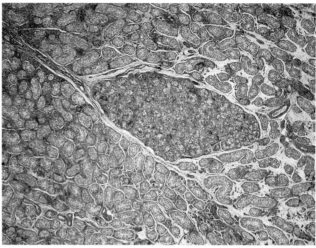

Fig. 6.170 Sertoli cell tumor, not otherwise specified. Tumor cells in some cases show very prominent cytoplasmic vacuolization

Fig. 6.172 Sertoli cell nodule. These small nodules enter the differential diagnosis of Sertoli cell tumor, not otherwise specified. They are microscopic and are only discovered incidentally in orchiectomy specimens; they may be more commonly found in excised cryptorchid testes, and are particularly common and often multiple in the excised gonads of patients with androgen insensitivity syndrome. They are nonencapsulated but discrete nodules consisting of seminiferous tubules lined by immature Sertoli cells. The tubules within the nodules are densely packed and are considerably smaller than the tubules in the adjacent testis

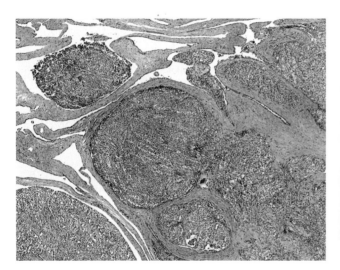

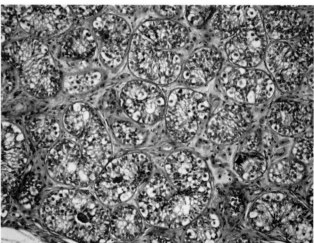

Fig. 6.171 Sertoli cell tumor, not otherwise specified. The tumor shows rather striking infiltration of the stroma of the rete testis and also has grown intraluminally in the channels of the rete testis

Fig. 6.173 Sertoli cell nodule. This is a closer view of the nodule shown in Fig. 6.172, which was found in one of the gonads excised from a patient with androgen insensitivity syndrome. Central aggregates of basement membrane material are often seen within Sertoli cell nodules. Leydig cells are present between the tubules (*arrow*), in contrast to Sertoli cell adenoma or Sertoli cell tumor not otherwise specified. Such lesions are regarded as hamartomas

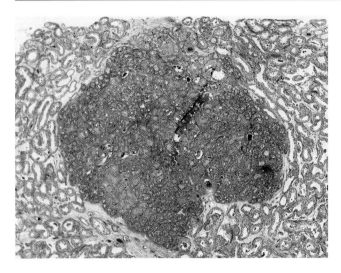

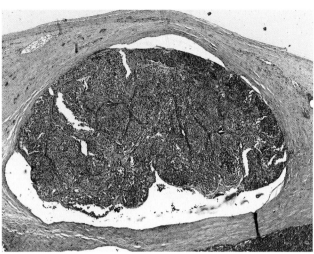

Fig. 6.174 Sertoli cell adenoma. These small nodules also enter the differential diagnosis of Sertoli cell tumor, not otherwise specified. This nodule was present in one of the gonads excised from a patient with androgen insensitivity syndrome. It is a well circumscribed compact aggregate of tubules lined by Sertoli cells

Fig. 6.176 Sertoli cell tumor, not otherwise specified, with vascular invasion. Malignancy in Sertoli cell tumor is defined by the occurrence of metastases. Malignant behavior is observed in about 10% of cases of Sertoli cell tumor. Vascular invasion, shown here, is a feature associated with malignant behavior; other features include tumor size larger than 5 cm, necrosis, pronounced cytologic atypia and pleomorphism, invasive borders, and the finding of more than five mitotic figures per ten high-power fields

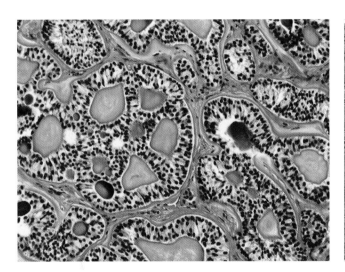

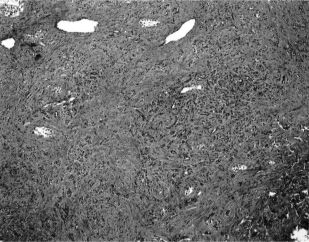

Fig. 6.175 Sertoli cell adenoma. On closer inspection of the lesion shown in Fig. 6.174, no Leydig cells are present between the tubules. Abundant deposits of basement membrane material are present. Sertoli cell adenomas are found in 25% of patients with androgen insensitivity syndrome (AIS), and in this setting they are multifocal, bilateral, and essentially indistinguishable from well-differentiated Sertoli cell tumor. It is unclear whether they are neoplastic or hamartomatous; regardless, there are no reports of malignant Sertoli cell tumors in patients with AIS

Fig. 6.177 Sertoli cell tumor, sclerosing type. The hallmark of this variant is that the cords, nests and hollow or solid tubules are arrayed in a densely collagenous stroma, which stands out prominently in this low-power view

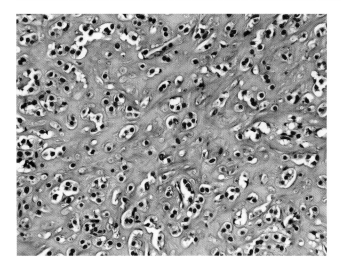

Fig. 6.178 Sertoli cell tumor, sclerosing type. The stroma is sclerotic, with limited vascularity. The tubules are small and solid. Tumor cells have small round uniform nuclei and lack mitotic activity

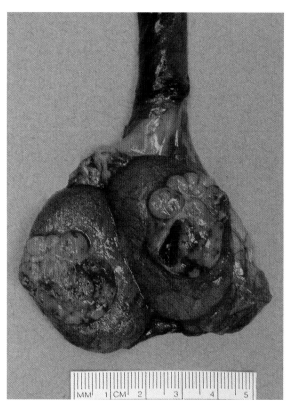

Fig. 6.180 Sertoli cell tumor, large cell calcifying type. This is an uncommon variant of Sertoli cell tumor, 60% of which are sporadic; the remainder are associated with endocrine syndromes, most often Carney's and Peutz-Jeghers syndromes, and an assortment of unusual clinical findings and associations. Tumors are usually less than 4 cm, well-circumscribed, yellow to tan and firm, sometimes with cystic degeneration, but rarely with necrosis (*Image courtesy of* Shams Halat, MD)

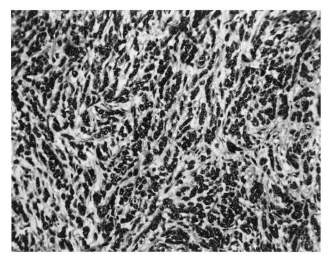

Fig. 6.179 Sertoli cell tumor, sclerosing type. The tumor cell nuclei in this case are slightly irregular and have small nucleoli. The sclerosing variant tends to occur in men averaging 35 years old, and lacking any hormonal symptoms; the outcome in such cases is favorable

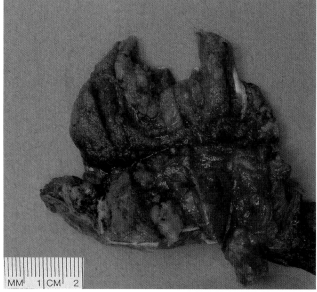

Fig. 6.181 Sertoli cell tumor, large cell calcifying type. Some are multifocal; the small tumor (*arrow*) was present in the testis shown in Fig. 6.180, but was spatially separate from the larger tumor. Tumors that are both multifocal and bilateral occur almost exclusively in Carney's syndrome (*Image courtesy of* Shams Halat, MD)

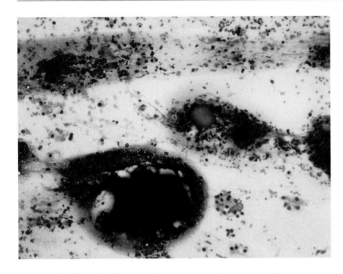

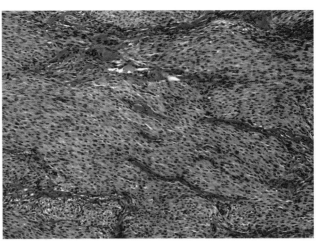

Fig. 6.184 Granulosa cell tumor, adult type. Tumor cells may grow in diffuse sheets, as in this case. Other architectural arrangements seen in this tumor include insular, gyriform, trabecular, macrofollicular, and microfollicular

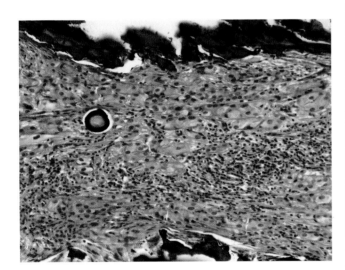

Fig. 6.182 Sertoli cell tumor, large cell calcifying type. The presence of intratumoral calcifications may produce a gritty sensation when the tumor is sectioned, as it was in this case, prompting a cytologic scrape prep, which showed abundant calcific structures admixed with the tumor cells

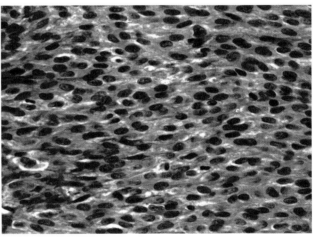

Fig. 6.185 Granulosa cell tumor, adult type. Tumor cells have scant-to-modest amounts of pale pink cytoplasm. Nuclei are round to oval, and some are grooved. Usually mitotic activity is limited or absent

Fig. 6.183 Sertoli cell tumor, large cell calcifying type. Tumor cells are arranged in sheets, nests, cords, ribbons, and trabeculae, set in a myxoid to collagenous stroma. Tumor cells are large due to the presence of abundant eosinophilic finely granular cytoplasm. Their nuclei are round with one or two small-to-medium nucleoli; mitotic figures are rare. A neutrophilic infiltrate can be seen, as in this case. Calcifications in the form of large laminated calcific nodules are scattered through the tumor; psammoma bodies and rarely ossified structures may be present

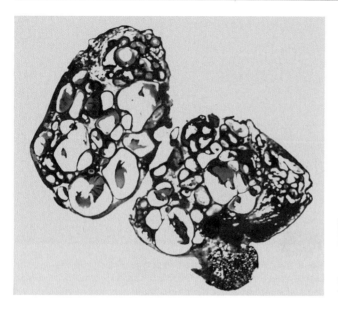

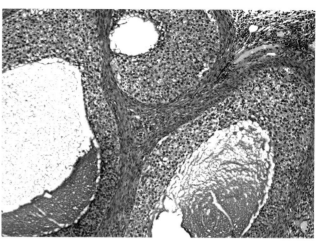

Fig. 6.188 Granulosa cell tumor, juvenile type. The follicles are surrounded by a spindle cell stroma and are lined by multiple layers of tumor cells surrounding a central lumen

Fig. 6.186 Granulosa cell tumor, juvenile type. Most patients with this testicular tumor are younger than 5 months old. The tumor is solid to cystic. The tumor shown here at very low power is remarkably cystic

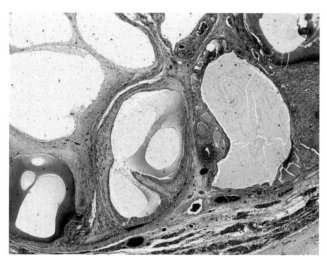

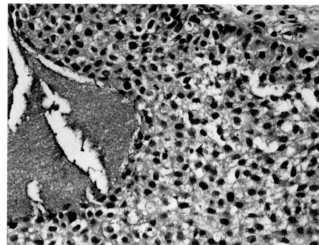

Fig. 6.187 Granulosa cell tumor, juvenile type. At low power, the tumor is composed of variably sized follicular spaces surrounded by solid tumor. The follicles contain basophilic fluid

Fig. 6.189 Granulosa cell tumor, juvenile type. The tumor cells have uniform round, dark nuclei and small nucleoli; they have abundant pale or light pink cytoplasm. The fluid in the follicles has mucinous properties and stains positively with mucicarmine stain. Apoptotic cells (*arrows*) are often present, and sometimes are abundant. Mitotic activity may be brisk

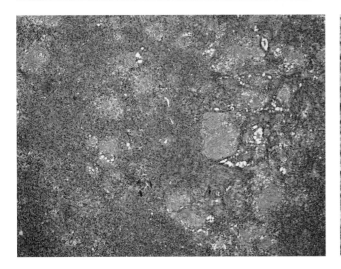

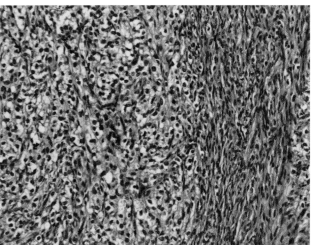

Fig. 6.190 Cellular fibroma. These tumors resemble ovarian fibroma. They are composed of short fascicles of densely packed uniform spindle cells at least focally arranged in a storiform pattern. It is unclear whether they are indeed of gonadal stromal origin or of tissue fibroblast origin. They are considered benign

Fig. 6.192 Sex cord-stromal tumor, unclassified. Tumors in this category display patterns that are typical of two or more of the well-recognized tumors in this group – Leydig cell tumors, Sertoli cell tumors, granulosa cell tumors, and fibroma. In the example shown here, sheets of nondescript sex cord cells are intermingled with fascicles of spindled cells. The findings defy a more specific categorization

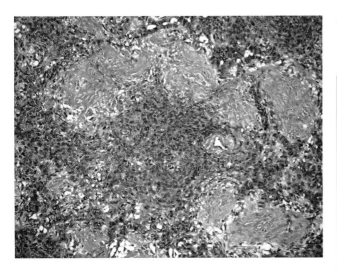

6.10 Tumors with Both Germ Cell and Sex Cord-Stromal Components

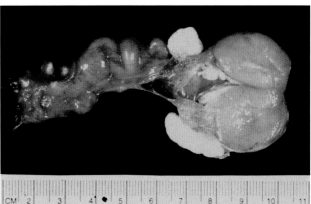

Fig. 6.191 Cellular fibroma. Plaques of acellular or paucicellular collagen are scattered through the tumor. Mitotic activity is usually limited

Fig. 6.193 Gonadoblastoma. Gonadoblastoma consists of both neoplastic germ cells and sex cord-stromal derivatives, and typically arises in the streak gonads of patients with pure or mixed gonadal dysgenesis, some of whom are phenotypic males with varying levels of feminization; the great majority are young phenotypic females with amenorrhea or virilization. Virtually all patients diagnosed with gonadoblastoma possess a Y chromosome. This gonad was removed from a phenotypic female patient with XO,XY karyotype and clinical features of Turner's syndrome. The gonad contained a light yellow-tan tumor with a shiny bulging cut surface

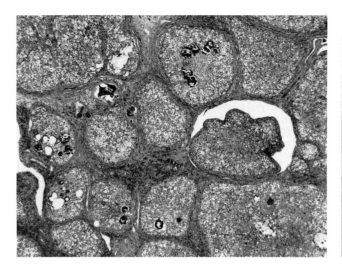

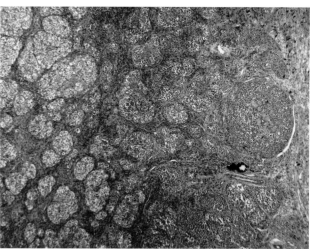

Fig. 6.194 Gonadoblastoma. The tumor is composed of nests of immature germ cells with clear cytoplasm resembling those of seminoma or dysgerminoma, admixed with smaller sex cord cells resembling immature Sertoli or granulosa cells, arranged in a background of dense connective tissue. Microcalcifications are very commonly present

Fig. 6.196 Gonadoblastoma. More than half of gonadoblastoma are overgrown by invasive germ cell tumors, as in the case shown here: a gonadoblastoma is at right center, and the remainder of the section consists of invasive dysgerminoma, corresponding to the large yellow-tan tumor shown in Fig. 6.193. Gonadoblastoma has never been identified in metastatic sites or in extragonadal locations; it is viewed as a form of in situ germ cell neoplasm, in view of its very frequent association with various types of invasive germ cell tumors

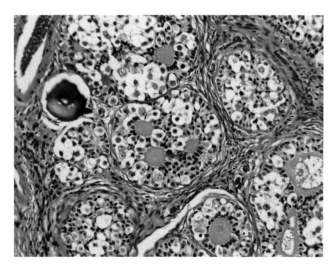

6.11 Ovarian-Type Epithelial Tumors

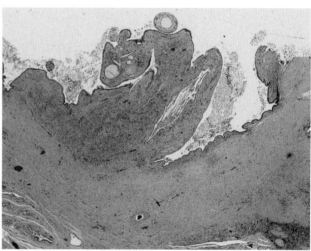

Fig. 6.195 Gonadoblastoma. Sex cord cells may surround individual germ cells, germ cell clusters, or small round aggregates of hyaline eosinophilic material. In some cases, they are arrayed only at the periphery of the cell nests

Fig. 6.197 Serous cystadenoma. This middle-aged man was found to have an asymptomatic testicular mass. There was an intratesticular cystic mass. The adjacent testis showed diffuse atrophy and Leydig cell hyperplasia. There were papillary-polypoid projections into the cavity of the cyst

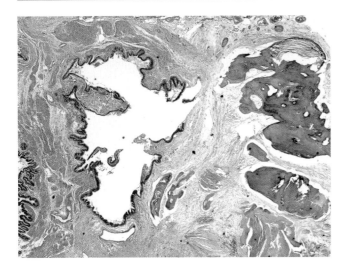

Fig. 6.198 Serous cystadenoma. The cyst was lined by tall columnar epithelium, and wispy mucin appeared to be present within the cystic spaces. Focally, metaplastic bone formation was evident in the stroma of the lesion

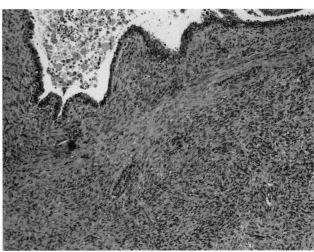

Fig. 6.200 Serous cystadenoma. The lesion also showed a substantial component of ovarian-type stroma, as shown here, a finding that is seen in other intratesticular papillary serous tumors. No evidence of intratubular germ cell neoplasia, unclassified, was noted in the uninvolved testis, supporting the notion that this lesion was unlikely to be an unusual form of teratoma

6.12 Soft Tissue Tumors

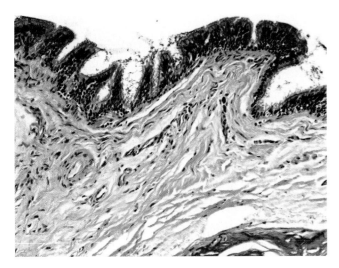

Fig. 6.199 Serous cystadenoma. The lining epithelium was predominantly of serous (ciliated) type, but some of the lining cells showed evidence of mucinous differentiation

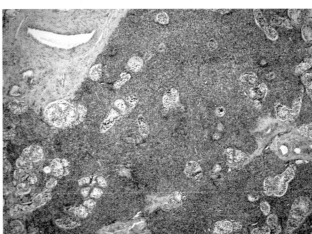

Fig. 6.201 Juvenile capillary hemangioma. Testicular hemangiomas are ill-defined unencapsulated masses, up to 3.7 cm, with a tan-pink to red homogeneous cut surface. Most are in young people; the tumor shown here was from an 18-year-old male who had a palpable testicular mass; at his insistence, it was excised with preservation of uninvolved adjacent testis, and did not recur. The interstitial space is replaced by a cellular proliferation that leaves native tubules intact

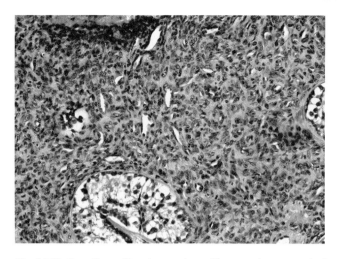

Fig. 6.202 Juvenile capillary hemangioma. The tumor is composed of plump endothelial cells lining small rather inconspicuous slit-like poorly canalized vascular spaces

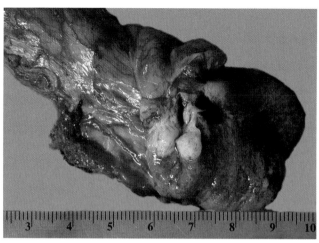

Fig. 6.204 Leiomyoma. Patient was a 74-year-old man with a non-tender palpable testicular mass, solid by ultrasound. A well-circumscribed, solid, light, tan lesion was found *(Image courtesy of* John Miedler, MD)

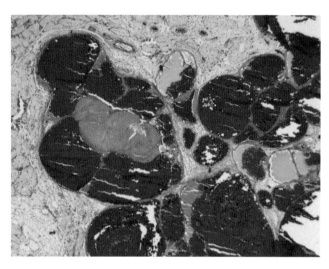

Fig. 6.203 Cavernous hemangioma. Most testicular hemangiomas are capillary, cavernous, or epithelioid. This cavernous hemangioma was found incidentally in one of two testes removed for hormonal treatment of advanced prostate cancer. It shows a roughly lobular arrangement of large dilated blood-filled vessels lined by inconspicuous endothelial cells. The blood vessel walls show irregular adventitial fibrosis

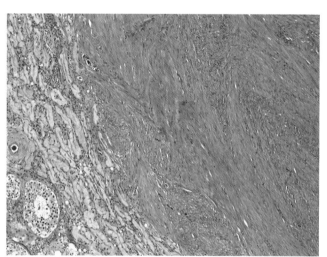

Fig. 6.205 Leiomyoma. The lesion in Fig. 6.204 was composed of intersecting fascicles of smooth muscle, lacking necrosis, mitotic activity or significant cytologic atypia

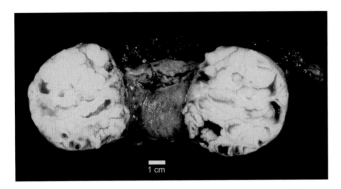

Fig. 6.206 Mesodermal adenosarcoma. Patient was a 76-year-old man who had noted swelling of one testis for about 20 years; the swelling had increased notably in the past 2 years. The orchiectomy showed a mass composed of multiple cystic spaces containing serous fluid and separated by firm fibrous septae; intracystic papillary-polypoid excrescences were noted (*see* Fleshman et al. 2005. With permission)

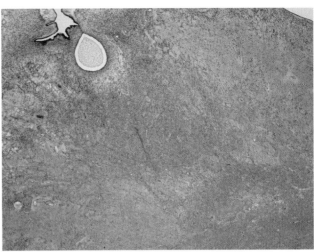

Fig. 6.208 Mesodermal adenosarcoma. The stromal component is composed of spindle cells in a fibrous and focally myxoid background. Variable cellularity is evident

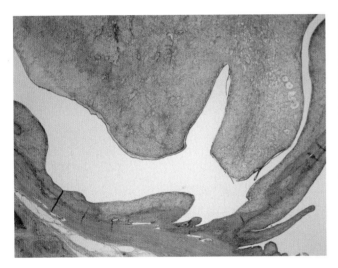

Fig. 6.207 Mesodermal adenosarcoma. At low power, the tumor is composed of cystically dilated or elongated and compressed luminal spaces that vary considerably in size and shape. Broad polypoid or leaf-like fronds of stroma project into the cysts, imparting a phyllodes-like appearance at low power. The tumor is morphologically similar to mesodermal (Müllerian) adenosarcoma of the uterus and ovary. In males, similar tumors have been described in the prostate and seminal vesicles under various names such as "müllerian adenosarcoma-like tumor"

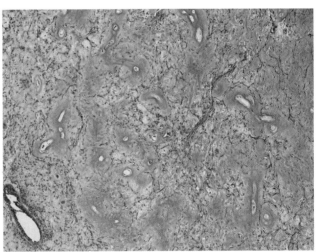

Fig. 6.209 Mesodermal adenosarcoma. Small thick-walled arterioles are scattered through the stroma, abundant in some areas and scant in other areas

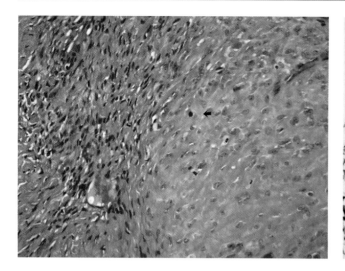

Fig. 6.210 Mesodermal adenosarcoma. Scattered mitotic figures are present (*arrow*); their numbers range from 0–1/50 high-power fields. Tumor cells are plump in some areas, and fusiform and spindled in other areas

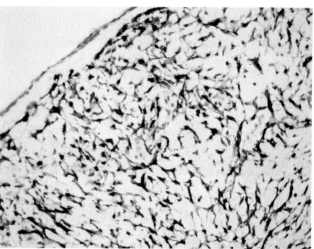

Fig. 6.212 Mesodermal adenosarcoma. Tumor cells showed diffusely positive immunostaining for CD10. This is consistent with an endometrial stromal phenotype. Adenosarcomas that arise in the female genital tract fall in the category of endometrioid neoplasms, and those arising outside the female genital tract usually arise within areas of endometriosis

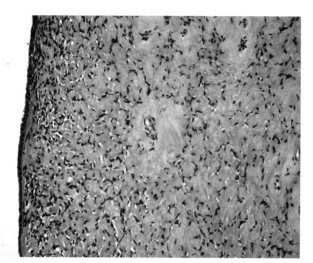

Fig. 6.211 Mesodermal adenosarcoma. The epithelium lining the cystic spaces is flattened to low cuboidal, and lacks malignant features. In many areas, the spindle cells show condensation immediately beneath the cyst lumen

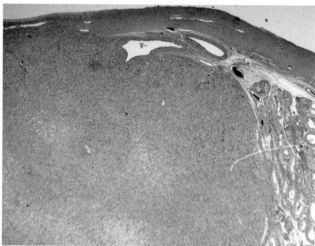

Fig. 6.213 Leiomyosarcoma of testis. Patient was a 58-year-old man with a testicular mass. The tumor was entirely intratesticular

6.13 Hematopoietic and Lymphoid Tumors

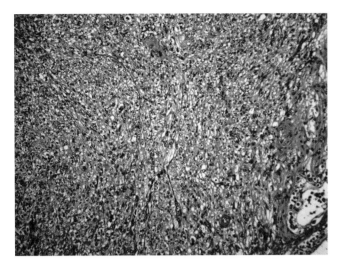

Fig. 6.214 Leiomyosarcoma of testis. Closer inspection of the lesion in Fig. 6.213 shows a tumor composed of spindled and epithelioid cells with considerable nuclear pleomorphism. Tumor cells showed positive immunostaining for desmin and muscle-specific actin

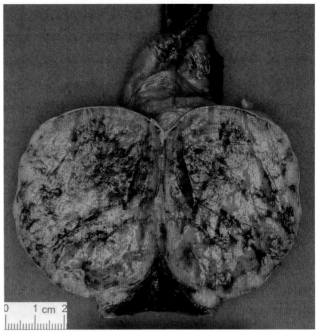

Fig. 6.216 Lymphoma. This 80-year-old man was treated for primary central nervous system Burkitt's lymphoma. During a period of about 3 weeks, he developed rapid enlargement of one testis, which was excised. All normal testicular parenchyma has been obliterated by a diffusely infiltrating neoplasm, which was found to be a B-cell lymphoma, unclassifiable, with features intermediate between diffuse large B-cell lymphoma and Burkitt lymphoma (2008 World Health Organization classification). A c-myc gene rearrangement was found *(Image courtesy of* Francisco Paras, MD)

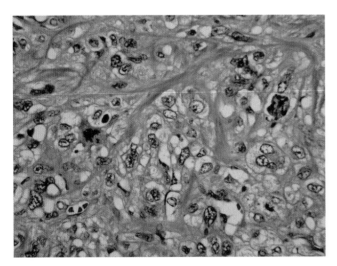

Fig. 6.215 Leiomyosarcoma of testis. Abundant apoptotic cells and mitotic figures, some of them markedly atypical as shown here, were present, supporting the diagnosis of leiomyosarcoma

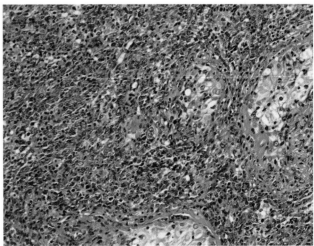

Fig. 6.217 Diffuse large B cell lymphoma. The testicular parenchyma shows diffuse intertubular infiltration by large-sized lymphoma cells. Occasional infiltration of seminiferous tubules by lymphoma cells is also present. The tumor cells are large-sized with a characteristic vesicular nuclear chromatin *(Case courtesy of* Alok Mohanty, MD)

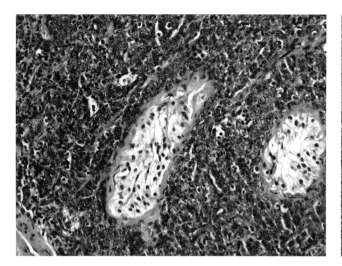

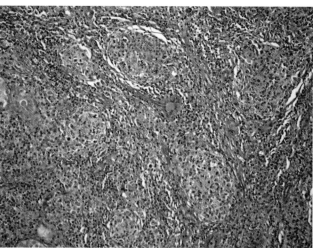

Fig. 6.218 Acute lymphoblastic leukemia. This 31-year-old man had a 21-month history of relentlessly recurrent acute lymphoblastic leukemia. He developed bilateral testicular masses. This is a section from one of the testes, showing diffuse pattern of infiltration by medium-sized cells with relative sparing of seminiferous tubules. The individual cells demonstrate an open nuclear chromatin and high mitotic rate, characteristic of blasts (*Case courtesy of* Alok Mohanty, MD)

Fig. 6.220 Prepubertal lymphoma. Closer inspection of the section shown in Fig. 6.219 reveals numerous small nodular aggregates, somewhat suggestive of granulomatous orchitis

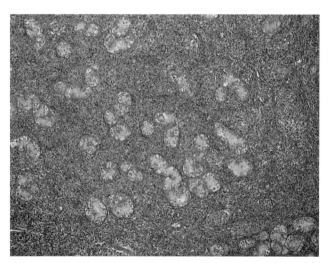

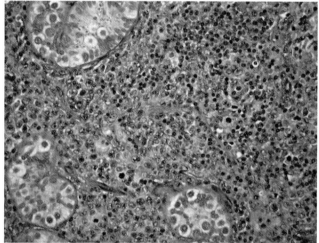

Fig. 6.219 Prepubertal lymphoma. This 11-year-old asymptomatic boy was noted to have an enlarged testis on routine well child care visit, and ultrasound confirmed that the testis was abnormal. Testis was excised. At low power, the interstitium shows a diffuse cellular infiltrate with preservation of seminiferous tubules

Fig. 6.221 Prepubertal lymphoma. The nodules contained large atypical lymphoid cells, many of which had multilobar nuclei. The atypical lymphoid cells, admixed with numerous small lymphocytes, infiltrated the interstitium extensively, as well as the rete testis, the tunica albuginea and the soft tissues adjacent to the epididymis. Diagnosis, based upon morphologic findings and results of a battery of immunostains, was follicular large cell lymphoma. The neoplasm was confined to the testis. He was treated with chemotherapy, and was in complete remission 59 months later

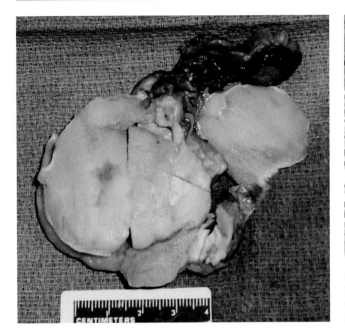

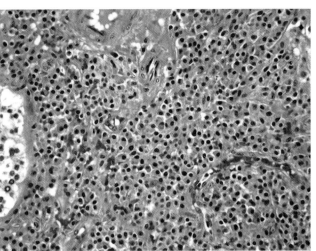

Fig. 6.224 Plasmacytoma of testis. The testis is extensively infiltrated by sheets of neoplastic plasma cells with abundant cytoplasm and eccentric nuclei, some of which have discrete nucleoli; mitotic activity is limited

Fig. 6.222 Plasmacytoma of testis. Patient was being followed for prostatism and developed a swelling in one testis, which was excised. The light tan lesion was quite well demarcated from the adjacent normal testis. Patient had a plasmacytoma excised from his tongue 9 years before the orchiectomy, but had been followed expectantly without intervening therapy (*Image courtesy of* Prabha Morthy, MD)

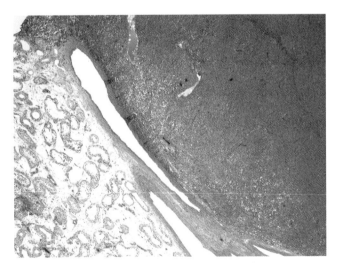

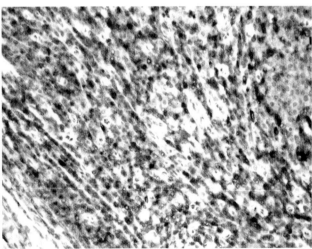

Fig. 6.223 Plasmacytoma of testis. A well-circumscribed, densely cellular mass is present adjacent to normal testicular parenchyma

Fig. 6.225 Plasmacytoma of testis. Tumor cells showed widespread diffusely positive immunostaining for CD79a

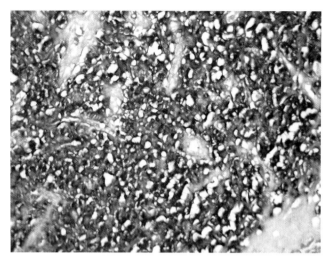

Fig. 6.226 Plasmacytoma of testis. In situ hybridization shows κ light-chain restriction

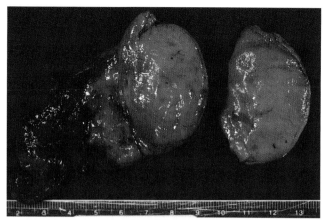

Fig. 6.228 Recurrent acute myelogenous leukemia. At age 22, patient had acute myelogenous leukemia; he was treated and underwent bone marrow transplant. He remained in remission for 12 years and then presented with enlargement and induration of one testis, which was excised. The testis was noted to be pink-tan with a slight greenish tinge, as well

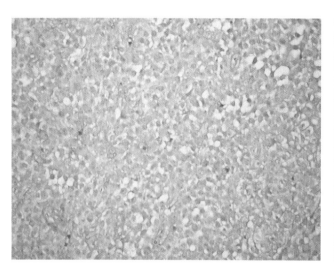

Fig. 6.227 Plasmacytoma of testis. In situ hybridization for λ light-chain is negative

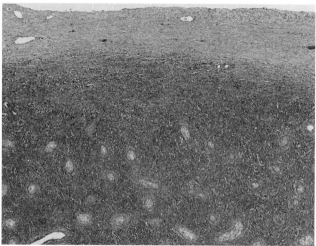

Fig. 6.229 Recurrent acute myelogenous leukemia. The interstitium is diffusely replaced by a densely cellular infiltrate. Seminiferous tubules are preserved

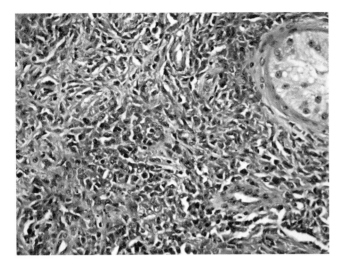

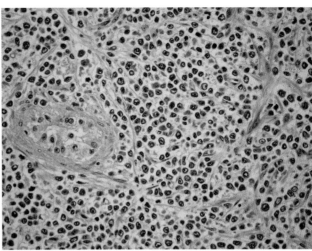

Fig. 6.230 Recurrent acute myelogenous leukemia. Higher power view of the image shown in Fig. 6.229 shows a leukemic infiltrate composed of medium-sized cells with open chromatin and convoluted nuclear contours. The tumor cells showed positive staining with CD34, CD43, muramidase, and Leder stain (*Case courtesy of* Alok Mohanty, MD)

Fig. 6.232 Granulocytic sarcoma. Histologic sections of the tumor showed a diffuse proliferation of medium to large atypical cells with a high nuclear–cytoplasmic ratio, indented or round nuclei, speckled chromatin, inconspicuous nucleoli, and fairly abundant cytoplasm. Tumor cells showed positive immunostaining for vimentin, lysozyme, and CD163, and focal weak immunostaining for CD43 and KP1 (weak granular positivity), and no immunostaining for a host of other relevant stains. Findings were considered diagnostic of granulocytic sarcoma

6.14 Metastases to Testis

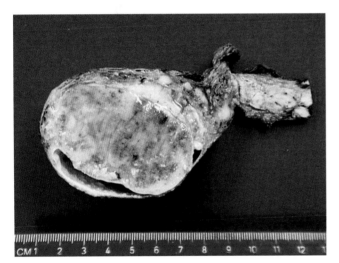

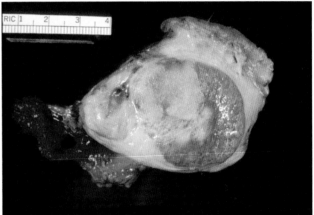

Fig. 6.231 Granulocytic sarcoma. Radical orchiectomy specimen from a 65-year-old man with a 2-month history of progressive testicular swelling and some abdominal lymphadenopathy on CT scan. The testicular parenchyma appears to have a diffusely infiltrative process. The testis and surrounding structures have a definite greenish tinge (*Image courtesy of* James A. MacDonald, MD)

Fig. 6.233 Metastases to testis. Testicular metastases occur in patients with and without known primary cancers. In adults, carcinomas of prostate, stomach, and lung, along with melanoma, are the commonest primaries; in children, neuroblastoma and rhabdomyosarcoma predominate. The image shown here illustrates metastatic urothelial carcinoma in a patient with known bladder cancer

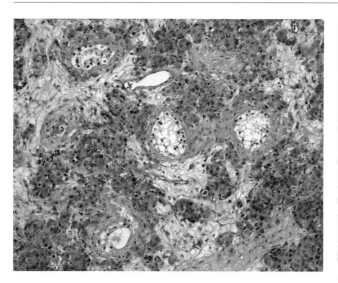

Fig. 6.234 Metastases to testis. This is metastatic prostate cancer. Extensive interstitial growth, multifocality, bilaterality, and extensive intravascular tumor favor the possibility of metastases; however, interstitial growth is also typical of lymphoid neoplasms

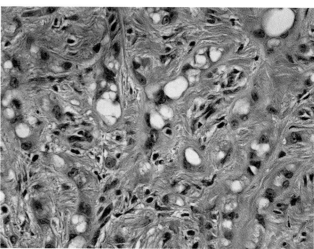

Fig. 6.236 Metastases to testis. High-power view of the testicular mass shown in Fig. 6.235 shows the presence of malignant cells with abundant cytoplasmic vacuolization. Patient was subsequently found to have linitis plastica of the stomach. The findings in this image are difficult to distinguish readily from adenomatoid tumor of tunica vaginalis, which can sometimes show intratesticular growth and commonly has prominent cytoplasmic vacuolization (*see* Figs. 7.70 and 7.71, Chap. 7)

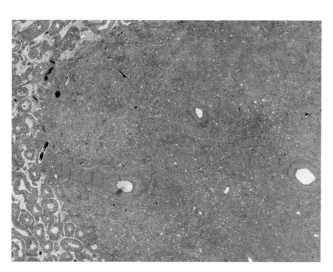

Fig. 6.235 Metastases to testis. In the absence of a known primary cancer, the differential can be challenging, as in this case of metastatic signet-ring cancer of the stomach. The testis shows an area of cellularity and stromal sclerosis

6.15 Lesions of Rete Testis

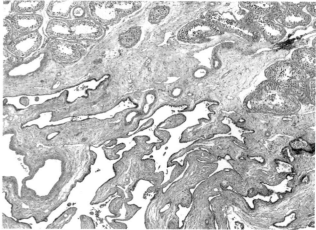

Fig. 6.237 Normal rete testis. About 1,500 seminiferous tubules empty into the rete testis in the hilum of the testis. The rete testis is a network of interconnecting irregular cavernous channels that begin within the testis, traverse the tunica albuginea and eventually anastomose together outside the testis to form 12–15 efferent ductules, which, as noted in Chap. 7, form a substantial portion of the head of the epididymis

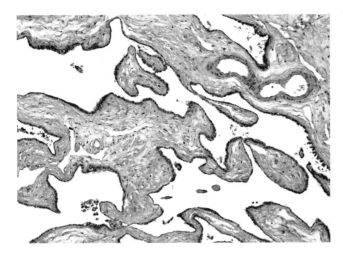

Fig. 6.238 Normal rete testis. The channels of the rete testis are lined by low columnar epithelium

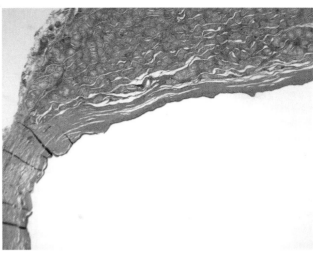

Fig. 6.240 Simple cyst of rete testis. This cystic structure, located in the hilum of the testis and lined by suniform low columnar epithelium like that of the normal rete testis, was found incidentally in an orchiectomy specimen from a patient with androgen insensitivity syndrome

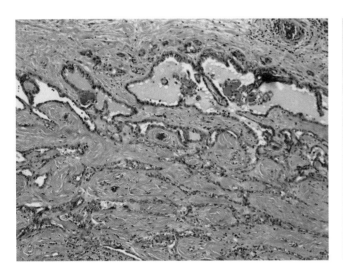

Fig. 6.239 Adenomatous hyperplasia of rete testis. This is a proliferation of rete testis tissue to form papillary or tubular structures, occasionally to an extent that it may appear neoplastic. It has been seen in all age groups. Its etiology is unknown, but it may simply represent disordered development. The epithelium shows no atypia, and no obstructive phenomena develop

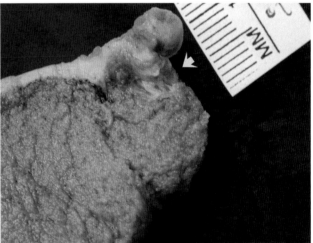

Fig. 6.241 Cystic transformation of rete testis. Patient was a 64-year-old man who developed a painful and tender 1.2 cm palpable testicular nodule, which was a complex cystic structure on ultrasound. Testis was excised, and a cystic nodule in the hilum of the testis was noted; after sectioning and decompression with drainage of clear fluid, it became much less prominent, having the appearance of interconnected tubular structures (*arrow*) (*Image courtesy of* Samantha Easley, MD)

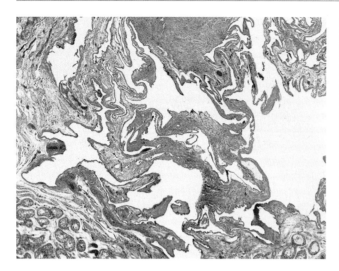

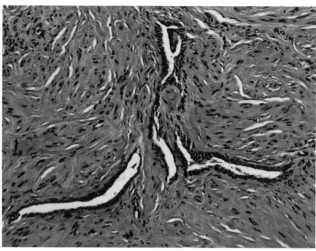

Fig. 6.242 Cystic transformation of rete testis. The lesion shown in Fig. 6.241 is consistent with simple acquired cystic transformation of the rete testis. It is characterized by the presence of dilated cavities lined by normal epithelium. It is probably the result of one of several forms of downstream obstruction, such as chronic epididymitis, varicocele, or prior epididymectomy

Fig. 6.244 Adenofibroma of rete testis. The lesion consists of a fibromatous stromal proliferation; the epithelium lining the rete testis channels is normal. Features of malignancy are absent

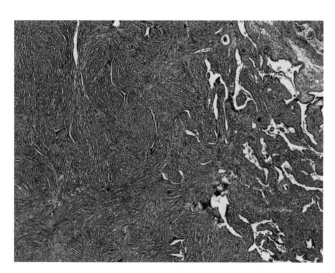

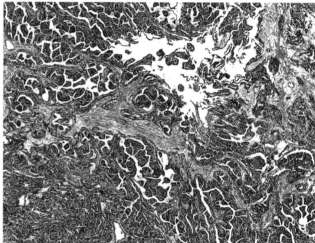

Fig. 6.243 Adenofibroma of rete testis. Benign tumors of the rete testis share the property of having benign epithelium, which may be associated with a fibromatous stromal component, in the case of adenofibroma, shown here, or may be arranged to form a solid aggregate of tubules (adenoma), conspicuous cystic structures (cystadenoma), or papillary structures (papillary cystadenoma). This image exemplifies an adenofibroma; it is predominantly a mesenchymal proliferation

Fig. 6.245 Papillary cystadenoma of rete testis. The lesion is an expansile proliferation of variably sized papillary structures, which appear to be within a cystic space

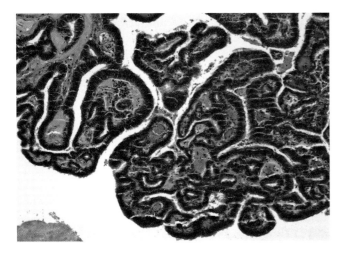

Fig. 6.246 Papillary cystadenoma of rete testis. The epithelium lining the papillary structures is bland, uniform and ciliated, consistent with rete testis epithelium. Features of malignancy are absent

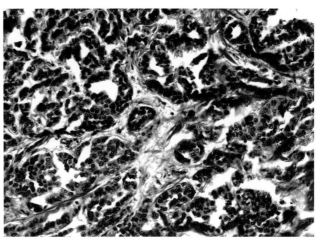

Fig. 6.248 Adenocarcinoma of rete testis. Tumor cells are small and cuboidal, with limited cytoplasm. Tumor cells have round-to-oval nuclei and prominent nucleoli

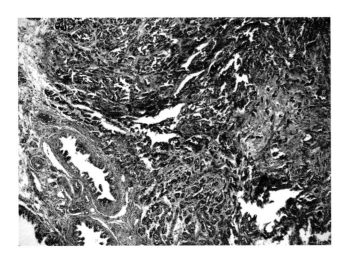

Fig. 6.247 Adenocarcinoma of rete testis. The tumor arose in the hilum of the testis, filled the rete testis and expanded to involve adjacent efferent ductules. The tumor has a tubulo-glandular appearance

The testicular tunics, appendix testis, appendix epididymis, efferent ductules, epididymis, vas deferens, and spermatic cord are regarded as paratesticular structures. This chapter discusses their normal histologic findings and the pathologic changes they undergo. The rete testis and its pathologic changes were discussed in Chap. 6.

7.1 Normal Findings

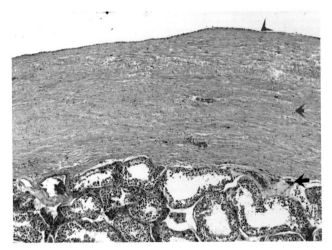

Fig. 7.1 Testicular tunics. A capsule encloses the testicular parenchyma. It consists of the outer tunica vaginalis (a thin layer of mesothelial cells) (*blue arrow*), the thick fibrous tunica albuginea (*red arrow*), and the inner tunica vasculosa, a loose fibroconnective tissue layer containing blood vessels and lymphatics (*black arrow*)

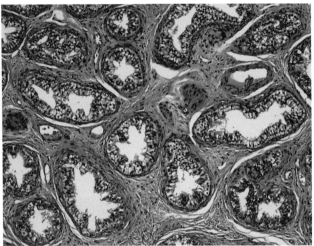

Fig. 7.2 Efferent ductules. Persistence of the caudal portion of the embryonic mesonephros forms the efferent ductules, and persistence of the Wolffian duct forms the epididymis, appendix epididymis, vas deferens, seminal vesicles, and ejaculatory ducts. About 12–15 efferent ductules emanate from the extratesticular portion of the rete testis and aggregate to form a significant portion of the head of the epididymis. Basal cells admixed with ciliated and nonciliated columnar cells line the efferent ductules, imparting a pseudostratified appearance

G. MacLennan and L. Cheng, *Atlas of Genitourinary Pathology*, DOI: 10.1007/978-1-84882-395-2_7,
© Springer-Verlag London Limited 2011

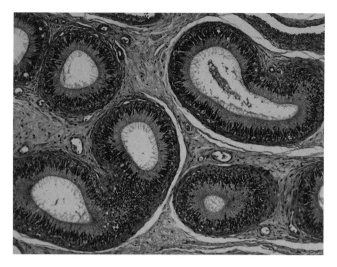

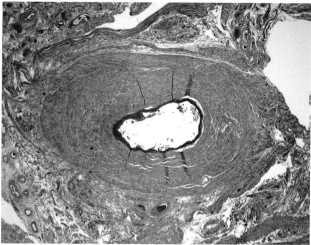

Fig. 7.3 Epididymis. This coiled tubular structure, 4–5 m in length, is regarded as having three regions: head, body, and caudal aspect. The tubules are surrounded by a prominent basement membrane and a distinct muscular coat. The epididymis is lined by tall columnar (principal) cells, narrow dark columnar cells, clear cells, and basal cells. The columnar cells have stereocilia that are tall, straight, and abundant in the proximal part of the epididymis, but are shorter and less prominent in the caudal aspect

Fig. 7.5 Vas deferens. The vas deferens is 30–40 cm long, enlarging in its distal 4–7 cm to form the ampulla of the vas, which joins the excretory duct of the seminal vesicle to form the ejaculatory duct. It is composed of three layers of smooth muscle – inner longitudinal, middle circular, and outer longitudinal, surrounding a small lumen lined by somewhat folded columnar epithelium

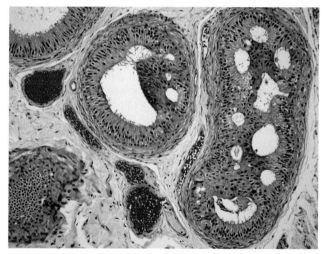

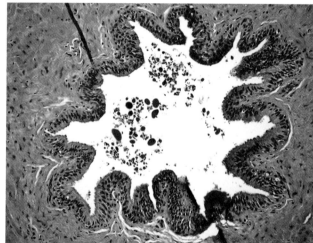

Fig. 7.4 Epididymis. Cribriform hyperplasia of the lining epithelium is a normal variant of no significance, except that it may raise concern for a neoplastic process

Fig. 7.6 Vas deferens. The vas deferens is lined by pseudostratified epithelium composed of a mixture of columnar cells and basal cells. The columnar cells bear stereocilia, which become shorter and more sparse near the ampulla

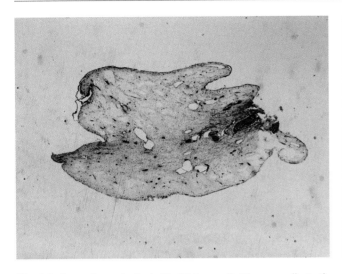

Fig. 7.7 Appendix testis (hydatid of Morgagni). The appendix testis and the prostatic utricle are müllerian remnants. The appendix testis is present in more than 90% of testes, as a sessile or polypoid mass, 2–4 mm in size, located at the superior pole of the testis near the epididymis. It consists of an epithelial-lined fibrovascular core, sometimes containing small tubular structures

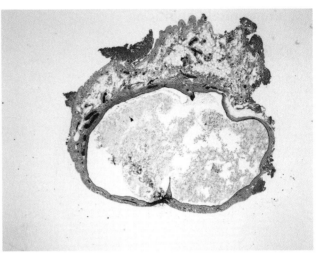

Fig. 7.9 Appendix epididymis. This is a remnant of Wolffian meso-nephric collecting tubules, found in about one third of testes. It is a pedunculated cystic epithelial-lined spherical or ovoid structure that arises from the anterosuperior pole of the head of the epididymis. The wall of the cyst is loose connective tissue; its outer surface is at least partially lined by cells of the tunica vaginalis

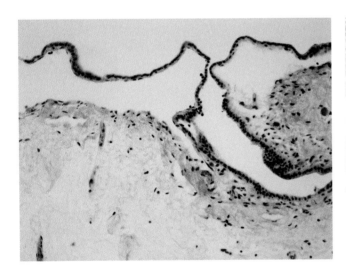

Fig. 7.8 Appendix testis. The loose connective tissue that forms the fibrovascular core is covered by simple cuboidal or low columnar mül-lerian-type epithelium, which merges with the adjacent tunica vaginalis

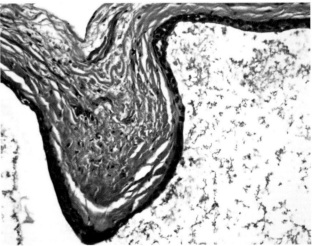

Fig. 7.10 Appendix epididymis. The cells lining the cystic structure are cuboidal or low columnar and sometimes ciliated. The cyst contains serous fluid and amorphous material

7.2 Congenital Conditions

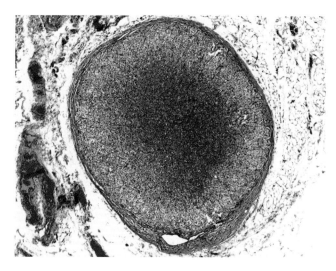

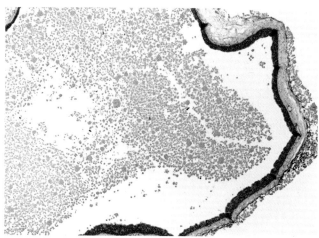

Fig. 7.13 Wolffian remnant in the spermatic cord. This cystic structure was found incidentally in spermatic cord tissue from a hernia repair. At low power, it is a thin-walled epithelial-lined cyst containing amorphous material, and bears a morphologic resemblance to an appendix epididymis (*see* Fig. 7.9)

Fig. 7.11 Ectopic adrenal in spermatic cord. Ectopic adrenal tissue is sometimes found along the path of testicular descent from the retroperitoneum to the scrotum, and as such it may appear as a small yellow-orange nodule, usually less than 5 mm in size, in the spermatic cord, epididymis, rete testis, or tunica albuginea. Such nodules are found in 1–2% of inguinal surgical specimens from pediatric patients. The nodule shown here was in tissue from a child undergoing hernia repair

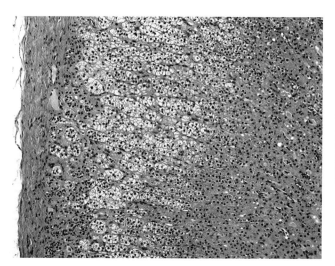

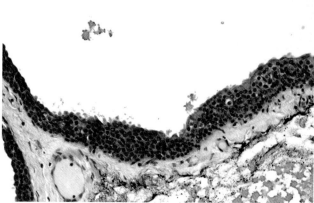

Fig. 7.12 Ectopic adrenal in spermatic cord. All cortical layers – glomerulosa, fasciculata, and reticularis – are represented. The presence of a medullary component in ectopic adrenal tissue is exceptional

Fig. 7.14 Wolffian remnant in the spermatic cord. On closer inspection, the cyst shown in Fig. 7.13 is lined by small cuboidal and low columnar cells, some of which appear to be ciliated, similar to those lining the appendix epididymis shown in Fig. 7.10

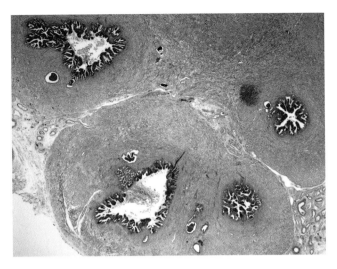

Fig. 7.15 Wolffian remnant in the spermatic cord. This lesion was an asymptomatic palpable nodule in a 35-year-old male; it was located in the upper aspect of the scrotum near the external ring. At low power, it bears a striking resemblance to seminal vesicle tissue

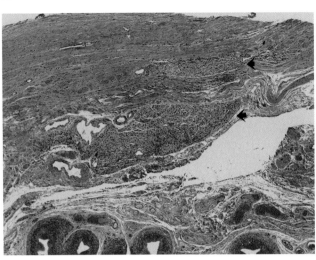

Fig. 7.17 Extratesticular steroid-type cells. Aggregates of steroid-type cells (*arrows*) are sometimes found in the hilar region of the testis, between the epididymis and the tunica vaginalis, adjacent to the tunica vaginalis and at other sites along the spermatic cord. In the case shown here, the finding was incidental, in a testis removed for other reasons

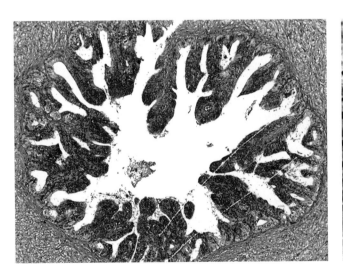

Fig. 7.16 Wolffian remnant in the spermatic cord. On closer inspection, the epithelium lining the luminal structures in the lesion shown in Fig. 7.15 shows complex papillary infoldings. The epithelium is tall columnar and predominantly ciliated. The overall findings in this unusual lesion were thought to best represent a Wolffian remnant

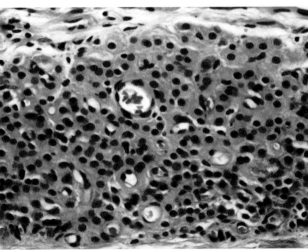

Fig. 7.18 Extratesticular steroid-type cells. On closer inspection of the cellular aggregates noted in Fig. 7.17, the cells bear some resemblance to Leydig cells. In some patients with untreated or inadequately treated adrenogenital syndrome, these cells undergo hyperplasia due to excessive adrenocorticotropic hormone stimulation and form palpable masses that can mimic neoplasia

7.3 Cysts and Celes

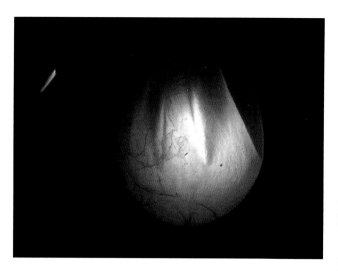

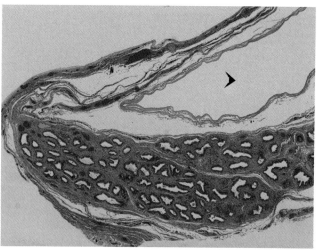

Fig. 7.21 Spermatocele. *Arrowhead* indicates the location of the sper-matocele, adjacent to the epididymis, and circumscribed by a thin fibrous wall. Spermatoceles may be unilocular or multilocular

Fig. 7.19 Spermatocele. This is a cystic dilatation of an efferent ductule, forming a mass adjacent to the head of the epididymis. Most are asymptomatic, and soft and nontender to palpation. In clinical prac-tice, transillumination of the lesion in a dark room, simulated in this image of a surgically resected specimen, provides some reassurance of its benign nature (*Image courtesy of* Annette Trivisonno)

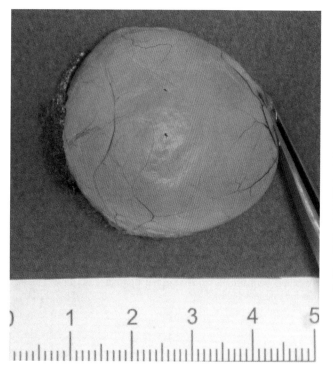

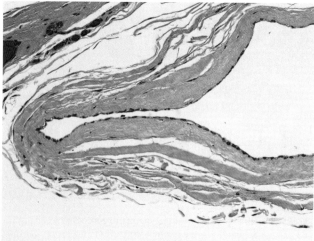

Fig. 7.22 Spermatocele. The cystic space is lined by a single layer of flattened or cuboidal cells, some of which may bear cilia

Fig. 7.20 Spermatocele. If the specimen is delivered intact, it is typi-cally cystic, with a smooth shiny wall, and contains milky fluid. If sought, spermatozoa are present in fluid aspirated from a spermatocele (*Image courtesy of* Annette Trivisonno)

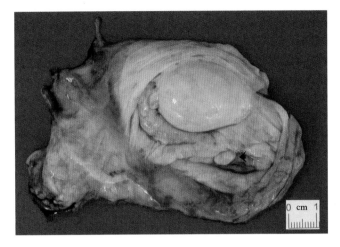

Fig. 7.23 Hydrocele. This is a collection of serous fluid within the tunica sac, lined by the mesothelial cells of the tunica vaginalis. The communicating type is characterized by a patent processus vaginalis that provides direct communication between the tunica sac and the peritoneal cavity. Much more common is the noncommunicating type, in which the tunica sac is a closed space because the processus vaginalis is no longer patent. Fluid accumulation within a hydrocele is usually an idiopathic process, thought to be related to an imbalance between the rate of fluid production by mesothelial cells and the rate of fluid reabsorption. This image shows a testis dwarfed by a large hydrocele sac. A small free-floating fibrous nodule was present (*arrow*) (*Image courtesy of* Douglas Hartman, MD)

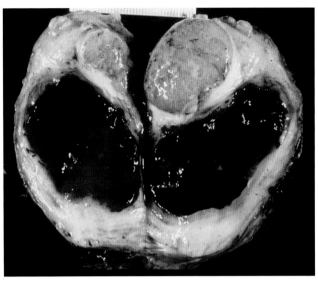

Fig. 7.25 Hydrocele, inflamed. Specimen is from a man with chronic urinary infection and recent epididymoorchitis. The walls of the hydrocele sac are markedly thickened, and the cavity of the hydrocele contains bloody fluid and fibrinous exudate

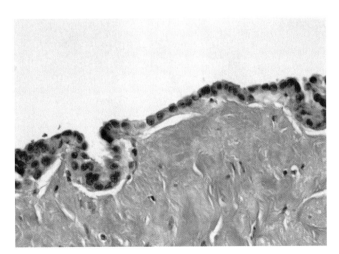

Fig. 7.24 Hydrocele. In the absence of inflammation, hydroceles are lined by a single layer of flat or cuboidal mesothelial cells that lack significant cytologic atypia

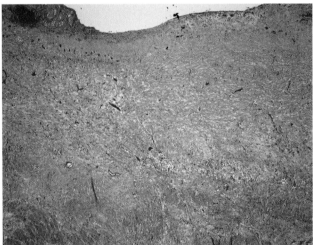

Fig. 7.26 Hydrocele, inflamed. Section from the specimen shown in Fig. 7.25. The wall of the hydrocele is thickened by fibrosis and is chronically inflamed. The surface lining is widely denuded and replaced by granulation tissue and fibrinous exudate

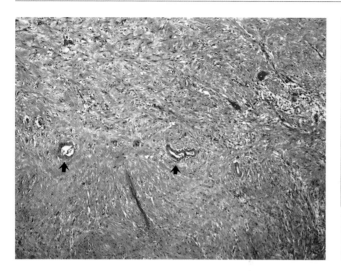

Fig. 7.27 Hydrocele, inflamed. Within the fibrotic wall of the chronically inflamed hydrocele, but near the surface, small tubular structures derived from mesothelium are present, representing portions of the tunica vaginalis entrapped by a reactive/reparative process

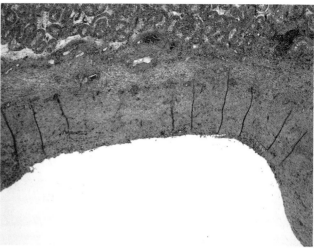

Fig. 7.29 Mesothelial cyst, intratesticular. The wall of the cyst consists mainly of hyalinized fibrous tissue, with areas of chronic inflammation. These cysts occur mainly in men older than 40 years old; their etiology is unknown

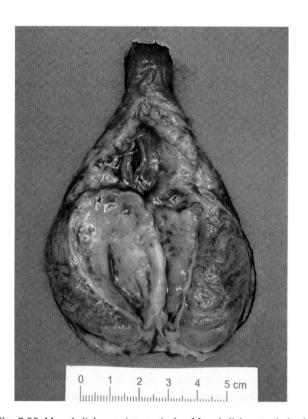

Fig. 7.28 Mesothelial cyst, intratesticular. Mesothelial cysts derived from the tunica vaginalis may involve the testis or epididymis. They contain serous or blood-tinged fluid. The cyst shown in this image was predominantly within the substance of the testis and was difficult to characterize clinically and radiologically, prompting orchiectomy (*Image courtesy of* Edmunds Reineks, MD)

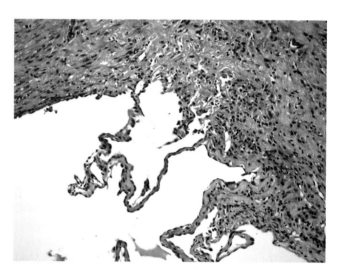

Fig. 7.30 Mesothelial cyst, intratesticular. The cavity of the cyst is lined by flattened or cuboidal mesothelial cells

7.4 Acquired and Inflammatory Conditions

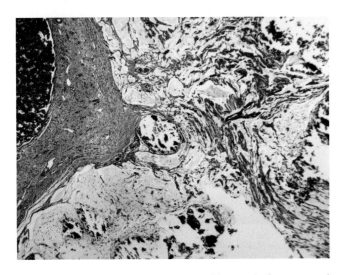

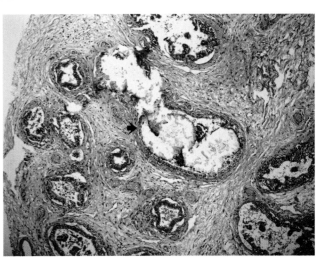

Fig. 7.33 Calcium oxalate deposition in efferent ductules. Hyperoxalemia and secondary oxalosis sometimes complicate chronic renal failure, due to decreased oxalate excretion, resulting in tissue deposition, typically in the kidney but also in other organs. Patients on dialysis for renal failure are sometimes found to have "cystic transformation of the rete testis and efferent ducts," characterized by oxalate crystal deposition in these structures, as exemplified in this image (*arrow*). Tissue reaction may result in formation of a clinically palpable nodule

Fig. 7.31 Meconium periorchitis. This condition results from antenatal or prenatal colon perforation. Meconium gains access to the peritoneal cavity and moves through the patent processus vaginalis into the tunica sac, inciting chronic inflammation, foreign body giant cell reaction and fibrosis of surrounding tissues. Grossly, the tunica sac contains one or more orange or green nodules. This image shows a testis at left; mucinous material and aggregates of calcific debris are present in the tunica sac

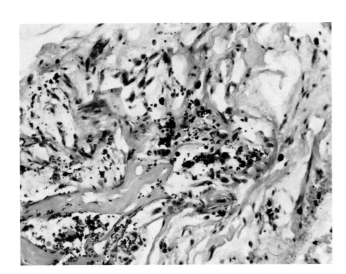

Fig. 7.32 Meconium periorchitis. The contents of the tunica sac include mucin, calcified amorphous material, pigment-laden macrophages and organizing granulation tissue

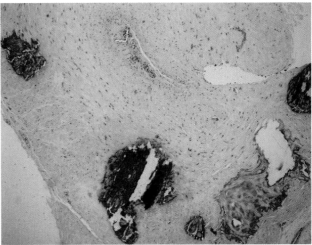

Fig. 7.34 Calcification of the vas deferens. This image of a vasectomy specimen from a diabetic man shows abundant calcifications in the wall of the vas. Vas deferens calcification is seen in patients with diabetes mellitus and in nondiabetic patients, but it is six times more common in the former. In nondiabetics, it is regarded as a manifestation of aging. It produces distinctive radiologic findings, appearing as bilateral symmetric parallel calcific lines on each side. This image also shows an area of ossification, which is reported less commonly in this setting

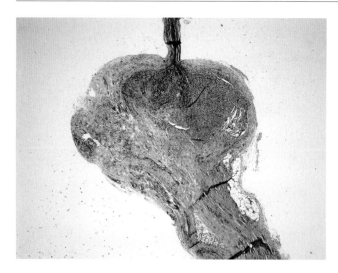

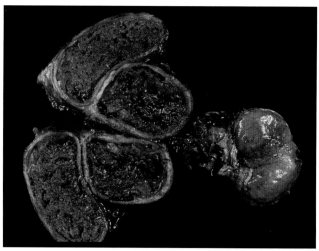

Fig. 7.35 Nodular mesothelial hyperplasia. This lesion is sometimes found incidentally in tissues removed at the time of inguinal hernia repair, as in the case shown here. It has been described in association with diverse lesions, such as hydrocele, hematocele, and fibrous pseudo-tumor. It consists of benign-appearing mesothelial cells arranged in solid nests

Fig. 7.37 Spermatic cord hematoma. An accumulation of blood in the tunica sac is designated as a hematocele. The image shown here is an orchiectomy specimen from a mentally challenged and institutionalized patient who developed a groin mass; radical orchiectomy was done due to concern for malignancy. The mass is composed of loculated collections of old blood enclosed within thick fibrotic walls

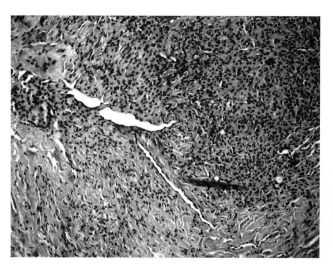

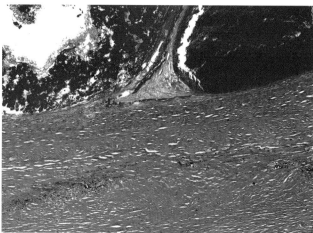

Fig. 7.36 Nodular mesothelial hyperplasia. The nodule shown in Fig. 7.35 is composed of sheets of uniform benign-appearing mesothelial cells. This process is regarded as a reactive proliferation in response to irritation or inflammation. Reactive mesothelium can also form simple papillary excrescences, as well as small tubules or cysts that lie beneath the surface mesothelium (*see* Fig. 7.27)

Fig. 7.38 Spermatic cord hematoma. Section from specimen shown in Fig. 7.37 shows only organizing hematoma. Extensive sampling showed no neoplasia. Cause of the hematoma was never ascertained. Findings may represent bleeding into a loculated noncommunicating hydrocele of the spermatic cord

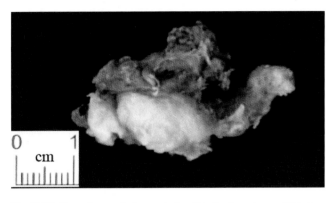

Fig. 7.39 Smooth muscle hyperplasia of testicular adnexa. This is a benign condition that presents clinically as an intrascrotal mass in adults, ranging up to 7 cm in size, indeterminate for neoplasia, prompting excision. The lesion shown here involved the epididymis and proximal vas deferens, producing a diffuse fusiform enlargement of these structures (*Image courtesy of* Pedro Ciarlini, MD)

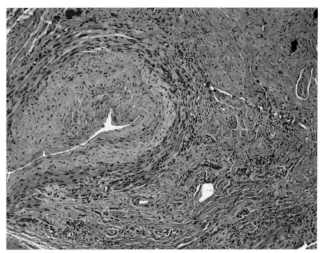

Fig. 7.41 Smooth muscle hyperplasia of testicular adnexa. The vas deferens is surrounded by a concentric proliferation of smooth muscle fibers. The etiology of this condition is unknown

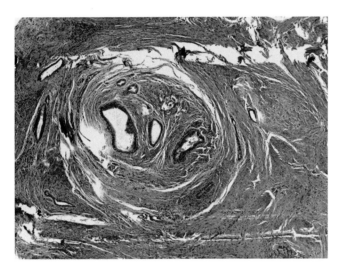

Fig. 7.40 Smooth muscle hyperplasia of testicular adnexa. Fascicles of smooth muscle are arranged concentrically around epididymal ducts and blood vessels, and expand the interstitium. Features of malignancy are absent

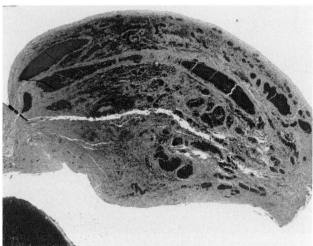

Fig. 7.42 Torsion of the appendix testis. The appendix testis, if it is pedunculated, may undergo torsion and ischemic necrosis. Clinically, this event may simulate torsion of the testis, resulting in surgical exploration, as in the case shown here. The appendix testis is hemorrhagic and edematous with areas of ischemic change

Fig. 7.43 Fibrous pseudotumor of tunica vaginalis. Fibrous pseudotumor is composed of one or more firm white nodules that may involve the tunica vaginalis of the testis, the epididymis and/or the spermatic cord. The nodules, which are usually between 0.5 and 8 cm in greatest dimension, may be as large as 25 cm. The nodules may be spatially separated or confluent; rarely, the entire testis may be encased by a diffuse fibrous proliferation (*see* Bhandari et al. 2008. With permission)

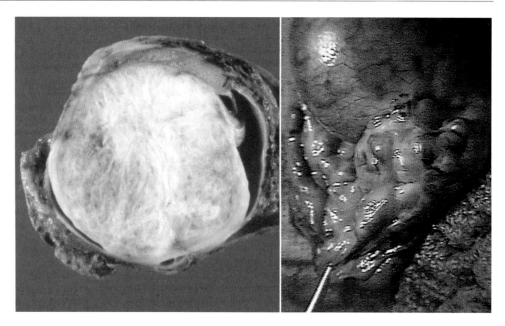

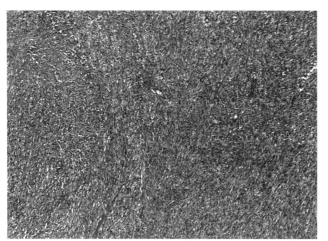

Fig. 7.44 Fibrous pseudotumor of tunica vaginalis. Fibrous pseudotumor arises in the connective tissues of the testicular tunics and paratesticular soft tissues, and is regarded as a reactive nonneoplastic lesion; however, its pathogenesis is unclear. It is composed of proliferating fibroblastic and myofibroblastic cells within a hyalinized collagenous stroma

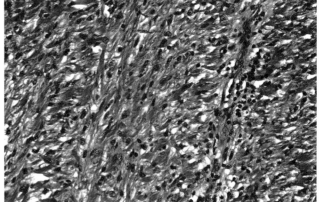

Fig. 7.45 Fibrous pseudotumor of tunica vaginalis. Mitotic figures are absent or very rare. There is no necrosis or significant cytologic atypia

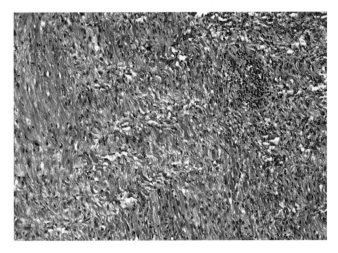

Fig. 7.46 Fibrous pseudotumor of tunica vaginalis. Patchy inflammation may be present most often as a mixed chronic inflammatory cell infiltrate of lymphocytes, plasma cells, and histiocytes, and sometimes scattered eosinophils and neutrophils. Additional findings may include calcification, ossification, myxoid change, and granulation tissue formation

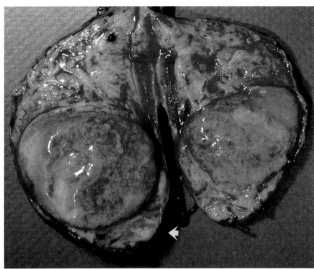

Fig. 7.48 Acute epididymoorchitis. The epididymis (*arrow*) contains abundant purulent material. The testis is edematous and its variegated cut surface reflects widespread inflammation, as well. In about half of cases of acute epididymitis, the testis is also involved. Bacterial infection accounts for most cases of acute epididymoorchitis – most often coliform organisms in children and older men, and sexually transmitted organisms in the remaining patients (*Image courtesy of* Hollie M. Reeves, MD)

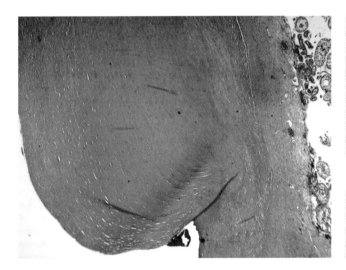

Fig. 7.47 Fibrous pseudotumor of tunica vaginalis. In some cases, the nodules may be composed of markedly paucicellular hyalinized fibroconnective tissue. This finding may reflect the later stages of a slowly evolving reactive/reparative process

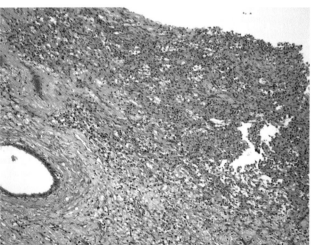

Fig. 7.49 Acute epididymoorchitis. Section from the epididymis in the specimen shown in Fig 7.48, showing a pronounced infiltrate of neutrophils

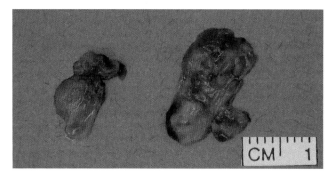

Fig. 7.50 Chronic epididymitis. The epididymis becomes scarred and fibrotic, with cystically dilated tubules. This epididymal lesion was palpably and radiologically abnormal, and indeterminate for neoplasia, prompting epididymectomy (*Image courtesy of* Samantha Easley, MD)

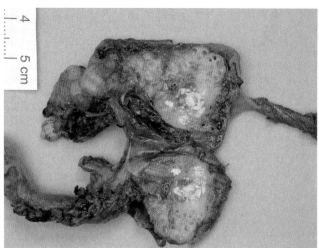

Fig. 7.53 Epididymal sperm granuloma. Patient had a palpable nodule in the epididymis. He had undergone bilateral vasectomy 9 years previously. An area of nodularity and fibrosis, with yellow tan aggregates of amorphous material are evident on cut section (*Image courtesy of* Diane Kidric, MD)

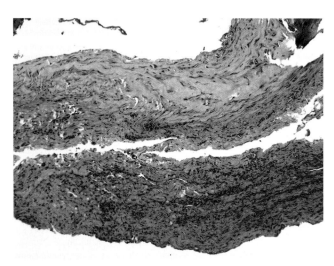

Fig. 7.51 Chronic epididymitis. Section from the specimen shown in Fig. 7.50. The lesion consists of chronically inflamed fibrous tissue. The lumens of the cystic spaces were devoid of epithelial lining, but mesothelium partially covered the external aspect of the lesion. Etiology of the lesion was indeterminate, but it was thought to be consistent with a reactive/reparative process associated with chronic epididymitis

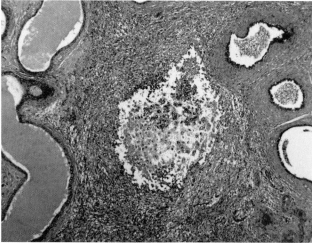

Fig. 7.54 Epididymal sperm granuloma. The small yellow nodules seen in Fig. 7.53 are aggregates of lipid-laden macrophages in the interstitium, between epididymal tubules

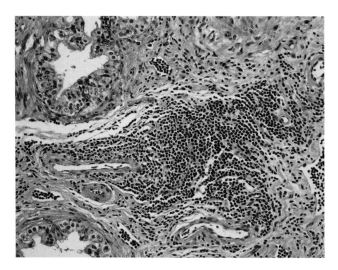

Fig. 7.52 Chronic epididymitis. Section from another case shows aggregates of lymphocytes, plasma cells, and macrophages in the interstitial tissue

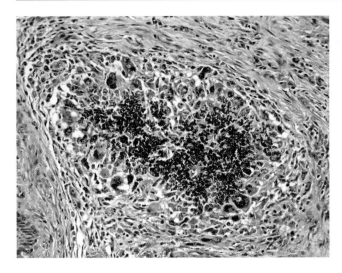

Fig. 7.55 Epididymal sperm granuloma. Extravasated spermatozoa are being engulfed by macrophages

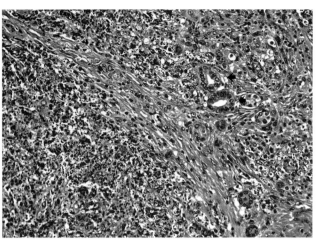

Fig. 7.57 Vasitis nodosa. Leakage of spermatozoa into the interstitial tissues secondary to tubular obstruction and increased luminal pressure causes a characteristic inflammatory reaction, designated sperm granuloma, characterized by spermatozoa admixed with epithelioid histiocytes and sometimes multinucleated giant cells, which engulf the extravasated spermatozoa. If this is accompanied by excessive regeneration of the epithelial lining, with formation of irregular small ductules which haphazardly infiltrate the wall of the vas (*arrows*) or the interstitium of the epididymis, the condition is designated vasitis nodosa or epididymitis nodosa, depending upon the location of the lesion

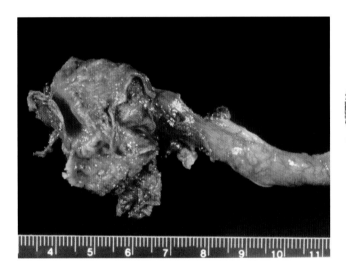

Fig. 7.56 Vasitis nodosa. Vasitis nodosa and epididymitis nodosa most often occur as late postvasectomy changes, but have also been described following trauma, herniorrhaphy, and radical prostatectomy. Vasitis nodosa is typically a nodule in the upper scrotum, superior to the testis along the course of the vas, exemplified in this image at the left end of the resected vas deferens segment. These nodules sometimes contain milky fluid

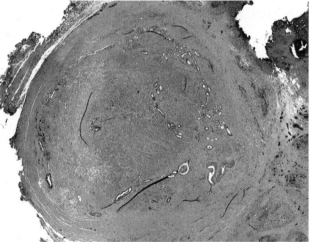

Fig. 7.58 Vasitis nodosa. In this low-power image, myriad small ductules are present within the wall of the vas deferens, following previous bilateral vasectomy. No sperm granuloma is apparent; sperm granulomas are found in only about 70% of cases of vasitis nodosa. Some tubules in this image contained spermatozoa, which is helpful in distinguishing this lesion from invasive adenocarcinoma, which may sometimes be considered in the differential

Fig. 7.59 Tuberculous epididymitis. Tuberculous epididymitis is a sequela in about 40% of cases of renal tuberculosis; secondary testicular infection complicates about 80% of cases of epididymal tuberculosis. The infection is characterized by caseating granulomas and fibrous thickening of the involved structures (*see*, "Spermatic Cord and Testicular Adnexae" [page 872] in Bostwick and Cheng 2008. With permission)

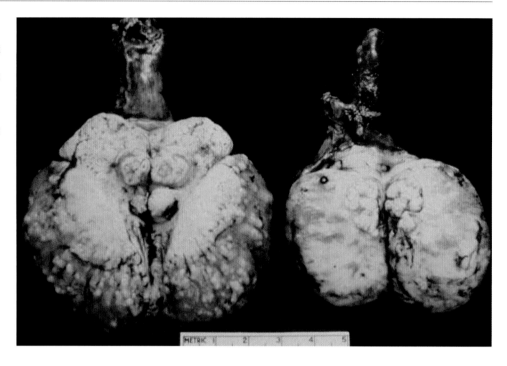

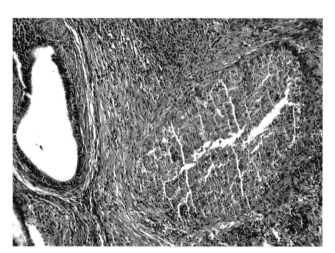

Fig. 7.60 Tuberculous epididymitis. In this image, a necrotizing granuloma is present in the interstitium of the epididymis

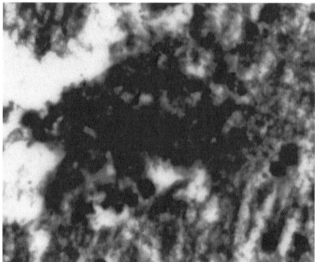

Fig. 7.61 Tuberculous epididymitis. Same case as in Fig. 7.60. Ziehl-Nielsen stain highlights acid-fast bacilli in the necrotizing granuloma

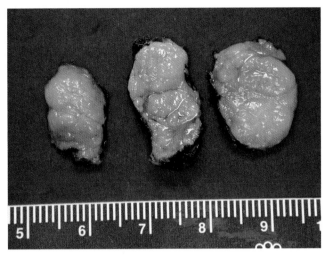

Fig. 7.62 Sarcoidosis of the epididymis. Involvement of the epididymis and/or testis by sarcoidosis can mimic a neoplastic condition because the men involved are commonly young, with genital lesions that cannot be distinguished clinically or radiologically from cancer, and often with radiologic pulmonary abnormalities; radical orchiectomy is done in one third of cases. The epididymis is expanded by firm elastic slightly bulging pale to tan nodules (*Image courtesy of* Edmunds Reineks, MD)

7.5 Benign Neoplasms

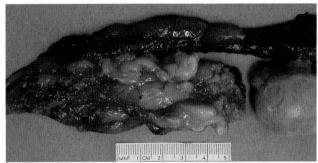

Fig. 7.64 Lipoma of spermatic cord. Lipoma accounts for up to 90% of spermatic cord tumors and is the commonest paratesticular tumor. Most are removed during hernia repairs. In the case shown here, part of the tumor was palpably indurated preoperatively and intraoperatively, raising concern for malignancy, and prompting radical orchiectomy. The lipoma (*bottom*) has been partially separated from the spermatic cord. The induration proved to be fat necrosis (*Image courtesy of* Anaibelith Del-Rio Perez, MD)

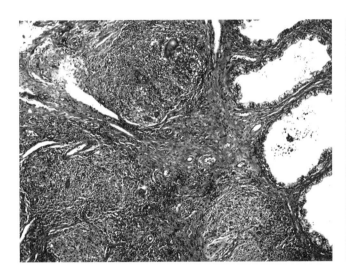

Fig. 7.63 Sarcoidosis of epididymis. The interstitium of the epididymis is occupied by abundant nonnecrotizing granulomas, in some cases of sarcoidosis, there may be minimal focal central necrosis in some granulomas. Special stains for fungal organisms and acid-fast bacilli are negative in this condition

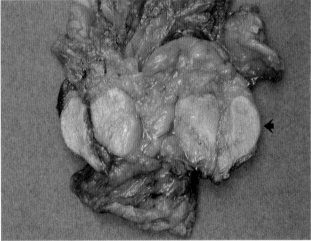

Fig. 7.65 Lipoma of spermatic cord, with fat necrosis. In this spermatic cord lipoma, there was an area of firm nodularity. Sectioning revealed two tan nodules (*arrow*), indistinctly circumscribed, in a background of adipose tissue (*Image courtesy of* Christine Lemyre and Allen Seftel, MD)

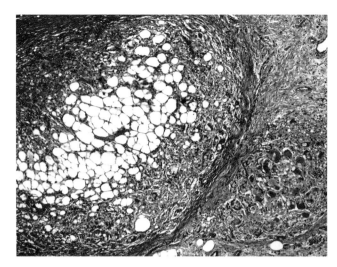

Fig. 7.66 Lipoma of spermatic cord, with fat necrosis. Section from one of the nodules shown in Fig. 7.65 shows necrotic adipose tissue being engulfed by macrophages and multinucleated giant cells

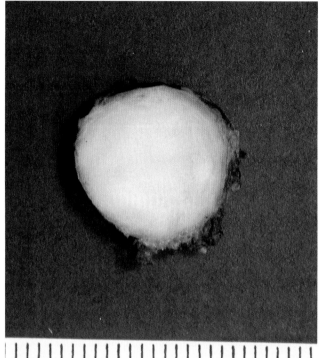

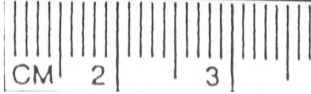

Fig. 7.68 Adenomatoid tumor. This lesion is second in frequency (by far) to lipoma, but accounts for about one third of nonlipomas in the paratesticular area. Being of mesothelial origin, it can arise virtually anywhere along the course of the spermatic cord, or in any area covered by tunica vaginalis. It is the most common benign epididymal neoplasm. It ranges from 0.4 to 5.0 cm, and is typically firm, tan or gray-white, and circumscribed, with a glistening cut surface

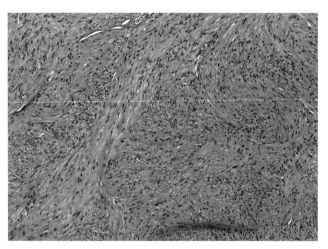

Fig. 7.67 Leiomyoma of epididymis. Leiomyoma of the epididymis is somewhat less common than adenomatoid tumor of the epididymis, and is quite rare in the spermatic cord proper. It forms a firm round gray-white mass up to 8 cm in diameter. Microscopically, it resembles leiomyoma at other sites; it is composing of intersecting fascicles of smooth muscle, lacking necrosis, cytologic atypia, or mitotic activity

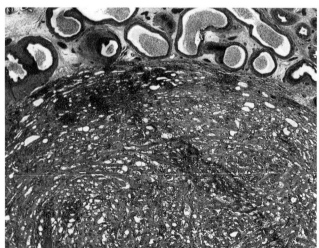

Fig. 7.69 Adenomatoid tumor. Tumor cells are typically arranged in the form of irregular tubules which may anastomose with one another, as is clearly evident in this low-power view

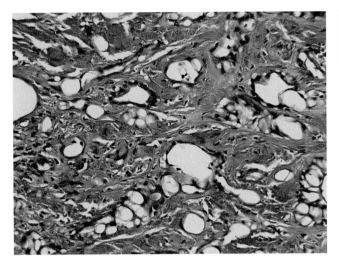

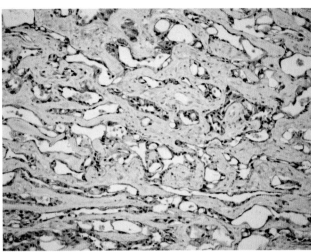

Fig. 7.70 Adenomatoid tumor. The tubules may be poorly formed or slit-like. Tumor cells are plump and eosinophilic

Fig. 7.72 Adenomatoid tumor. Tumor cells show positive immunostaining for markers of mesothelial origin, such as calretinin, as in the image shown here

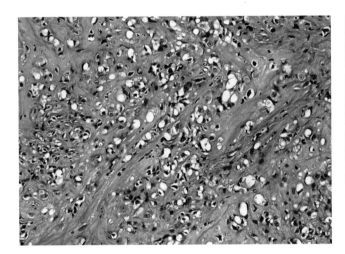

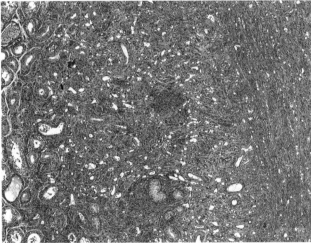

Fig. 7.71 Adenomatoid tumor. Tumor cells may also be arranged in nests or trabecular structures; they commonly contain intracytoplasmic vacuoles, and may have a signet ring appearance. The stroma is typically fibrous and is often hyalinized. Adenomatoid tumor may appear locally infiltrative, but it does not metastasize, and is cured by complete surgical excision

Fig. 7.73 Adenomatoid tumor involving testis. Although most adenomatoid tumors are located external to the tunica albuginea, infrequently an adenomatoid tumor may involve the testicular parenchyma, as in the case shown here, in which the tumor diffusely insinuates itself between seminiferous tubules

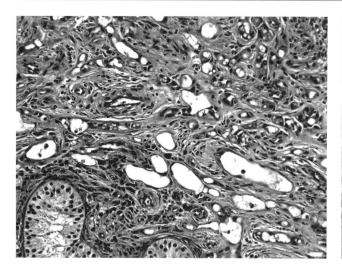

Fig. 7.74 Adenomatoid tumor involving testis. The tumor cells, many of which show cytoplasmic vacuolization, form clusters and irregular tubules in the interstitium adjacent to seminiferous tubules. Intratesticular growth of adenomatoid tumor may be difficult to differentiate from sex cord-stromal tumors of the testis

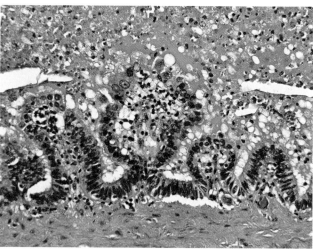

Fig. 7.76 Papillary cystadenoma of the epididymis. The papillae consist of fibrovascular cores lined by a single or double layer of bland cuboidal or columnar cells. The lining epithelial cells often have vacuolated or clear cytoplasm, and are sometimes ciliated

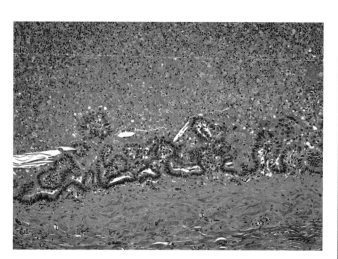

Fig. 7.75 Papillary cystadenoma of the epididymis. This is the second most common benign epidymal neoplasm, and is often bilateral. It is typically circumscribed, tan-yellow to gray-brown, solid, cystic, or solid-cystic, and often contains green, yellow or blood-tinged fluid. Microscopically, it consists of tubules and dilated cystic spaces into which papillary structures project

7.6 Malignant Neoplasms

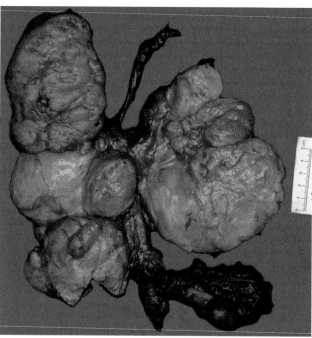

Fig. 7.77 Liposarcoma of spermatic cord. This is the most common type of paratesticular sarcoma in adults. It ranges up to 30 cm in size and sometimes dwarfs the testis, shown here at bottom. Cord liposarcomas are lobulated and nodular, gray-white, or yellow-tan, and often have fibrous septa in the lobules. Necrosis and hemorrhage appear in some (*see* Fitzgerald and MacLennan 2009. With permission)

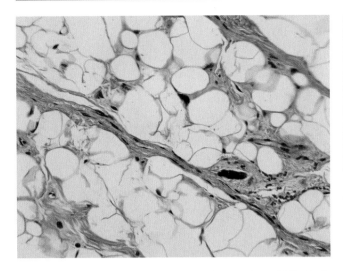

Fig. 7.78 Well-differentiated liposarcoma of spermatic cord. Histologic types of liposarcoma include well differentiated, dedifferentiated, and myxoid/round cell types. In the lipoma-like variant of well-differentiated liposarcoma, the findings may be subtle; the neoplastic adipose cells with enlarged hyperchromatic irregular nuclei may be widely scattered in a background of bland adipose tissue

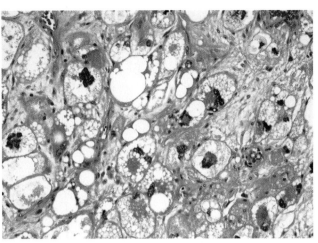

Fig. 7.80 Well-differentiated liposarcoma of spermatic cord. Well-differentiated liposarcoma showing lipoblasts at varying stages of development in a background of myxoid change. The delicately arborizing capillary architecture that characterizes myxoid liposarcoma is not present

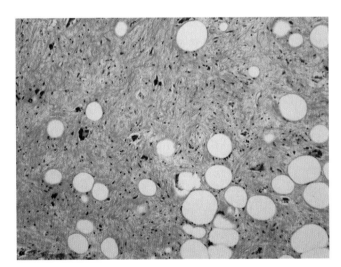

Fig. 7.79 Well-differentiated liposarcoma of spermatic cord. Section from a well-differentiated liposarcoma showing lipoblasts with pleomorphic and sometimes spindled hyperchromatic nuclei in a variably sclerotic background

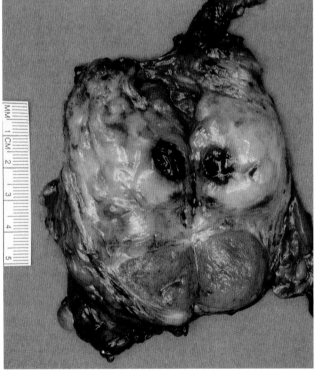

Fig. 7.81 Dedifferentiated liposarcoma of spermatic cord. Patient had previously undergone resection of retroperitoneal liposarcoma. Recurrences were noted in retroperitoneum, omentum, inguinal region, and upper scrotum. The mass superior to the testis is firm and fibrous and does not resemble fat (*Image courtesy of* Christina M. Bagby, MD)

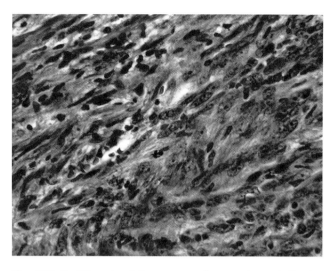

Fig. 7.82 Dedifferentiated liposarcoma of spermatic cord. Section from the tumor shown in Fig. 7.81 shows high-grade undifferentiated spindle cell neoplasm. A bizarre mitotic figure is evident near the center of the image

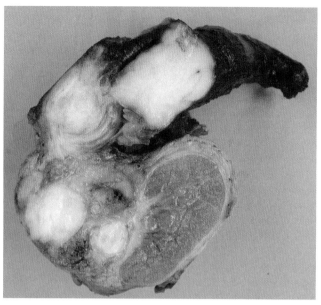

Fig. 7.84 Rhabdomyosarcoma, paratesticular. Tumor from a postpubertal male forms multiple gray-white nodules in the spermatic cord and soft tissues adjacent to the testis. Paratesticular rhabdomyosarcomas are particularly prone to develop in patients between ages 7 and 18 years

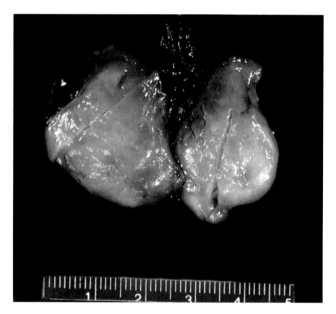

Fig. 7.83 Rhabdomyosarcoma, paratesticular. This paratesticular rhabdomyosarcoma was excised from a 6-year-old male. Tumor was an embryonal rhabdomyosarcoma with focal anaplastic/pleomorphic features (*see* MacLennan GT, Resnick MI, Bostwick DG, 2003. With permission)

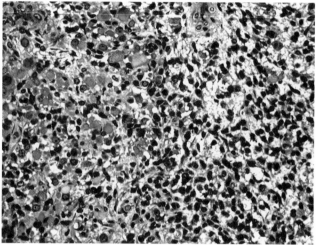

Fig. 7.85 Rhabdomyosarcoma, paratesticular. Although any type of rhabdomyosarcoma may occur in this location, the embryonal subtype, especially the spindle cell variant of the embryonal subtype, is likely to be found here. This image shows embryonal rhabdomyosarcoma, composed of primitive dark round cells, short spindled cells, and large rhabdomyoblasts with copious eosinophilic cytoplasm

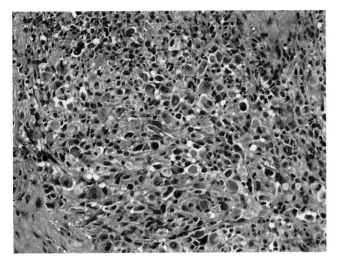

Fig. 7.86 Rhabdomyosarcoma, paratesticular. Another area of embryonal rhabdomyosarcoma, composed predominantly of large round-to-ovoid rhabdomyoblasts and elongated "strap" cells. Only a few small dark blue cells are present

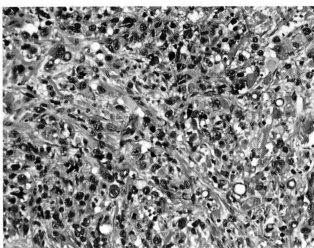

Fig. 7.88 Rhabdomyosarcoma, paratesticular. Pleomorphic rhabdomyosarcoma is the rarest form of rhabdomyosarcoma, occurring most often in adults, and consisting of sheets and poorly formed fascicles of round to polygonal cells with hyperchromatic and markedly pleomorphic nuclei and often abundant brightly eosinophilic cytoplasm

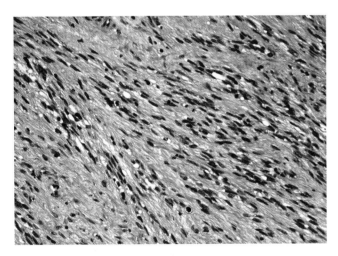

Fig. 7.87 Rhabdomyosarcoma, paratesticular. This is the spindle cell variant of embryonal rhabdomyosarcoma. It is composed of a fascicular arrangement of fusiform elongated cells with eosinophilic cytoplasm. Numerous mitotic figures are present. Special studies are often needed to distinguish this entity from leiomyosarcoma and fibrosarcoma

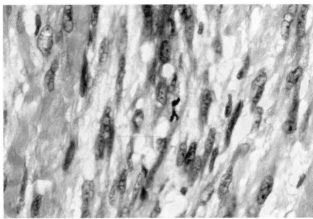

Fig. 7.89 Leiomyosarcoma, paratesticular. Leiomyosarcoma accounts for about one-third of adult paratesticular sarcomas, forming firm rubbery gray-tan masses. Histologically, it consists of intersecting fascicles of elongated spindle cells with eosinophilic cytoplasm and moderately pleomorphic cigar-shaped blunt-ended nuclei that often have perinuclear vacuoles. Mitotic figures, sometimes bizarre as shown here, are compelling evidence of malignancy in smooth muscle neoplasms in this area

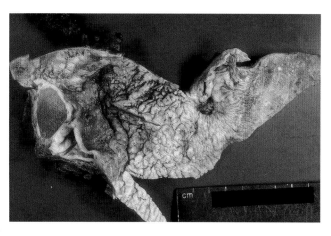

Fig. 7.90 Mesothelioma of tunica vaginalis. The surface of a large hydrocele sac is studded with yellow-tan nodular excrescences (*Image courtesy of* David G. Bostwick, MD)

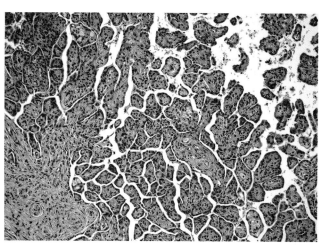

Fig. 7.92 Well-differentiated papillary mesothelioma. The fibrovascular cores are lined by a single layer of bland uniform cuboidal mesothelial cells lacking significant nuclear atypia or mitotic activity. The abundance and complexity of the papillary proliferation are beyond that seen in a reactive/reparative process. If completely excised, such neoplasms generally do not recur

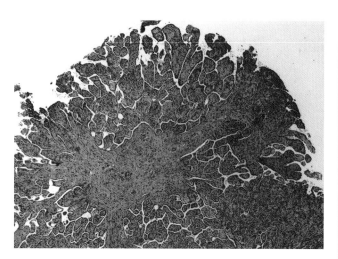

Fig. 7.91 Well-differentiated papillary mesothelioma. The tumor has an exophytic complex papillary architecture

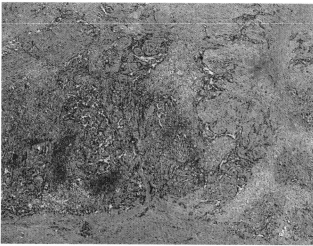

Fig. 7.93 Malignant mesothelioma. The tumor is composed of clearly invasive tubules and papillae. Focal necrosis is evident

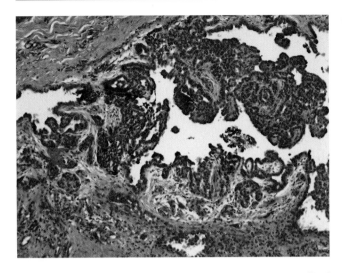

Fig. 7.94 Malignant mesothelioma. The fibrovascular cores are lined by multiple layers of atypical mesothelial cells. There is unequivocal stromal invasion by tumor cells

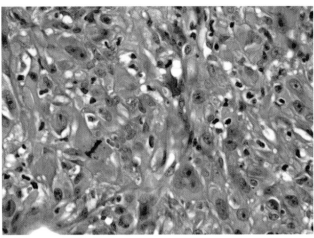

Fig. 7.96 Malignant mesothelioma. In areas where tumor cells grow in solid sheets rather than forming papillary or tubular structures, the tumor cells are often much more pleomorphic or even anaplastic in appearance, with very prominent nucleoli and frequent mitotic figures, frequently accompanied by areas of necrosis

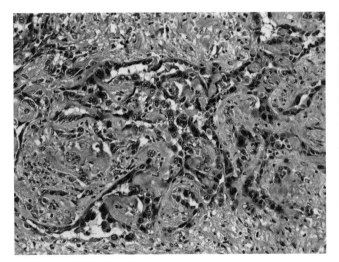

Fig. 7.95 Malignant mesothelioma. Tumor cells are of epithelial type. They have moderate to abundant eosinophilic cytoplasm, moderately pleomorphic vesicular nuclei and readily visible nucleoli

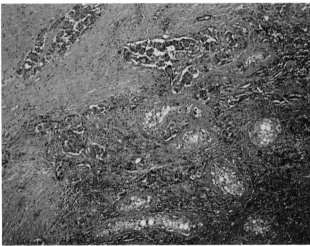

Fig. 7.97 Malignant mesothelioma. The tumor has infiltrated adjacent testicular parenchyma

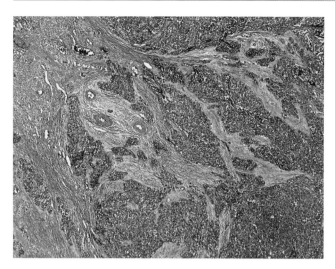

Fig. 7.98 Desmoplastic small round cell tumor. These rare polyphenotypic tumors tend to arise in areas where mesothelium is present, including the paratesticular region. Tumors grow in variably sized sheets and nests in a background of cellular fibrous or fibromyxoid stroma

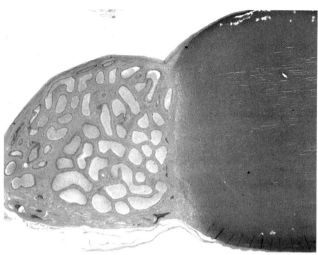

Fig. 7.101 Plasmacytoma. Soft tissues adjacent to the epididymis are diffusely infiltrated and expanded by a monotonous population of dark cells

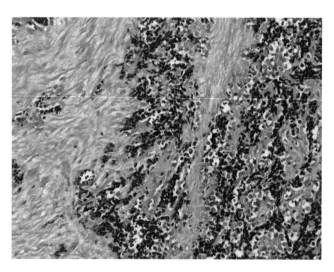

Fig. 7.99 Desmoplastic small round cell tumor. Tumor cells are small, dark, and undifferentiated, and have very little cytoplasm. Definitive diagnosis is facilitated by the use of immunohistochemical and molecular studies, necessary to distinguish this lesion from entities such as rhabdomyosarcoma and primitive neuroectodermal tumor

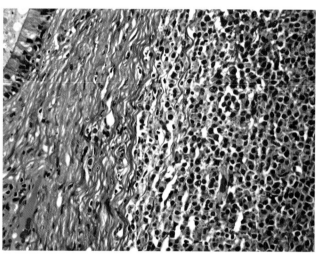

Fig. 7.102 Plasmacytoma. Tumor cells are morphologically similar to plasma cells. They showed positive immunostaining for CD79a and were monoclonal for κ light chains by in situ hybridization

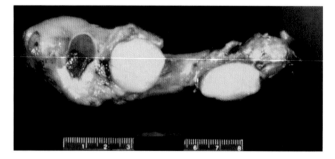

Fig. 7.100 Plasmacytoma. Plasmacytoma sometimes involves the epididymis or spermatic cord, sometimes in association with testicular involvement. It forms circumscribed tumor nodules in the soft tissues (*see* MacLennan GT, Resnick MI, Bostwick DG, 2003. With permission)

Fortunately, many of the disorders that affect the penis and scrotum (e.g., various skin conditions, certain infections, and Peyronie's disease) are managed without the need for biopsy or excision. At times, surgical pathologists are asked to examine lesions to clarify a diagnosis, and in some circumstances, surgical excision is clearly unavoidable.

8.1 Nonneoplastic Penile Lesions

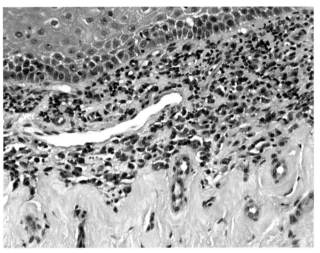

Fig. 8.2 Plasma cell balanitis (Zoon's balanitis). A higher magnification of Fig. 8.1 showing the inflammatory infiltrate, composed predominantly of plasma cells, with scattered lymphocytes

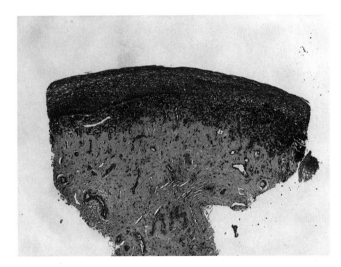

Fig. 8.1 Plasma cell balanitis (Zoon's balanitis). This lesion of unknown etiology is seen most often in elderly uncircumcised men. It forms a moist bright-red patch on the glans or inner foreskin, clinically mimicking squamous cell carcinoma in situ and prompting biopsy. Microscopically, the upper dermis is infiltrated by a variable number of plasma cells, often arranged in a band. Numerous dilated capillaries are evident in the dermis, and the overlying squamous epithelium is usually thin and sometimes absent

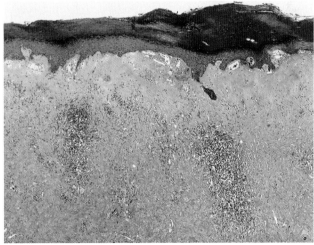

Fig. 8.3 Balanitis xerotic obliterans. Lichen sclerosus et atrophicus is an atrophic disorder of the genital or perianal skin in both sexes; when it involves the glans penis or foreskin, it is called balanitis xerotica obliterans. Its cause is unknown. It presents as a circumscribed firm gray-white patch on the foreskin or glans. It can result in phimosis or urethral meatal stenosis. The epidermis becomes thin, with overlying hyperkeratosis. The rete pegs become progressively shortened, and the basal layer of the epidermis becomes inconspicuous

G. MacLennan and L. Cheng, *Atlas of Genitourinary Pathology*, DOI: 10.1007/978-1-84882-395-2_8,
© Springer-Verlag London Limited 2011

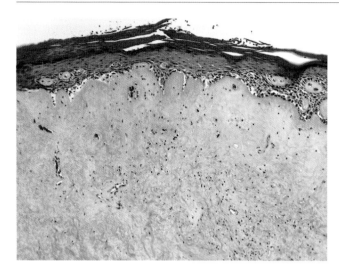

Fig. 8.4 Balanitis xerotic obliterans. The upper dermis is at first edematous, with a prominent band-like lymphocytic infiltrate. Over time, the dermal edema changes to dermal collagenization. Basal cell vacuolization is common. The inflammatory cell infiltrate in later stages becomes chiefly concentrated beneath the layer of homogeneous collagen in the upper dermis

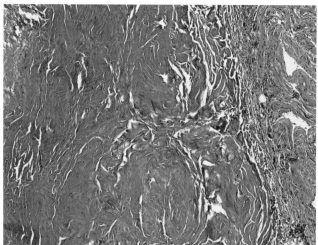

Fig. 8.6 Peyronie's disease. The microscopic findings in mature plaques resemble fibromatosis in other sites, such as Dupuytren's contracture. The plaque consists of hypocellular and extensively hyalinized fibrous tissue. The collagen bands are haphazardly arranged

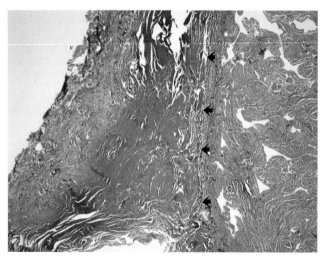

Fig. 8.5 Peyronie's disease. This condition affects men older than age 40; the cause is unknown. Erection is associated with pain and deformity. Dorsal penile plaques are palpable. The plaques are composed of fibrous tissue localized in the tunica albuginea (*arrows*), sometimes with associated calcification or bone formation

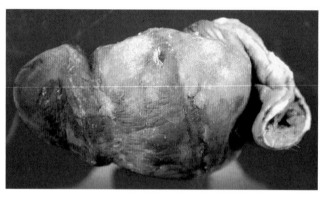

Fig. 8.7 Penile strangulation and infarction. The patient was a bedridden quadriplegic with a long-term indwelling bladder catheter. The catheter inadvertently became wrapped around the base of the penis for several hours, restricting its blood flow. The penis was deemed nonviable and was excised

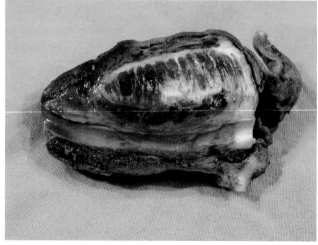

Fig. 8.8 Penile strangulation and infarction. Sectioned parallel to the urethra, the penis shows hemorrhage and ischemic changes

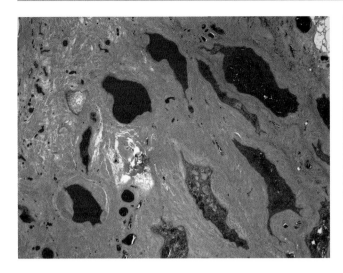

Fig. 8.9 Penile strangulation and infarction. Microscopic examination reveals coagulative necrosis and prominent vascular dilation

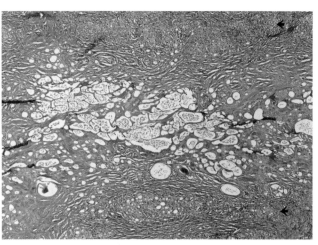

Fig. 8.11 Lipogranuloma. This condition results from injection of foreign materials (wax, silicone or paraffin) into the penis, and in some cases, the scrotum as well. Nodules develop at the site of foreign material placement, sometimes causing penile deformity and sometimes raising concern for neoplasia. The central portion of the image (*blue arrows*) consists of sclerotic fibroconnective tissue with numerous unlined cystic spaces of variable size. At top and bottom, there is evidence of a granulomatous tissue reaction (*black arrows*) (*see* MacLennan GT, Resnick MI, Bostwick DG, 2003. With permission)

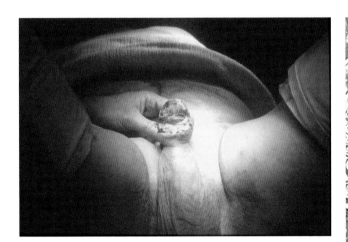

Fig. 8.10 Penile radiation necrosis. Patient had localized penile radiation for treatment of non-Hodgkin lymphoma. He was brought to the operating room for debridement of nonviable tissue

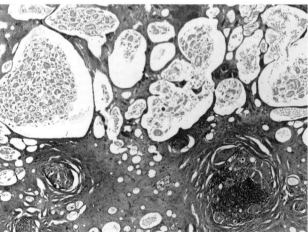

Fig. 8.12 Lipogranuloma. Numerous cystic spaces of variable size are present, unlined by epithelial cells or endothelial cells, representing the sites of deposition of amorphous foreign material. Granulomatous inflammation is present

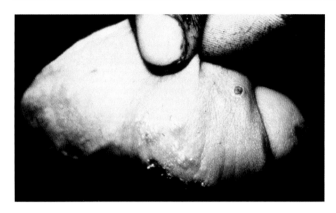

Fig. 8.13 Genital herpes. Genital herpes is a sexually transmitted viral infection caused by herpes simplex virus, types 1 and 2. Primary genital herpes may involve the glans, prepuce, shaft, sulcus, and scrotum. The classical clinical appearance is grouped vesicles that evolve to pustules, which become small ulcers that heal in 2–4 weeks. This image illustrates vesicles and ulcers in different phases of healing (*see* MacLennan GT, Resnick MI, Bostwick DG, 2003. With permission)

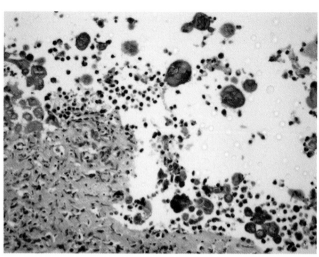

Fig. 8.15 Genital herpes. Closer view of the contents of a vesicle shows enlarged infected keratinocytes exhibiting multiple intranuclear inclusions, which have a homogeneous ground-glass appearance

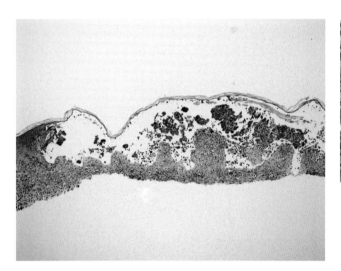

Fig. 8.14 Genital herpes. This biopsy includes an intact vesicle. The vesicle is intraepidermal; it is populated by multinucleated squamous cells with viral inclusions. The overlying squamous epithelium is intact

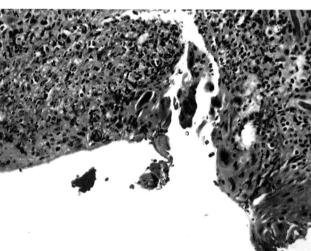

Fig. 8.16 Genital herpes. This is a biopsy taken during the ulcer phase. An ulcer bed consisting of acutely inflamed granulation is at left. The residual squamous epithelium (*right*) shows characteristic large keratinocytes with typical intranuclear inclusions

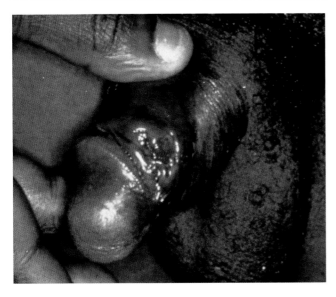

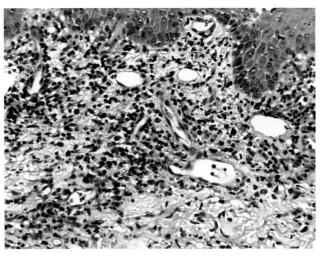

Fig. 8.19 Syphilis. The infiltrate is composed predominantly of plasma cells. Numerous small blood vessels are present, some of which are lined by large endothelial cells with prominent nuclei

Fig. 8.17 Syphilitic chancre. Syphilis, a sexually transmitted infection caused by the spirochete *Treponema pallidum*, is characterized by a firm painless ulcer or chancre at the site of inoculation, typically the prepuce, the coronal sulcus of the glans, or the penile shaft. The chancre may range from a few millimeters to 2 cm in diameter, with indurated raised rolled edges and a red, meaty color (*see* MacLennan GT, Resnick MI, Bostwick DG, 2003. With permission)

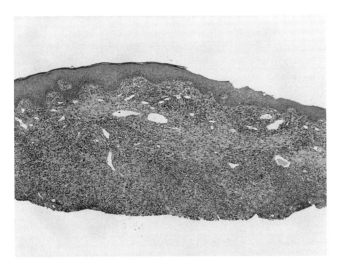

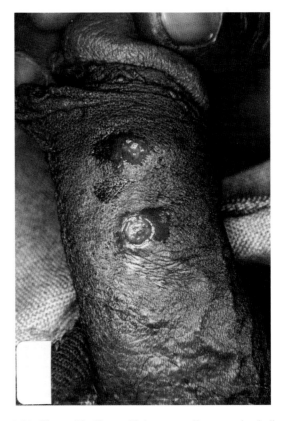

Fig. 8.18 Syphilis. A lesional biopsy demonstrates a dense inflammatory cell infiltrate in the dermis, and an abundance of small blood vessels

Fig. 8.20 Chancroid. Chancroid is a sexually transmitted disease caused by a Gram-negative bacillus, *Hemophilus ducreyi*. The primary lesions may appear on the prepuce, frenulum, coronal sulcus, glans, or penile shaft. Typically, one or more very painful nonindurated ulcers with sharp, undermined borders appear. Though chancroid may mimic syphilis clinically, these lesions are tender and the border of the ulcer is not indurated (*Image courtesy of* Allan Ronald, MD)

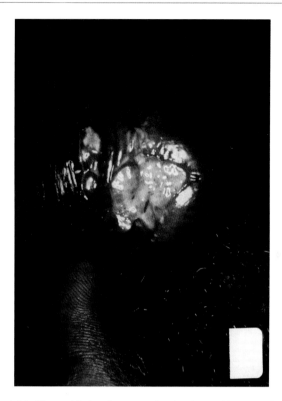

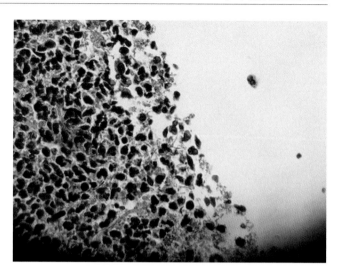

Fig. 8.23 Chancroid. Bacteria are present on the surface of the ulcer. Accurate diagnosis of chancroid depends upon culture of *Haemophilus Ducreyi*, which requires specialized growth media; sensitivity is only about 80% using this media. The most reliable results are obtained by inoculating the exudate directly onto the culture plate

Fig. 8.21 Chancroid. Another example of a chancroid ulcer, this one on the frenulum of the glans. Nearby, there are two smaller satellite lesions (*Image courtesy of* Allan Ronald, MD)

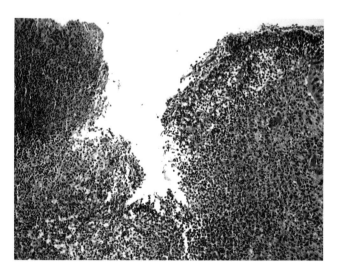

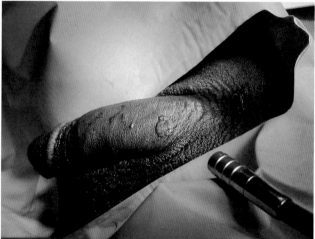

Fig. 8.22 Chancroid. This biopsy shows ulceration with florid acute and chronic inflammation. Classically, three distinct zones of reactive/reparative change are described: surface ulceration with necrosis, fibrin deposition, and neutrophil infiltrate (as shown here); a middle zone of vascular proliferation; and a deep zone of plasma cell and lymphocyte infiltrate

Fig. 8.24 Condyloma acuminatum. Condyloma acuminatum is most often caused by infection of squamous cells by human papillomavirus, types 6 and 11; dysplastic lesions are caused by types 16, 18, 31, 33, and 35. Condyloma acuminatum most often appears on the glans and foreskin, but may also appear on any part of the penis, or the skin of the scrotum or perineum. Some condyloma are flat and relatively inconspicuous, as is the lesion shown here (*see* MacLennan GT, Resnick MI, Bostwick DG, 2003. With permission)

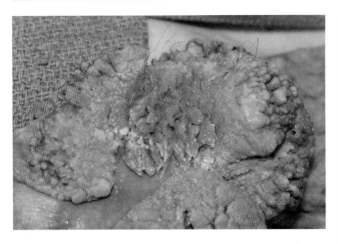

Fig. 8.25 Condyloma acuminatum. The majority of condyloma have a papillary or cauliflower-like appearance, as exemplified in this image. The multiple condyloma shown here involved the skin at the base of the penis (*Image courtesy of* Kenneth Angermeier, MD, and Hadley Wood, MD)

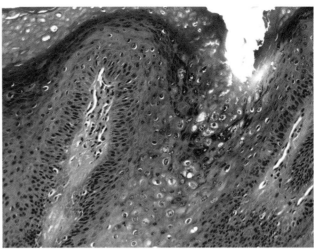

Fig. 8.27 Condyloma acuminatum. Hyperkeratosis and parakeratosis are often present. Many squamous cells show "koilocytosis," characterized by wrinkled, pleomorphic, and hyperchromatic nuclei, cytoplasmic retraction away from the nucleus, and frequent binucleation. Usually, mitotic figures are confined to the basal layer. In moderately or severely dysplastic lesions, there is progressive loss of normal maturation toward the surface, and mitotic figures appear in the upper levels of the dysplastic epithelium

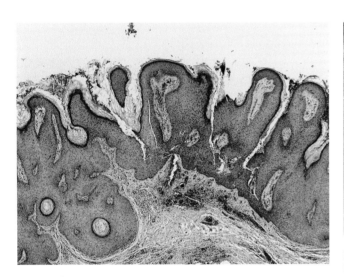

Fig. 8.26 Condyloma acuminatum. The lesion is a proliferative papillomatous squamous lesion. The squamous epithelium is thickened but exhibits orderly maturation

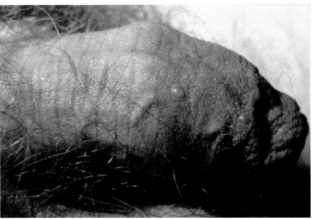

Fig. 8.28 Molluscum contagiosum. Molluscum contagiosum, caused by infection of squamous cells by a DNA pox virus, is characterized by the presence of numerous dome-shaped papules, 3–6 mm in diameter, on the skin of the penile shaft. The papules often have a central dimple (*see* MacLennan GT, Resnick MI, Bostwick DG, 2003. With permission)

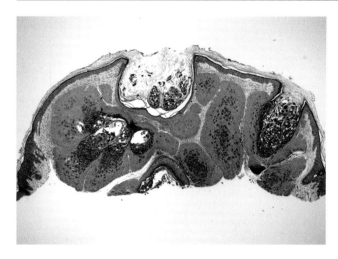

Fig. 8.29 Molluscum contagiosum. Microscopically, the papules take the form of cup-shaped squamous proliferations which bulge downward into the dermis

8.2 Neoplastic Penile Lesions

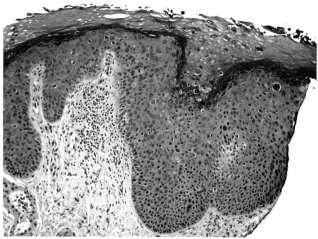

Fig. 8.31 Bowenoid papulosis. This lesion, probably caused by human papillomavirus infection (types 16 and 18), is indistinguishable from squamous cell carcinoma in situ histologically, but differs from that entity clinically and biologically. It presents as numerous papules, usually on the penile shaft, and rarely on the glans, foreskin, or perineum, in men between 20 and 40 years old. Individual papules may measure up to 10 mm, but coalesced lesions may be larger. This penile biopsy from a 20-year-old man shows a proliferative squamous lesion with delayed maturation, parakeratosis and hyperkeratosis

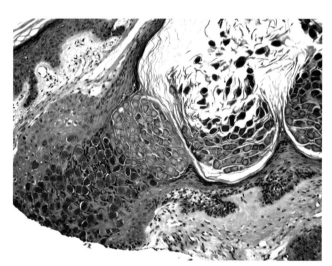

Fig. 8.30 Molluscum contagiosum. The basal cell layer is unremarkable. The infected keratinocytes of the stratum malpighii acquire eosinophilic cytoplasmic inclusions (Molluscum bodies), which become basophilic in the upper layers and in the cells extruded into the cup-shaped crater. The underlying dermis is unremarkable, unless the contents of the epidermal papule rupture into it

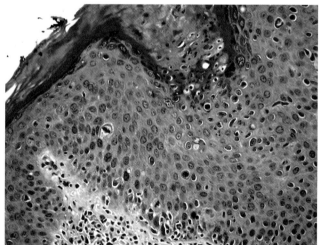

Fig. 8.32 Bowenoid papulosis. A higher-power view of Fig. 8.31 shows markedly dysplastic squamous cells with nuclear enlargement, pleomorphism, and hyperchromasia. There is a loss of polarity and dyskeratotic cells in the upper epidermis. Mitotic figures are well above the basal layer. Keratinocyte maturation, although delayed, is evident in the surface layers. Despite its appearance, bowenoid papulosis is biologically indolent: it responds to conservative local therapy or regresses spontaneously if untreated

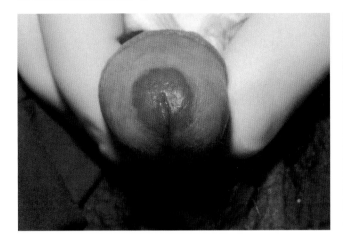

Fig. 8.33 Squamous cell carcinoma in situ. An erythematous lesion is noted in the glans. This appearance can be mimicked by Zoon's balanitis and candidal balanitis. Squamous cell carcinoma in situ in the glans and prepuce has traditionally been designated clinically as "erythroplasia of Queyrat" (*Image courtesy of* Kenneth Angermeier, MD)

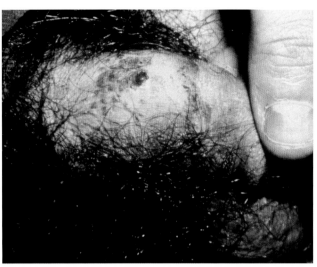

Fig. 8.35 Squamous cell carcinoma in situ. This lesion arose on the shaft of the penis, as a scaly plaque with an area of ulceration. Histologically, it is indistinguishable from "erythroplasia of Queyrat," but lesions such as this (remote from the head of the penis and lacking the distinctive appearance of histologically similar lesions in that site) are designated clinically as "Bowen's disease" (*see* MacLennan GT, Resnick MI, Bostwick DG, 2003. With permission)

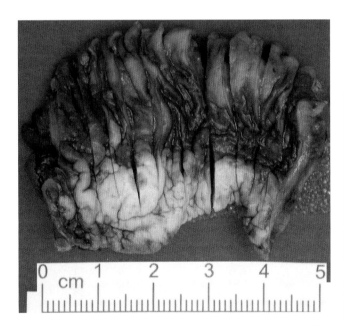

Fig. 8.34 Squamous cell carcinoma in situ. This is a circumcision specimen from a patient with AIDS. The white lesion was squamous cell carcinoma in situ. By its location, it would qualify for the designation "erythroplasia of Queyrat"

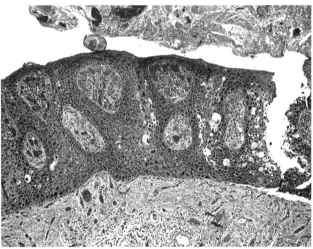

Fig. 8.36 Squamous cell carcinoma in situ (Bowen's disease). Full-thickness involvement of the epidermis by neoplastic keratocytes. There is prominent vascular proliferation immediately below the epidermis. The proliferative process is confined to the surface epithelium

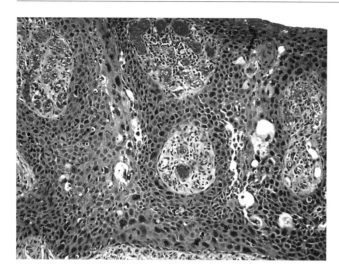

Fig. 8.37 Squamous cell carcinoma in situ (Bowen's disease). The neoplastic cells have bizarre, pleomorphic nuclei with clumped chromatin. There is lack of maturation. Abundant mitotic figures are present, well above the basal layer

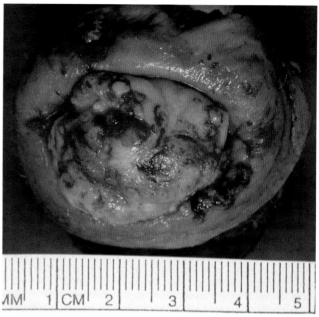

Fig. 8.39 Squamous cell carcinoma (gross). This invasive cancer obliterated much of the glans penis (*Image courtesy of* Ed Reineks, MD)

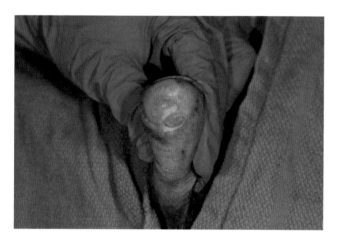

Fig. 8.38 Squamous cell carcinoma. The lesion near the frenulum was small and proved to be only superficially invasive (*Image courtesy of* Dave Rowe, MD)

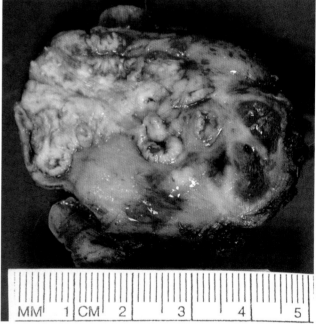

Fig. 8.40 Squamous cell carcinoma (gross). Midsagittal section of the lesion shown in Fig. 8.39. The lesion is deeply invasive. Urethral meatus is at left; resection margin is at right

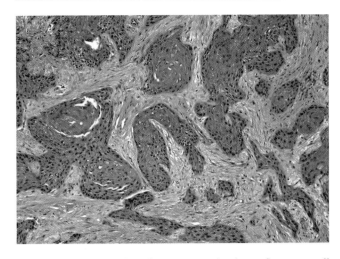

Fig. 8.41 Squamous cell carcinoma, conventional type. Squamous cell carcinoma of conventional type is typically well or moderately differentiated, composed of irregular fingers and nests of malignant squamous cells that infiltrate underlying tissues. Stromal desmoplasia and infiltrates of chronic inflammatory cells are commonly present. Keratin pearls are present

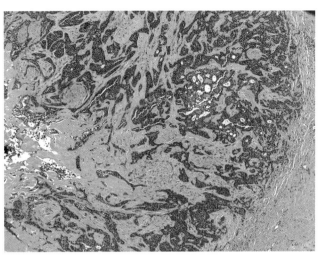

Fig. 8.43 Squamous cell carcinoma, basaloid type. Infiltrating nests and cords are composed of small basophilic neoplastic cells with minimal cytoplasm

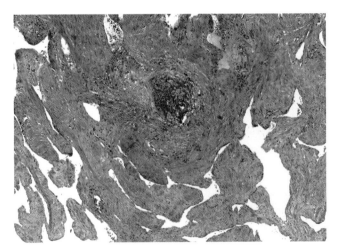

Fig. 8.42 Squamous cell carcinoma. Tumor involves the erectile tissues of the corpus cavernosum

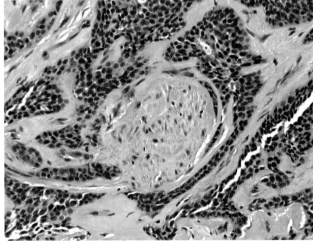

Fig. 8.44 Squamous cell carcinoma, basaloid type. Perineural invasion is noted. Nucleoli are absent or inconspicuous. Numerous apoptotic cells are present

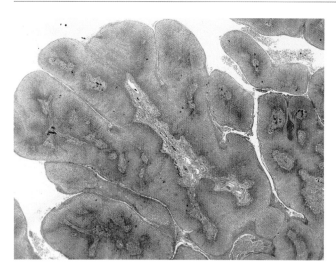

Fig. 8.45 Squamous cell carcinoma, warty type. The tumor is composed of a papillary exophytic component and an infiltrative basal component. The papillae are complex, long, and undulating with prominent central fibrovascular cores

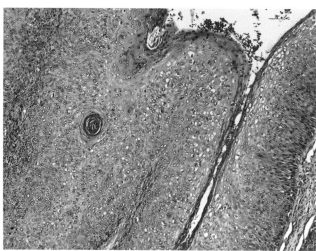

Fig. 8.47 Squamous cell carcinoma, warty type. Tumor cells show nuclear pleomorphism, koilocytic atypia and parakeratosis. Human papillomavirus DNA is present in up to 45% of cases of warty type of squamous cell carcinoma

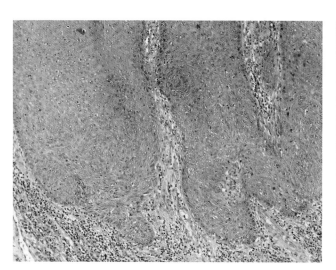

Fig. 8.46 Squamous cell carcinoma, warty type. The base of the tumor is irregular and somewhat pushing in appearance

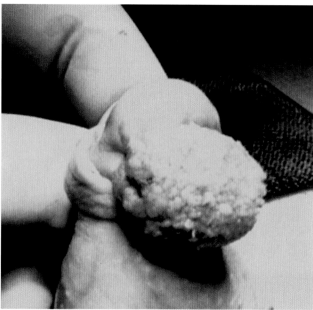

Fig. 8.48 Squamous cell carcinoma, verrucous type. The base of this large exophytic tumor was near the frenulum of the glans (*see* MacLennan GT, Resnick MI, Bostwick DG, 2003. With permission)

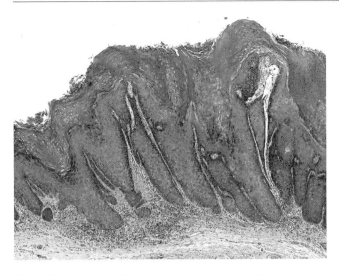

Fig. 8.49 Squamous cell carcinoma, verrucous type. Tumor demonstrates both exophytic and endophytic papillary growth. The fibrovascular cores are relatively delicate and inconspicuous. The infiltrative interface at the base of the tumor is broad-based and pushing in appearance

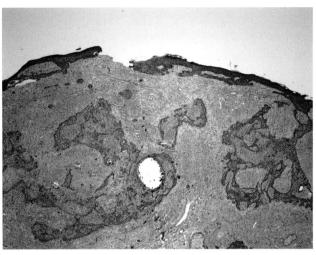

Fig. 8.51 Basal cell carcinoma (fibroepithelioma of Pinkus type). The tumor is composed of anastomosing, reticular cords of basal cells connecting to the overlying epidermis

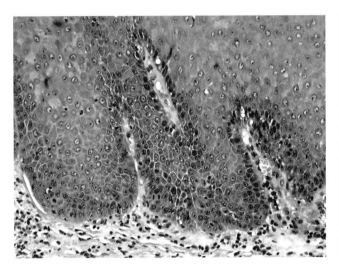

Fig. 8.50 Squamous cell carcinoma, verrucous type. The tumor has a smooth regular interface with underlying stroma. The tumor cells appear well differentiated, with no significant cytologic atypia. Koilocytic atypia is not seen

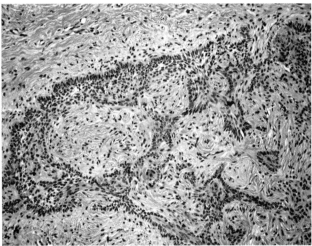

Fig. 8.52 Basal cell carcinoma (fibroepithelioma of Pinkus type). Tumor is composed of interconnecting nests of small uniform basaloid cells with peripheral palisading. The stroma is loose with paucity of inflammatory cells. Intercellular bridges and keratin formation are inconspicuous. Mitotic activity is limited or absent

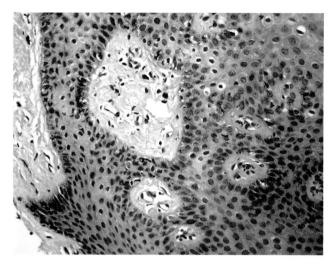

Fig. 8.53 Melanosis. There is hyperpigmentation of the basal cell layer that is accentuated at the tips of the rete ridges. There are numerous melanophages in the papillary dermis. This lesion is not related to melanoma

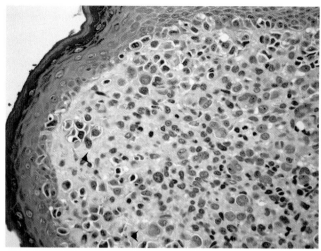

Fig. 8.55 Melanoma. The infiltrating atypical melanocytes show marked pleomorphism. Some are small and hyperchromatic, and some contain melanin (*arrows*). A mitotic figure is present at the dermalepidermal junction

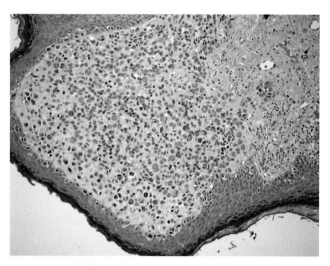

Fig. 8.54 Melanoma. Penile skin lesion in a 45-year-old man. Atypical melanocytes are present at the dermalepidermal junction and have infiltrated the dermis

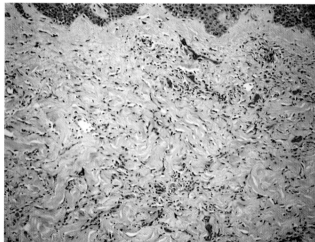

Fig. 8.56 Kaposi sarcoma. This is the patch stage of Kaposi sarcoma. There is a subtle infiltration of the dermis by numerous slit-like vascular channels dissecting bundles of dermal collagen

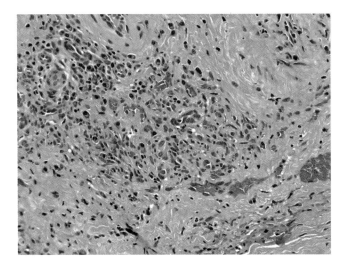

Fig. 8.57 Kaposi sarcoma. Cytologic atypia is noted in the spindled cells lining some of the small vascular spaces. The dermis also contains aggregates of plasma cells, and there are abundant extravasated erythrocytes

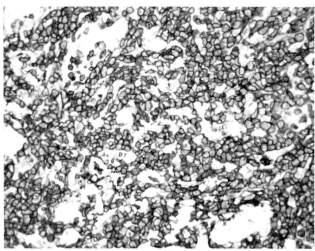

Fig. 8.59 Lymphoma. The tumor cells shown in Fig. 8.58 showed strong diffusely positive immunostaining for CD45RB (shown here) and also for T-cell markers CD3 and CD45RO

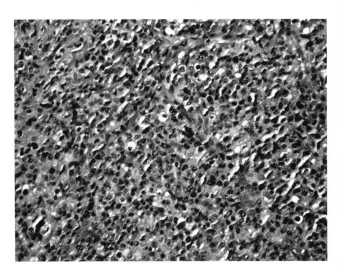

Fig. 8.58 Lymphoma. Patient was a 70-year-old man who had been followed for cutaneous T-cell lymphoma. He developed a mass at the base of his penis, which was biopsied. Tumor consisted of large undifferentiated atypical cells with prominent nucleoli and abundant mitotic Fig.s

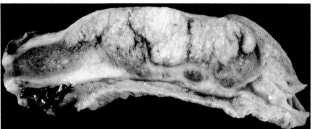

Fig. 8.60 Metastasis to the penis. Penile metastasis from a distant cancer is rare, and usually a late phenomenon. Prostatic adenocarcinoma and urothelial carcinoma of the bladder account for about 70% of cases; other common primaries are colonic adenocarcinoma and renal cell carcinoma. This is an example of metastatic urothelial carcinoma, which is forming nodules in the corpora cavernosa of the penis

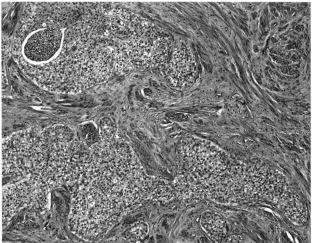

Fig. 8.61 Metastasis to the penis. Metastatic urothelial carcinoma invades into the corpus cavernosum

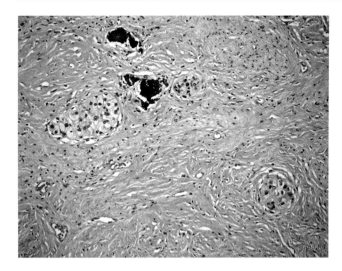

Fig. 8.62 Metastasis to the penis. Metastatic prostatic adenocarcinoma involved the penis. The microcalcifications may represent tumor necrosis

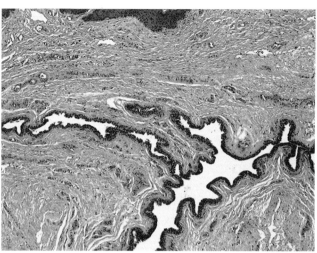

Fig. 8.64 Median raphe cyst. The cyst is lined by pseudostratified columnar epithelium and contains mucinous material

8.3 Nonneoplastic Scrotal Lesions

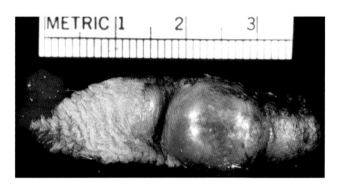

Fig. 8.63 Median raphe cyst. This cyst may be unilocular or multilocular. It is a midline developmental cyst that presents as a solitary nodule on the ventral surface of the penis, or in the midline median raphe of the scrotal skin (see MacLennan GT, Resnick MI, Bostwick DG, 2003. With permission)

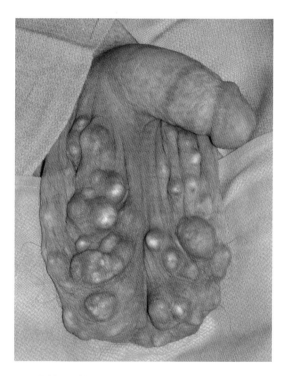

Fig. 8.65 Epidermoid cyst. Epidermoid cyst begins as an epidermal inclusion, and occurs commonly in the skin of the penis and scrotum. Some become infected, or cause a local inflammatory reaction to extravasation of cyst contents into the surrounding soft tissues. Sometimes multiple epidermoid cysts form, as in this case (Image courtesy of Kenneth Angermeier, MD)

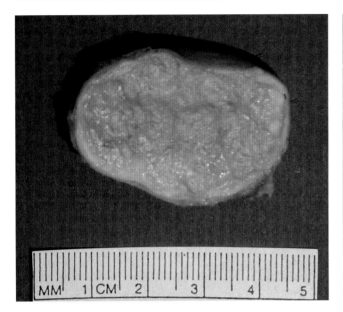

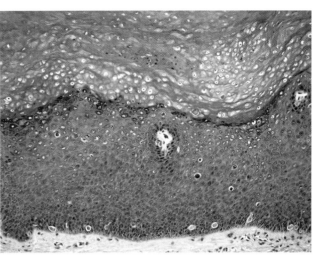

Fig. 8.68 Epidermoid cyst. Squamous cell carcinoma in situ focally lined the cavity of this scrotal epidermoid cyst

Fig. 8.66 Epidermoid cyst. Most are less than 1 cm in diameter, but they can be much larger, as evidenced by the lesion shown here. The cyst enlarges as gray or pearly-white desquamated keratin accumulates within the cyst cavity. A fibrous wall typically encloses the cyst

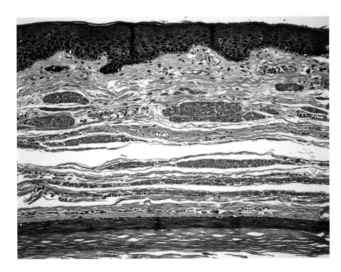

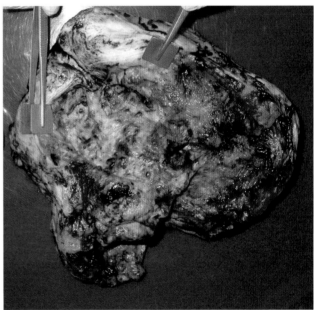

Fig. 8.67 Epidermoid cyst. The cyst wall (if identifiable) is lined by keratinizing squamous epithelium; in this image, the skin is at top, and the cyst wall epithelium is shown at bottom. Keratin debris is usually present. In cases in which cyst contents have extravasated into surrounding soft tissues, only a residual foreign-body giant cell reaction with evidence of acute and chronic inflammation may be evident

Fig. 8.69 Scrotal abscess. This thick-walled abscess developed after hernia repair with mesh. This was the last of several surgical procedures to manage relentlessly recurrent abscess formation in the scrotum. The cavity contained purulent material and old blood. Some of the tissue was ischemic (*Image courtesy of* Christine Lemyre)

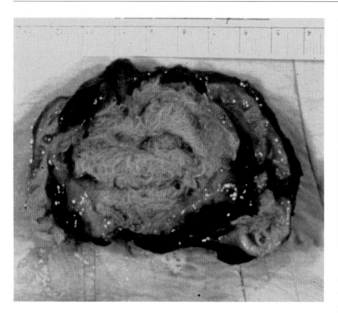

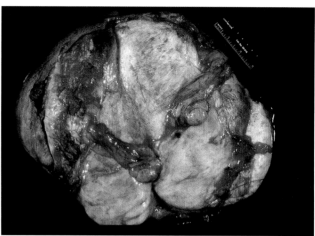

Fig. 8.72 Massive scrotal lymphedema. In most instances, surgical treatment entails excision of the involved subcutaneous genital tissue, with skin grafting. In some instances, such as this one, the testes are included in the resection specimen

Fig. 8.70 Foreign body in scrotum. Patient developed a painful mass following orchiectomy. The mass had a thick fibrous wall, and contained a surgical sponge

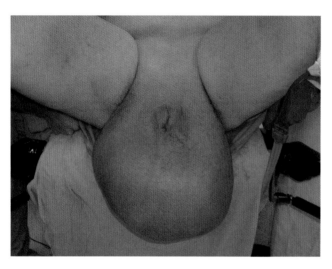

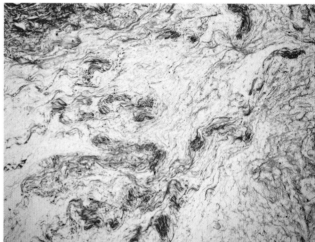

Fig. 8.71 Massive scrotal lymphedema. Pronounced scrotal lymphedema presents in two ways: as a rare congenital deficiency of lymphatic drainage, or as an acquired condition, such as in filariasis. The scrotum can become extraordinarily enlarged, as exemplified in this image (*Image courtesy of* Kenneth Angermeier, MD, and Hadley Wood, MD)

Fig. 8.73 Massive scrotal lymphedema. Sections from the resection specimen show variability in the degree of tissue edema and tissue fibrosis; areas of loose acellular edematous stroma account for much of the bulk of the lesion

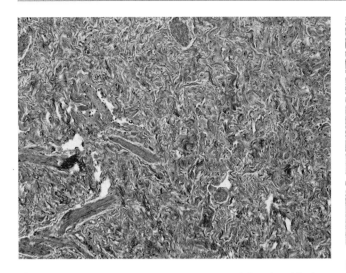

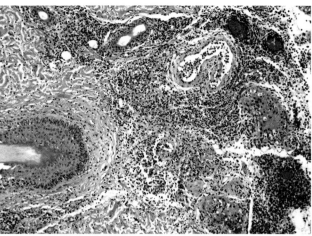

Fig. 8.74 Massive scrotal lymphedema. Areas of fibrosis, with abundant collagen deposition, comprise part of the specimen

Fig. 8.76 Hidradenitis suppurativa. Follicular hyperkeratosis is shown at lower left. Apocrine and eccrine glands are involved by acute and chronic inflammation

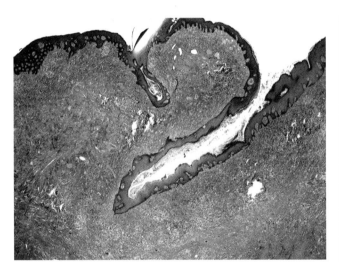

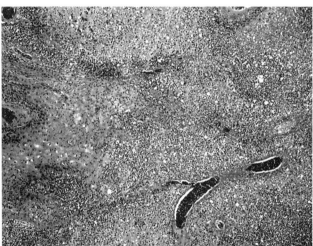

Fig. 8.75 Hidradenitis suppurativa. This lesion results from obstruction of the drainage system of apocrine and eccrine glands by keratin plugs. Pilosebaceous units become distended, and infection with a variety of bacteria supervenes. The pilosebaceous units rupture, releasing their contents into the surrounding dermis and inciting necrotizing and granulomatous inflammation with abscess formation. The process becomes diffuse as lesions coalesce to form plaques. This image shows a sinus tract that provides drainage of inflammatory exudate to the skin surface

Fig. 8.77 Hidradenitis suppurativa. The base of a sinus tract lined by squamous epithelium is present at left; it appears to communicate with an abscess

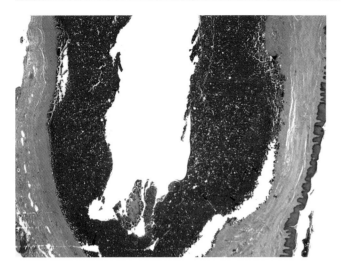

Fig. 8.78 Scrotal calcinosis. Some cases of scrotal calcinosis represent calcification of preexisting epidermoid and pilar cysts. Idiopathic scrotal calcinosis is characterized by calcification of dermal connective tissue of the scrotum without evidence of a preexisting cyst, although it is hypothesized that this condition develops within eccrine units, with progressive loss of lining epithelial cells as the calcific deposits slowly accumulate. Nodules form in the scrotal skin, measuring up to 3 cm in diameter. Microscopically, rounded aggregates of granular calcific debris are present in the dermis. The skin overlying the nodules is usually unremarkable, but sometimes ulcerates

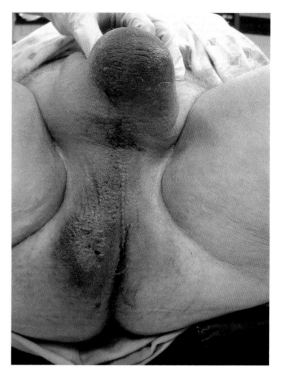

Fig. 8.80 Fournier's gangrene. This is an idiopathic polymicrobial necrotizing fasciitis that involves the soft tissues of the genitals and perineum. In its early phase, it appears as cellulitis with overlying edema (*Image courtesy of* Donald Bodner, MD)

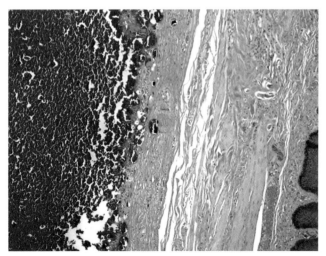

Fig. 8.79 Scrotal calcinosis. A cystic space is present in the dermis, filled with granular calcified debris. The fibrous capsule surrounding the nodule of calcinosis is devoid of inflammatory cells

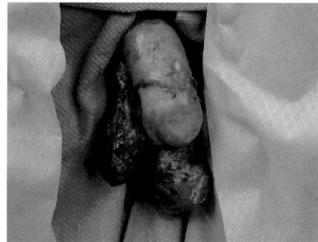

Fig. 8.81 Fournier's gangrene. If medical attention is not sought the lesion progresses to skin ulceration and necrosis and gangrenous necrosis of the local tissues (*Image courtesy of* Allen Seftel, MD)

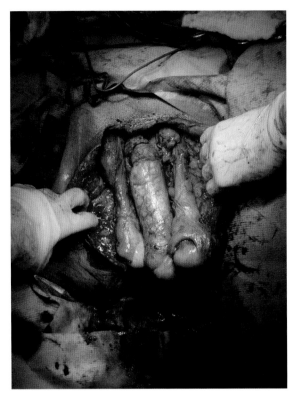

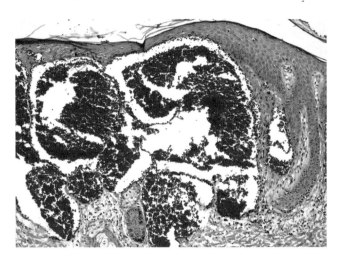

8.4 Neoplastic Scrotal Lesions

Fig. 8.84 Angiokeratoma. In one clinical form of this disorder (Fordyce type), angiokeratomas are localized to the scrotum. They present as 2–5 mm red papules in the scrotal skin. Microscopically, the dermal papillae are expanded by ectatic thin-walled blood vessels in the superficial dermis, with overlying epidermal hyperplasia

Fig. 8.82 Fournier's gangrene. The condition is potentially life-threatening and requires aggressive therapy, including aggressive debridement of devitalized tissues (*Image courtesy of* Howard Goldman, MD)

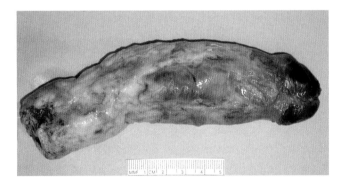

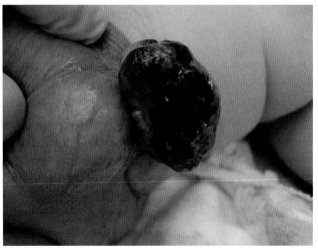

Fig. 8.83 Fournier's gangrene. Debridement may even include penectomy, as in this case. Despite aggressive therapy and prior debridement, the head of the penis became gangrenous, and a urethral fistula developed, possibly related to the presence of an indwelling catheter. Microscopy confirmed widespread tissue necrosis (*Image courtesy of* Christine Lemyre and Ed Cherullo, MD)

Fig. 8.85 Hemangioma. Hemangiomas are the most common benign soft tissue tumors during infancy and childhood, but only about 1–2% arise in the genital region. Capillary hemangiomas, the commonest type, are flat, bright-red to blue lesions resulting from proliferation of immature capillary vessels. They grow rapidly during infancy, but the great majority involute by age 7 years. Shown here is a scrotal capillary hemangioma in a 2-month-old male that was present at birth

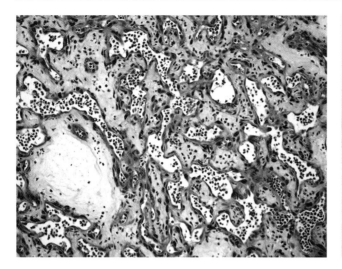

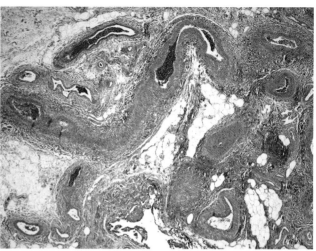

Fig. 8.86 Hemangioma. Hemangiomas are composed of myriad tiny vessels encircled by connective tissue fibers. As they mature and blood flow increases, vascular lumens are more readily apparent and the lining endothelial cells change from plump to flattened. Section from the lesion shown in Fig. 8.85 shows a vasoproliferative lesion of capillary-sized blood vessels lined by plump round to cuboidal endothelial cells

Fig. 8.88 Arteriovenous malformation. Section from the lesion shown in Fig. 8.87 shows that it is composed of tortuous ectatic blood vessels of varying wall thickness

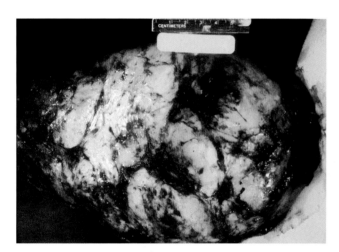

Fig. 8.87 Arteriovenous malformations. Arteriovenous malformations are congenital vascular anomalies that grow with the child, sometimes associated with an audible bruit, and exhibiting distinctive diagnostic radiologic findings. This large soft tissue mass was a scrotal arteriovenous malformation in a 26-year-old man (*see* MacLennan GT, Resnick MI, Bostwick DG, 2003. With permission)

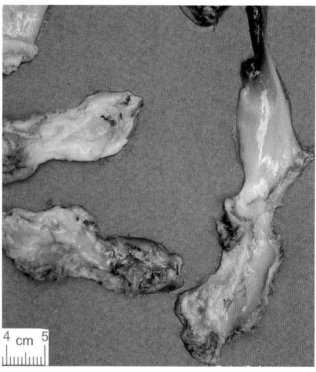

Fig. 8.89 Aggressive angiomyxoma. This lesion uncommonly arises in the male genital area. The lesion shown here was an ill-defined and poorly circumscribed soft tissue abnormality in the scrotum of a 14-year-old boy. It has a shiny and somewhat gelatinous appearance (*Image courtesy of* Sean Fitzgerald, MD)

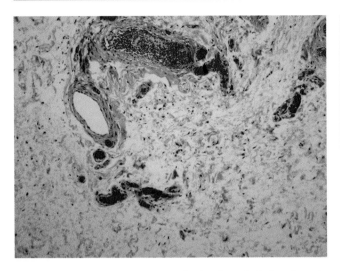

Fig. 8.90 Aggressive angiomyxoma. Section from the lesion shown in Fig. 8.89 shows a hypocellular myxoid stroma sparsely populated by evenly dispersed spindled and stellate cells with small oval uniform nuclei with dense chromatin and indistinct nucleoli. Numerous randomly distributed blood vessels of varying caliber and type are present, including arteries, veins, venules, arterioles, and capillaries

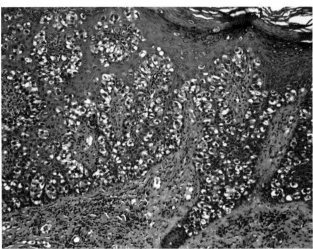

Fig. 8.92 Extramammary Paget's disease (EMPD). The epidermis is populated and irregularly infiltrated by atypical large cells with abundant pale clear cytoplasm and vesicular nuclei, arrayed singly or in small nests. Tumor cells tend to cluster at the tips of the rete ridges. Hyperkeratosis, parakeratosis, and papillomatosis are commonly present

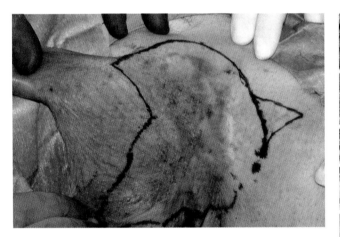

Fig. 8.91 Extramammary Paget's disease (EMPD). This is a rare genitourinary malignancy that most often arises in men older than age 60 years, presenting with pruritus and pain associated with an erythematous, eczematous, or ulcerated plaque-like lesion with well-defined borders. The most frequent site of involvement is the penoscrotal junction, as shown here (*Image courtesy of* Kenneth Angermeier, MD)

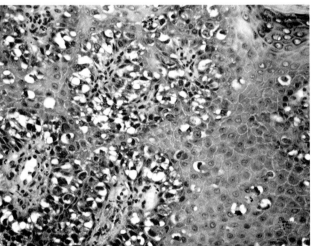

Fig. 8.93 Extramammary Paget's disease (EMPD). The cytoplasmic clarity in the tumor cells of EMPD is due to intracytoplasmic accumulation of mucin, which is readily demonstrable with histochemical stains for mucin, such as mucicarmine, as illustrated here

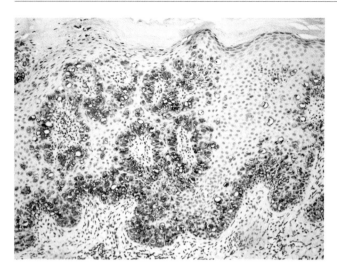

Fig. 8.94 Extramammary Paget's disease (EMPD). The tumor cells of EMPD show positive immunostaining for cytokeratin 7, as shown here, and also express carcinoembryonic antigen

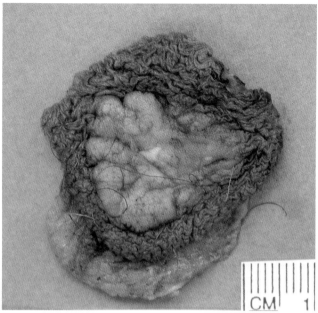

Fig. 8.96 Squamous cell carcinoma. This small scrotal skin lesion was well differentiated and only minimally invasive

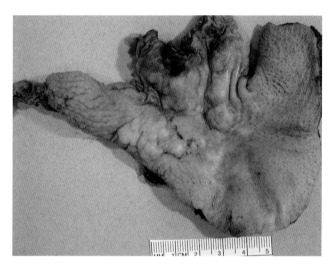

Fig. 8.95 Squamous cell carcinoma in situ. This was a wide local excision of elevated pale skin lesions at the penoscrotal junction that showed squamous cell carcinoma in situ; no invasive component was identified

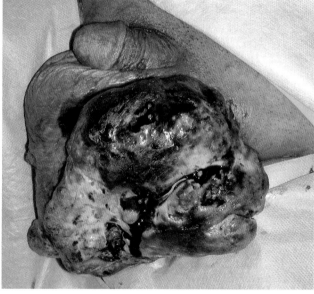

Fig. 8.97 Squamous cell carcinoma. A bulky nodular hemorrhagic and partially necrotic squamous cell carcinoma of the scrotum, immediately prior to excision (*Image courtesy of* Kenneth Angermeier, MD)

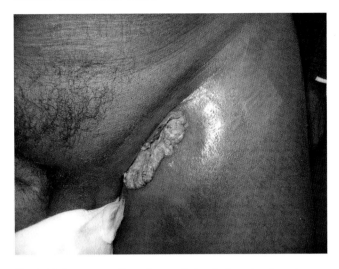

Fig. 8.98 Squamous cell carcinoma. Patient had previously undergone excision of a scrotal squamous cell carcinoma, as well as inguinal lymphadenectomy. The tumor recurred locally in the inguinal region

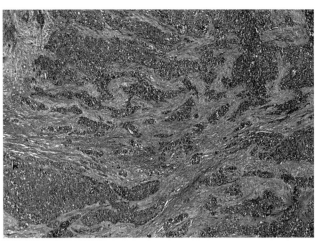

Fig. 8.100 Desmoplastic small round cell tumor. Tumor is composed of irregular nests and sheets of undifferentiated tumor cells surrounded by dense desmoplastic stroma

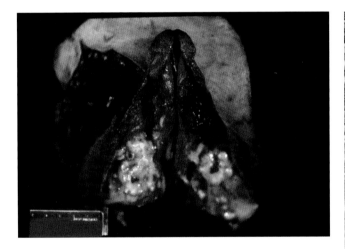

Fig. 8.99 Desmoplastic small round cell tumor. The tumor formed multinodular tan-yellow masses scattered through the soft tissues of the inguinal canal, scrotum and perineum, requiring extensive local excision, including the penis, as shown here

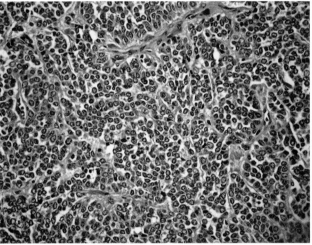

Fig. 8.101 Desmoplastic small round cell tumor. Tumor is composed of undifferentiated small cells with minimal cytoplasm, and hyperchromatic round or oval nuclei with inconspicuous nucleoli

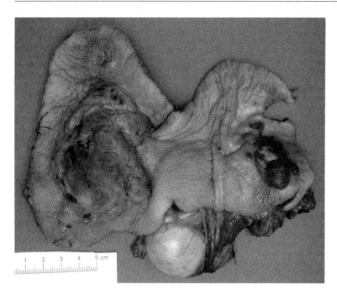

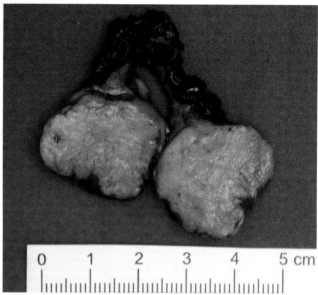

Fig. 8.102 Malignant fibrous histiocytoma. Patient had previously undergone excision of a malignant fibrous histiocytoma that arose in the inguinal canal. The tumor recurred in the scrotum, as shown here, necessitating wide local excision (*Image courtesy of* Hollie Reeves, MD)

Fig. 8.103 Metastasis to the scrotum. Patient had a known history of squamous cell carcinoma of the lung. He developed a scrotal nodule, which was excised and proved to be squamous cell carcinoma, consistent with a metastatic lesion. No squamous lesions were present in the skin of the genital region (*Image courtesy of* Christine Wojewoda, MD)

Suggested Readings

1 Amin MB, Grignon DJ, Humphrey PA, Srigley JR. *Gleason Grading of Prostate Cancer: a Contemporary Approach*. Lippincott Williams & Wilkins, Philadelphia, PA, 2004.

2 Bostwick DG, Cheng L. *Urologic Surgical Pathology* (Second edition). Elsevier, New York, NY, 2008.

3 Bostwick DG, Dundore PA. *Biopsy Pathology of the Prostate*. Chapman and Hall, New York, NY, 1997.

4 Bostwick DG, Lopez-Beltran A. *Bladder Biopsy Interpretation*. United Pathologists Press, Tampa, FL, 1999.

5 Cheng L, Bostwick DG. *Essentials of Anatomic Pathology* (Third edition). Springer, New York, NY, 2010.

6 Eble JN, Sauter G, Epstein JI, Sesterhenn IA. *World Health Organization Classification of Tumours: Pathology and Genetics of Tumours of the Urinary System and Male Genital Organs*. International Agency for Research on Cancer (IARC) Press, Lyon, France, 2004.

7 Epstein JI, Amin MB, Reuter VE. *Bladder Biopsy Interpretation. Biopsy Interpretation Series*. Lippincott Williams & Wilkins, Philadelphia, PA, 2004.

8 Epstein JI, Netto GJ. *Biopsy Interpretation of the Prostate. Biopsy Interpretation Series* (Fourth Edition). Lippincott Williams & Wilkins, Philadelphia, PA, 2008.

9 Foster CS, Bostwick DG. Pathology of the prostate. In: *Major Problems in Pathology*. (Volume 4). LiVolsi VA (ed). WB Saunders, Philadelphia, PA, 1998.

10 Foster CS, Ross JS. *Pathology of the Urinary Bladder: Major Problems in Pathology*. Saunders/Elsevier, Philadelphia, PA, 2004.

11 Humphrey PA. *Prostate Pathology*. AJCP Press, Chicago, IL, 2003.

12 Koss LG, Melamed MR. *Koss' Diagnostic Cytology And Its Histopathologic Bases* (Fifth Edition). Lippincott Williams & Wilkins, Philadelphia, PA, 2005.

13 Lack EE, American Registry of Pathology. *Tumors of the Adrenal Glands and Extraadrenal Paraganglia* (Fourth edition). Armed Forces Institute of Pathology, Washington, DC, 2007.

14 MacLennan GM, Bostwick DG, Cheng L. *Renal Tumors: Clinics in Laboratory Medicine*. WB Saunders/Elsevier Inc, Philadelphia, PA, 2005.

15 MacLennan GT, Resnick MI, Bostwick DG. *Pathology for Urologists*. Saunders/Elsevier, Philadelphia, PA, 2003.

16 Mikuz G. *Clinical Pathology of Urologic Tumors*. Informa UK Ltd., London, UK, 2007.

17 Mostofi FK, Sobin LH, Torloni H. *Histological Typing of Urinary Bladder Tumours*. World Health Organization, Geneva, 1973.

18 Murphy WM, Grignon DJ, Perlman EJ, American Registry of Pathology. *Tumors of the Kidney, Bladder, and Related Urinary Structures* (Fourth edition). Armed Forces Institute of Pathology, Washington, DC, 2004.

19 Petersen RO, Sesterhenn IA, Davis CJ. *Urologic Pathology* (Third Edition). Lippincott Williams & Wilkins, Philadelphia, PA, 2009.

20 Ro JY, Grignon DJ, Amin MB, Ayala A, Day L. *Atlases in Diagnostic Surgical Pathology Series: Atlas of Surgical Pathology of the Male Reproductive Tract*. WB Saunders, Philadelphia, PA, 1997.

21 Tannenbaum M, Madden JF. *Diagnostic Atlas of Genitourinary Pathology*. Churchill Livingston/Elsevier, Philadelphia, PA, 2006.

22 Young RH, Scully RE. *Testicular Tumors*. ASCP Press, Chicago, IL, 1990.

23 Young RH, Srigley JR, Amin MB, Ulbright TM, Cubilla AL. *Atlas of Tumor Pathology: Tumors of the Prostate Gland, Seminal Vesicles, Male Urethra, and Penis* (Third edition, Fascicle 28). Armed Forces Institute of Pathology, Washington, DC, 2000.

24 Zhou M, Magi-Galluzzi C. *Foundations in Diagnostic Pathology Series: Genitourinary Pathology*. Churchill Livingstone/Elsevier, Philadelphia, PA, 2007.

Index